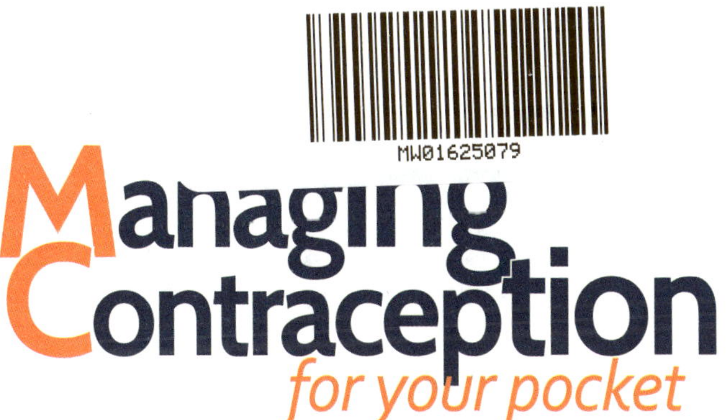

Managing Contraception

for your pocket

Mimi Zieman
Robert A. Hatcher
Ariel Z. Allen
Lisa Haddad

Order copies on
www.ManagingContraception.com

COPYRIGHT INFORMATION

Second Printing 2022

Suggested formal citation:
Zieman M, Hatcher RA., Allen A. Z., Haddad L, Managing Contraception 16th ed.

IMPORTANT DISCLAIMER

The authors remind readers that this book is intended to educate health care providers, not guide individual therapy. The authors advise a person with a particular problem to consult a primary-care clinician or a specialist in obstetrics, gynecology, or urology (depending on the problem or the contraceptive) as well as the product package insert and other references before diagnosing, managing, or treating the problem. Under no circumstances should the reader use this handbook in lieu of or to override the judgment of the treating clinician. The order in which diagnostic or therapeutic measures appear in this text is not necessarily the order that clinicians should follow in each case. The authors and staff are not liable for errors or omissions.

Sixteenth Edition
ISBN 978-1-7329884-4-6
Printed in the United States of America
Managing Contraception, LLC
Second Printing

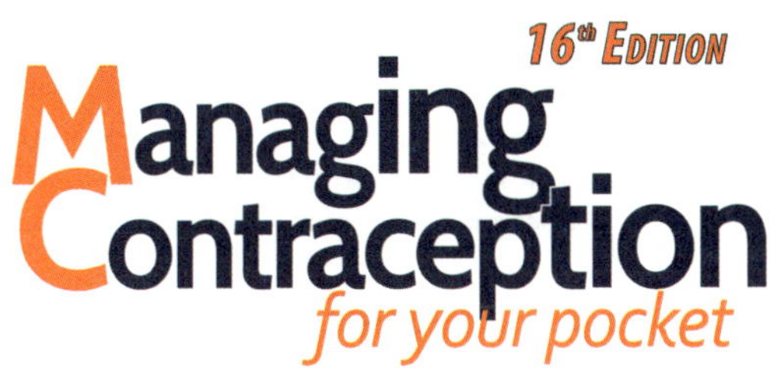

Mimi Zieman, MD
President, SageMed, LLC
Founding Director, Fellowship in Family Planning
Emory University School of Medicine

Robert A. Hatcher, MD, MPH
Professor Emeritus of Gynecology and Obstetrics
Emory University School of Medicine

Ariel Z. Allen, MD
Urology, Albert Einstein College of Medicine

Lisa B. Haddad, MD, MS, MPH
Medical Director
Center for Biomedical Research
Population Council

Kelly Cleland, MPA, MPH
Proofreader

Technical and Computer Support for *Managing Contraception:*
DID Media, LLC., Cornelia, Georgia
Jason Blackburn
706-776-2918
jason@didmedia.com

Check out the Q&A archives on
www.managingcontraception.com

New questions may be submitted to
www.mimizieman md.com

OUR MISSION

The mission of Bridging The Gap Foundation is to improve reproductive health and contraceptive decision-making of women and men by providing up-to-date educational resources to the physicians, nurses and public health leaders of tomorrow.

OUR VISION

Our vision is to provide educational resources to the health care providers of tomorrow, to help ensure informed choices, better service, access to effective contraceptive methods, happier and more successful contraceptors, competent clinicians, fewer unintended pregnancies and disease prevention.

We hope this book will make important information accessible to more people.

Please consider making a contribution to this 501-C-3 organization:

The Bridging the Gap Foundation • Atlanta, Georgia • PO Box 79299 • Atlanta, GA 30357

The extent to which we can make this 16th edition of *Managing Contraception* available to medical students, residents and family planning programs internationally depends on contributions from people like you. Since the first edition of Managing Contraception, over 1,115,000 copies of this book have been given away at no cost to medical students, residents, nursing and nurse midwifery students and nurse practioners through the support of both the David and Lucille Packard Foundation and an anonymous foundation.

NOTE:

We use the term "women" and the pronouns "she / her" in this book to describe those seeking female contraceptive methods or other healthcare. When possible, we also use "individual" to be inclusive. We recognize that not all people capable of pregnancy or seeking gynecological care identify as women.

On 256 pages, we cannot possibly provide you with all the information you might want or need about contraception. However, many of the questions clinicians ask are answered in this book, *Managing Contraception* 16th edition.

DEDICATION

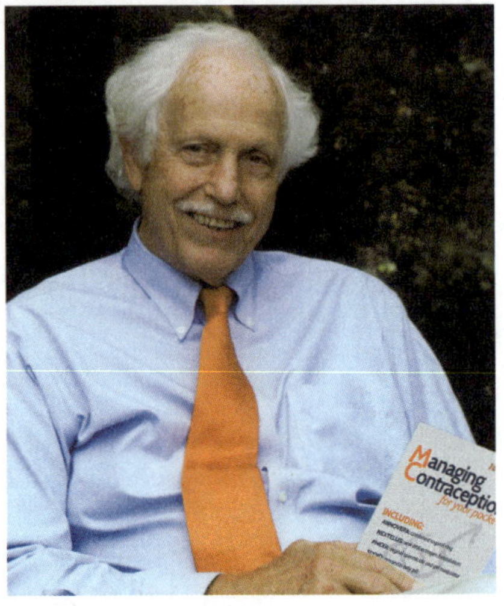

The authors of *Managing Contraception* other than Dr. Hatcher, dedicate this edition to him: Dr. Robert A. Hatcher for his outstanding accomplishments in Family Planning and his commitment to disseminating evidence-based information. Dr. Bob, as he is fondly called, has mentored scores of health care providers including all three of us personally, and he continues to inspire us with his dedication, warmth, creativity, and enthusiasm.

Dr. Bob first had the idea for Managing Contraception as a pocket-sized Family Planning resource for health care providers to carry into clinical settings. He enlisted Mimi Zieman, then Director of the Division of Family Planning at Emory, and a student, Rachel Blankstein, to draft the first pilot edition published in 1999. Rachel is now an assistant professor at the University of Maryland School of Nursing, and conducts research in maternal health. We have continued to publish updated, timely editions ever since. Dr. Hatcher's vision was that every medical student and resident in OB/GYN, nursing students and others would receive a free copy of this book, to compensate for the little time spent teaching contraception and Family Planning in medical, nursing, and other schools. Several years of grants from the David and Lucille Packard Foundation and others helped us distribute over one million copies of *Managing Contraception* to professionals in training over the years. Now available at a low cost, we continue to aim for wide access to this portable source of up-to-date information.

Dr. Hatcher began his remarkable career of scholarship and service at Williams college, graduating Phi Beta Kappa. He was also a fierce athlete– serving as co-captain of the Williams track team, was New England wrestling champion in 1957 and 1959, and was tight end and fullback on the football team.

He received his medical degree from Cornell University, with the "Good Physician Award," bestowed by his classmates. He completed a residency in pediatrics at Grady Hospital in Atlanta, then served as an Epidemic Intelligence Officer with the CDC, and received an MPH from University of California, Berkeley.

Dedicated to educating future leaders, he created the Emory University Summer Program in Family Planning and Human Sexuality which ran from 1966-1998. Many students who studied with him went on to have successful scientific careers. He served as Professor of Gynecology and Obstetrics, Emory University School of Medicine and Director of Family Planning. He was devoted to helping shape "humane and responsible reproductive health policies," and he provided expert and compassionate care for thousands of patients, educated generations of physicians, and published extensively.

Dr. Hatcher became known internationally for authoring the comprehensive textbook on family planning, *Contraceptive Technology*, now in its twenty-first edition. He has done extensive international work including as a senior author of two editions of Family Planning Methods and Practices: Africa.

He has served on numerous boards including the Planned Parenthood Federation of America, the National Family Planning and Reproductive Health Association, and the Center for Populations Options. In addition to his many professional affiliations, he is a tireless citizen in his North Georgia community, has many friends, and is active in the Rotary Club and Faith, an organization that offers programs addressing the needs of victims of abuse and violence. One of his proudest achievements is that he is one of two individuals who founded the first Atlanta chapter of the "I have a Dream," nonprofit. An entire class of students adopted in fifth grade were guaranteed college funding.

He has received countless awards including the Rockefeller Public Service Award in 1981 for service to Families and Youth. As recipients of his kind mentorship, we are most proud of the award created in his honor by the Society of Family Planning: The Robert A. Hatcher Award for Outstanding Mentorship.

Dr. Hatcher's creativity knows no bounds whether making connections with his complex thinking, writing, or designing blooming flowers in his garden. He keeps a large journal to write ideas, to scribble, and to count things. He loves numbers. And we love nothing more than an escape to visit Bob, his wife Maggie, their dog Jack, and to take a walk on the trail he built with his bare hands and hear updates about their children and grandchildren. Sometimes we're lucky enough to eat a fresh apple straight from the tree, or berries from his bushes. He bubbles with optimism and enthusiasm discussing the natural world around him with its magnificent scenery, or his community in Tiger Georgia, or how we can work together for a better world. Bob is so committed to positivity, he accumulated stories of people caring for others and compiled them in an annual calendar / book called *Something Nice to Do 365 Days a Year*. He is a loving and dedicated family man, and we consider ourselves fortunate to be part of his extended family.

IMPORTANT CONTACTS AND WEBSITES

TOPIC	ORGANIZATION	PHONE NUMBER	WEBSITE
Abortion	National Abortion Federation	202-667-5881	www.prochoice.org
	Abortion Hotline	800-772-9100	
			www.ipas.org
			www.earlyoptionpill.com
Abstinence			www.sexrespect.com
	Managing Contraception		www.managingcontraception.com
Abuse / Rape	National Domestic Violence Hotline	800-799-SAFE	www.thehotline.org
			www.ndvh.org
	Prevent Child Abuse America	312-663-3520	www.preventchildabuse.org
Adolescent Reproductive Health			www.teenpregnancy.org
			www.advocatesforyouth.org
Adoption	Adopt a Special Kid-America	800-4-A-CHILD	
	Adoptive Families Magazine	800-372-3300	
Breastfeeding	La Leche League	800-LA-LECHE	www.lalecheleague.org
			www.ilca.org
Cancer / HPV			www.asccp.org
			www.cancer.org
COCs	Managing Contraception		www.managingcontraception.com
	Planned Parenthood Federation of America	800-230-PLAN	www.plannedparenthood.org
Condoms			condomania.com
			askdurex.com
			www.ppfa.org
Contraception			www.conrad.org
	Contraceptive Technology		www.contraceptivetechnology.com
	Managing Contraception		www.managingcontraception.com
	Planned Parenthood Federation of America	800-230-PLAN	www.plannedparenthood.org
	Family Health International	919-544-7040	www.fhi360.org
	World Health Organization		www.who.int
	Assoc. of Reproductive Health Professionals (ARHP)	202-466-3825	
	Contemporary Forums	800-377-7707	www.cforums.com
			www.ippfwhr.org
			www.engenderhealth.org
			www.bedsider.org
Counseling	Depression and Bipolar Support Alliance	800-826-3632	www.dbsalliance.org
			www.gmhc.org
Education			www.siecus.org
			www.cdc.gov
Emergency contraception			www.planbonestep.com
Female Barrier Methods			www.femalehealth.com
			www.femcap.com
	Planned Parenthood Federation of America	800-230-PLAN	www.plannedparenthood.org
Fertility Awarenes Methods			www.cyclebeads.com
			www.irh.org

TOPIC	ORGANIZATION	PHONE NUMBER	WEBSITE
HIV/AIDS	Ntl. HIV/AIDS Clinicians' Consultation Center	800-933-3413	www.nccc.ucsf.edu
			www.cdc.gov/hiv
			www.cdc.gov/nchstp/dstd/dstdp.htm
IUC			www.popcouncil.org
			www.engenderhealth.org
			www.bayer.com
			www.paragard.com
Menopause			www.menopause.org
			www.nams.org
Natural Family			www.canfp.org
Ordering Devices			www.nexplanon.com
			www.mirena-us.com
			www.paragard.com
POPs	Managing Contraception		www.managingcontraception.com
Pregnancy	Lamaze International	202-367-1128	www.lamaze.org
	Depression After Delivery	800-944-4773	www.postpartum.net
Pregnancy Planning			www.irh.org
			www.ccli.org
			www.aidsinfo.nih.gov
			www.nichd.nih.gov
	Planned Parenthood Federation of America	800-230-PLAN	www.plannedparenthood.org
Pregnancy Testing	Planned Parenthood Federation of America	800-230-PLAN	www.plannedparenthood.org
			www.ovulation.com
Postpartum Contraception			www.avsc.org
			www.fhi.org
Public Health / Population Organizations			www.popcouncil.org
			www.prb.org
			www.undp.org
			www.population.org
Professional Organizations			www.acog.org
			www.fda.gov
			www.fhi.org
			www.jsi.com
			www.NPWH.org
	Planned Parenthood Federation of America	800-230-PLAN	www.plannedparenthood.org
			www.societyfp.org
			www.who.int
Reproductive Health Research			www.guttmacher.org
			www.fhi.org
STIs	CDC Sexually Transmitted Disease Hotline	800-CDC-INFO	www.cdc.gov
Sterilization			www.engenderhealth.org
	Planned Parenthood Federation of America	800-230-PLAN	www.plannedparenthood.org
			www.essure.com
Withdrawal			www.managingcontraception.com

ABBREVIATIONS USED IN THIS BOOK

ACOG	American College of Obstetricians & Gynecologists
AIDS	Acquired immunodeficiency syndrome
AMA	American Medical Association
ASAP	As soon as possible
BBT	Basal body temperature
BCA	Bichloroacetic acid
BID	Twice daily
BMI	Body Mass Index
BP	Blood pressure
BTB	Breakthrough bleeding
BTL	Bilateral tubal ligation
BV	Bacterial vaginosis
Bx	Biopsy
CA	Cancer (if not California)
CDC	Centers for Disease Control and Prevention
COC	Combined oral contraceptives (estrogen & progestin)
CHC	Combined Hormonal Contraceptives
CMV	Cytomegalovirus
CT	Chlamydia trachomatis
CuIUD	Copper containing IUD
CVD	Cardiovascular disease
D & C	Dilation and curettage
D & E	Dilation and evacuation
DCBE	Double contrast barium enema
DM	Diabetes Mellitus
DMPA	Depot-medroxyprogesterone acetate (Depo-Provera)
DUB	Dysfunctional uterine bleeding
DVT	Deep vein thrombosis
Dx	Diagnosis
Dz	Disease
E	Estrogen
EC	Emergency contraception
ECPs	Emergency contraceptive pills ("morning-after pills")
ED	Erectile dysfunction
E_2	Estradiol
EE	Ethinyl estradiol
ENG	Etonorgestrel
EPA	Environmental Protection Agency
EPT	Estrogen-progestin therapy
ET	Estrogen therapy
EVA	Ethylene vinyl acetate
FAM	Fertility awareness methods
FDA	Food and Drug Administration
FH	Family History
FSH	Follicle stimulating hormone
GAPS	Guidelines for Adolescent Preventive Services
GC	Gonococcus/gonorrhea
GI	Gastrointestinal
GnRH	Gonadotrophin-releasing hormone
H/O	History of
HBsAg	Hepatitis B surface antigen
HAV	Hepatitis A virus
HBV	Hepatitis B virus
HCG	Human chorionic gonadotrophin
HCV	Hepatitis C virus
HDL	High density lipoprotein
HIV	Human immunodeficiency virus
HMB	Heavy menstrual bleeding
HPV	Human papillomavirus
HSG	Hysterosalpingogram
HSV	Herpes simplex virus (I or II)
H(R)T	Hormone (replacement) therapy
Hx	History
IM	Intramuscular
IPPF	International Planned Parenthood Federation
IUC	Intrauterine contraceptive
IUD	Intrauterine device
IUP	Intrauterine pregnancy
IUS	Intrauterine system
IV	Intravenous
KOH	Potassium hydroxide
LARC	Long acting reversible contraception

LAM	Lactational amenorrhea method
LARC	Long acting reversible contraceptives
LDL	Low-density lipoprotein
LGV	Lymphogranuloma venereum
LH	Luteinizing hormone
LMP	Last menstrual period
LNG-IUD	Levonorgestrel IUD
MEC	Medical Eligibilty Criteria
MI	Myocardial infarction
MIS	Misoprostol
MMG	Mammogram
MMPI	Minnesota Multiphasic Personality Inventory
MMR	Mumps Measles Rubella
MMWR	Mortality and Morbidity Weekly Report
MPA	Medroxyprogesterone acetate
MPT	Multipurpose Prevention Technology
MRI	Magnetic resonance imaging
MSM	Men who have sex with men
MTX	Methotrexate
MVA	Manual vacuum aspiration
N-9	Nonoxynol-9
NFP	Natural family planning
NSAID	Nonsteroidal anti-inflammatory drug
OA	Overeaters Anonymous
OB/GYN	Obstetrics & Gynecology
OC	Oral contraceptive
OR	Operating Room
OTC	Over the counter
P	Progesterone or progestin
Pap	Papanicolaou
PCOS	Polycystic ovarian syndrome
PE	Pulmonary embolism
PET	Polyesther (fibers)
PG	Prostaglandin
pH	Hydrogen ion concentration
PCO	Polycystic ovarian syndrome
PID	Pelvic inflammatory disease
PLISSIT	Permission giving Limited information Simple suggestions Intensive Therapy
PMDD	Premenstrual dysphoric disorder
PMS	Premenstrual syndrome
po	Latin: "per os"; orally, by mouth
POCs	Progestin-only contraceptives
POP	Progestin-only pill (minipill)
PP	Postpartum
PPFA	Planned Parenthood Federation of America
PRN	As needed
PUL	Pregnancy of Unknown Location
Q	Every
qd	Once daily
qid	Four times a day
R/O	Rule out
RR	Relative risk
Rx	Prescription or therapy
SAB	Spontaneous abortion
SHBG	Sex hormone binding globulin
SPR	Selected Practice Recommendations
SPT	Spotting
SSRI	Selective Serotonin Reuptake Inhibitors
STD	Sexually transmitted disease
STI	Sexually transmitted infection
Sx	Symptoms
TAB	Therapeutic abortion/elective abortion
TB	Tuberculosis
TCA	Trichloroacetic acid
TFT	Thyroid function test
tid	Three times a day
TSS	Toxic shock syndrome
TVU	Transvaginal ultrasound
UPA	Ulipristal acetate
URI	Upper respiratory infection
U.S. MEC	U.S. Medical Eligibility Criteria
USPSTF	U.S. Preventive Services Task Force
UTI	Urinary tract infection
VTE	Venous thromboembolism
VVC	Vulvovaginal candidiasis
WHO	World Health Organization
Y/O	Years old
ZDV	Zidovudine

FIGURE 1.1 MENSTRUAL CYCLE EVENTS - IDEALIZED 28 DAY CYCLE

[Hatcher 2018]

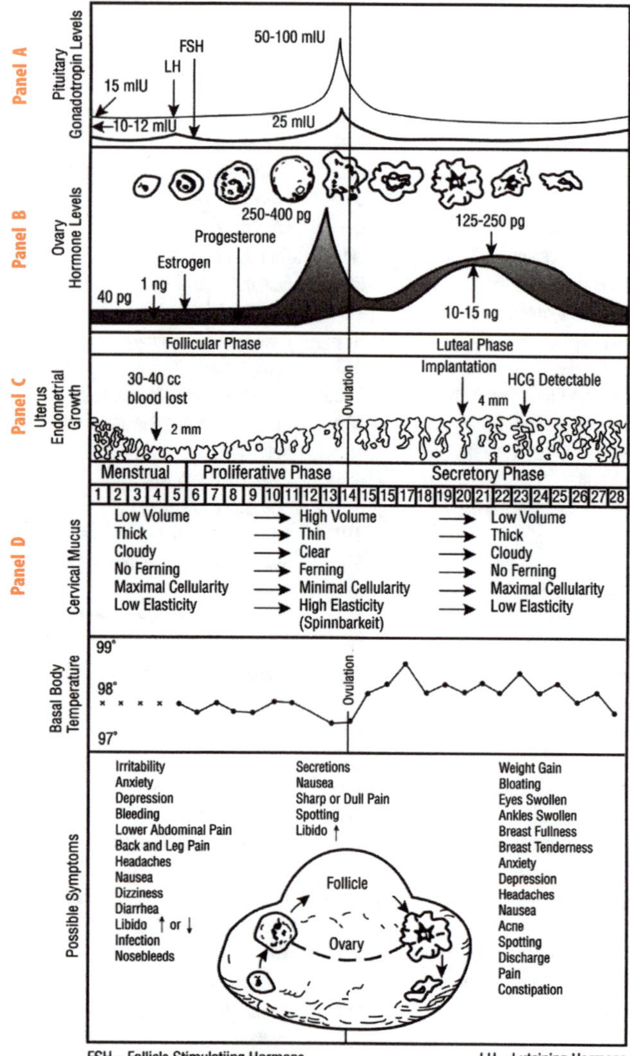

CHAPTER 1

THE MENSTRUAL CYCLE

The natural menstrual cycle is the vital sign of a woman's reproductive system, i.e., regular cyclic periods, in the absence of exogenous hormones, convey health.

Use of exogeneous hormonal contraception disrupts the natural cycle and may alter the natural bleeding pattern. When use of oral contraceptive pills mimics monthly bleeding, this results in a "pill period."

THE MENSTURAL CYCLE

Results from a complex orchestration between the hypothalamic -pituitary-ovarian (H-P-O) axis

Hypothalamus:

- Secretes GnRH to stimulate the pituitary

Pituitary: *(see panel A of Fig. 1.1)*

- Secretes FSH to stimulate the ovaries to produce follicles and secrete estradiol
- Secretes LH to stimulate ovulation and progesterone secretion

Estradiol:

- Causes endometrium to proliferate *(see panel C of fig. 1.1)*
- Causes thinning of cervical mucus, at the time of the LH surge, to facilitate sperm transport *(see panel D of Fig. 1.1)*

Initiation of each menstrual cycle is due to atrophy of the corpus luteum, days 26-28 previous cycle *(see panel B of Fig. 1.1)*:

- Decreased estrogen secretion from ovary
- Increased FSH secretion from pituitary, which causes a new group of follicles to develop
- The follicles secrete estradiol, which raises serum levels again
- The follicles also secrete inhibin B which is a negative feedback to decrease FSH

A dominant follicle emerges:

- It has more granulosa cells and more FSH receptors per granulosa cell, and increased blood flow
- Therefore it "escapes" the effects of falling FSH before ovulation (caused by inhibin B)
- The dominant follicle secretes estradiol
- When E2 sustained at about 200 pg/ml for more than 50 hours, negative feedback of E2 on LH reverses to positive feedback, resulting in the LH surge *(see panel A, B of Fig. 1.1)*
- The dominant follicle grows with the LH surge and 10-12 hours later extrudes an oocyte, known as ovulation *(see panel B of Fig. 1.1)*
- The other non-dominant follicles undergo atresia
- The dominant follicle collapses and transforms into the corpus luteum, which secretes estrogen and progesterone to promote implantation / support pregnancy

If no implantation occurs, hormone levels fall and the endometrium sloughs resulting in menstrual bleeding

TO ORDER ADDITIONAL COPIES OF MANAGING CONTRACEPTION OR OTHER CONTRACEPTIVE RESOURCES

go to *managingcontraception.com* or
email info@managingcontraception.com or call 404-875-5001

CHAPTER 2

COUNSELING AND CHOOSING A METHOD

THE BEST METHOD IS THE ONE THAT IS MEDICALLY APPROPRIATE AND IS USED EVERY TIME BY SOMEONE SATISFIED WITH THE METHOD

- Each contraceptive method has both advantages and disadvantages
- Be prepared to discuss all methods, even those you may not use in your own practice
- When counseling someone, be aware of your own biases
- Ask client their choice of pronoun and add this question to your intake form

ATTRIBUTES OF METHODS THAT INFLUENCE CLIENT'S CHOICE OF METHOD:

- ***Safety***. U.S. Medical Eligibility Criteria (MEC) rates appropriateness of method based on health conditions
- ***Effectiveness:*** motivation to prevent pregnancy
- ***Convenience*** and ability to use method correctly. This also influences effectiveness
- ***Protection against STIs / HIV*** for individuals at risk
- ***Menstrual effects*** of method
- ***Ability to negotiate*** use of method with partner
- ***Cost:*** insurance status and access
- ***Personal influences:*** religion, privacy, friend's advice, mother's opinion, frequency of sex, involvement and support of partner
  For example: Will partner help pay for contraceptives, sterilization, or abortion if needed?

HOW TO USE U.S. MEC

MEC categories for methods:

1	No restrictions (method can be used)
2	Advantages generally outweigh theoretical or proven risks
3	Theoretical or proven risks usually outweigh the advantages
4	Unacceptable health risk (method not to be used)

Simplified 2-category system for methods

To make clinical judgment, the MEC 4-category classification system can be simplified into a 2-category system.

MEC Category	With Clinical Judgment	With Limited Clinical Judgment
1	Use the method in any circumstances	Use the method
2	Generally use the method	
3	Use of the method not usually recommended unless other, more appropriate methods are not available or acceptable	Do not use the method
4	Method not to be used	

To download most recent 2016 Medical Eligibility Criteria go to: www.cdc.gov

2020 U.S. MEC UPDATE: Depo-Provera injection and all IUDs are safe for use without restrictions by women at high risk for HIV infection. U.S. MEC 1

When counseling about the safety of method use, assess risk of method against risk of pregnancy. Recognize medical conditions that pose high risks if an individual becomes pregnant and CDC recommendation that long-acting reversible contraception (LARC) might be the best choice.*

Conditions associated with increased risk for adverse health events as a result of pregnancy*

- Breast cancer
- Complicated valvular heart disease
- Cystic fibrosis
- Diabetes: insulin dependent; with nephropathy, retinopathy, or neuropathy or other vascular disease; or of >20 years' duration
- Endometrial or ovarian cancer
- Epilepsy
- Hypertension (systolic ≥160 mm Hg or diastolic ≥100 mm Hg)
- History of bariatric surgery within the past 2 years
- HIV: not clinically well or not receiving antiretroviral therapy
- Ischemic heart disease
- Gestational trophoblastic disease
- Hepatocellular adenoma and malignant liver tumors (hepatoma)
- Peripartum cardiomyopathy
- Schistosomiasis with fibrosis of the liver
- Severe (decompensated) cirrhosis
- Sickle cell disease
- Solid organ transplantation within the past 2 years
- Stroke
- Systemic lupus erythematosus
- Thrombogenic mutations
- Tuberculosis

**Long-acting, highly effective contraceptive methods might be the best choice for women with conditions that are associated with increased risk for adverse health events as a result of pregnancy. These women should be advised that sole use of barrier methods for contraception and behavior-based methods of contraception might not be the most appropriate choice because of their relatively higher typical-use rates of failure.*

APPROACHES TO COUNSELING:

Personalized counseling with shared decision-making: collaborative approach where the best available evidence is integrated with client's values and preferences.

- Consider the specific counseling needs of transgender and nonbinary individuals
- The goal of contraceptive counseling is to help individuals reach their desired reproductive outcomes
- If interested primarily in effectiveness, use the tiered-efficacy model *(see page 6)*

May use the GATHER guide to structure counseling visit:

- **Greet** client in a friendly manner and establish rapport *(see page 18)*
- **Ask** open questions to discover what client is looking for and listen closely
- **Tell** the client relevant information about methods
- **Help** the client think through her choice and reflect what she is saying back to her as a question to make sure everything is clear
- **Explain** how to use the method and explain side effects. Ask client to repeat back method instructions
- **Return:** Encourage client to return if she has any questions or for any other needs
- For assessing client's contraceptive needs, consider the questions below:

KEY QUESTIONS while counseling about method choice start with "one key question"

Option 1: "Would you like to become pregnant in the upcoming year?" This question identifies the need for contraception and / or preconception health as stated from the CDC Reproductive Life Plan approach.

OR

Option 2: "Do you want to prevent pregnancy now?" This question identifies those at risk who want to discuss options.

Method Related Questions:

- What method are you using, if any?
- What have you used in the past?
- Have you ever used emergency contraception (EC)?
- Did you use birth control at last sexual encounter?
- What difficulties have you experienced with prior methods (if any)?
- Do you have a specific method in mind?
- Have you discussed method with your partner, and does he/she have any preferences?
- ***Last Question:*** What is important to you about your method? This helps provider counsel about noncontraceptive benefits, side effects and effectiveness, etc.

Regardless of the patient's final choice for birth control, mention using condoms during every act of intercourse to avoid the transmission of STIs if at risk and provide further contraceptive benefit.

Tiered-Efficacy Model: presents birth control options from the most effective to least

- ***Key question:*** When individual identifies protection against pregnancy as her most important goal.
- LARCs (IUDs and implants) are given priority / discussed first.
- Studies have found patients find efficacy-based visual aids to be the most easily understandable.

  Example of success with this model is **The Contraceptive CHOICE Project:**
  - a prospective cohort study of 9,256 women in St. Louis
  - contraceptives given at no cost, and LARCs were promoted as first-line (a LARC first script).

  Results:
  - 75% of women chose LARC methods (vs. the national average of ~10% in 2011).
  - teen pregnancy rate fell to 3.4% and abortion rate dropped.
  - Satisfaction and continuation with each method in the CHOICE Cohort

Method	Continuation 1 year (%)	Satisfaction 1 year (%)	Continuation 2 year (%)	Continuation 3 year (%)
Copper IUD	84	>80	77	70
LNG-IUD	88	>80	79	70
Implant	83	80	69	56
Short acting (Pills, Patch, Ring)	50-60	53	40-43	31

Criticism / pitfalls of tiered effectiveness counseling:

- Potential to be coercive. Providers should be aware of biases such as thinking LARC is best for everyone
- If a provider wants to promote LARC use, patients may feel pressured to satisfy the provider's first choice
- LARC more difficult to terminate on own, decreasing autonomy over method
- Important to be aware of history of contraceptive provision, which, at times, has been coercive, especially towards people of color and low-income communities.

WHAT WE MEAN BY EFFECTIVENESS:

It is important for patients to understand how we determine effectiveness.

Effectiveness may be measured in 2 ways *(see Table 2.1 page 9)*:

1. ***Typical use first year failure rates:*** The percentage of women who become pregnant during their first year of use. This number reflects pregnancies in both couples who use the method perfectly and of those who do not. Most contraceptors are "typical" not "perfect" users.

   The typical use failure rate is generally the number to use when counseling new start users.
2. ***Perfect (or correct and consistent) use first year failure rate:*** The percentage of women who become pregnant during their first year of use when they use the method **perfectly.**

- In spite of very effective options, the U.S. has a high rate of unintended pregnancy.
- Just under 50% of all pregnancies in the U.S. are not planned. This is because most people are typical users or non-users of contraceptives.

Counseling about effectiveness:

- Methods are divided into 3 groups:
  A. Highly effective: female and male sterilization, implants, and IUDs (LARC)
  B. Moderately effective: pills (COCs and POPs), ring, patch, and Depo injections
  C. Less effective: male latex condoms, female condoms, diaphragm, cervical cap, spermicides (gel, foam, suppository, film), withdrawal, and natural family planning (calendar, temperature, cervical mucus)

Caution in comparing effectiveness between methods using different efficacy indices.
In this book we cite effectiveness from various sources that may not be directly comparable, e.g., the Trussell chart *(page 9)***, package inserts or recent clinical trials. Recent trials may have higher failure rates due to inclusion of more diverse populations and other methodological factors.**

Figure 2.1 Effectiveness of family planning methods

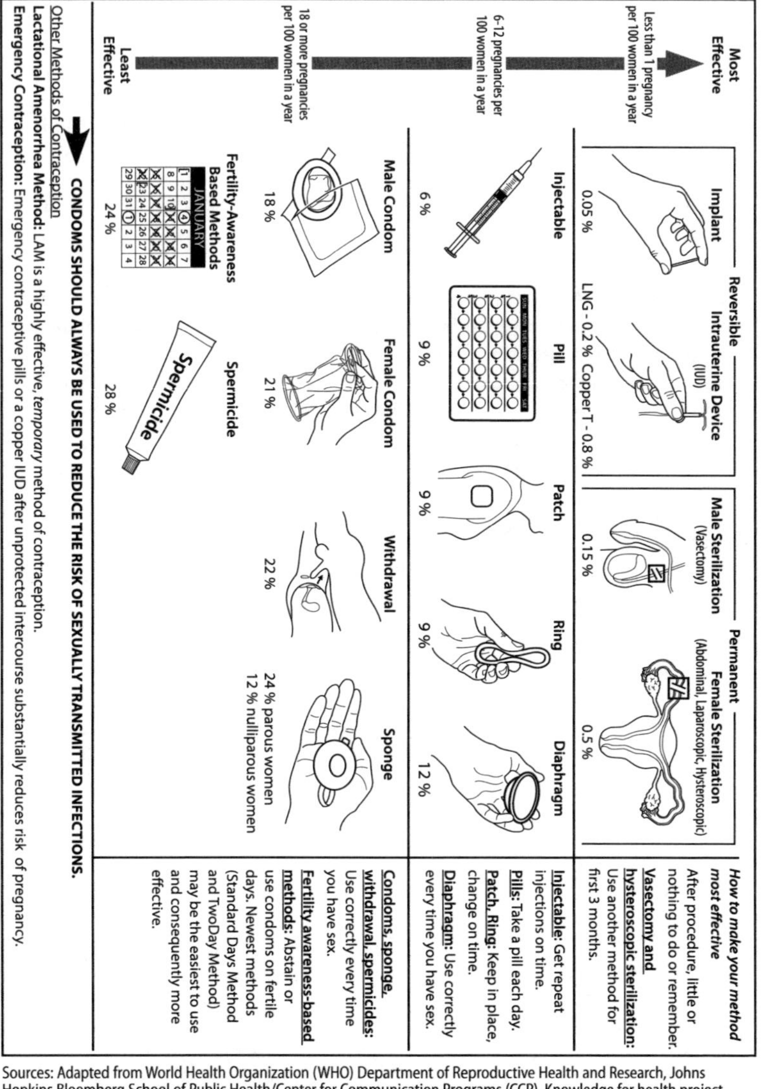

Sources: Adapted from World Health Organization (WHO) Department of Reproductive Health and Research, Johns Hopkins Bloomberg School of Public Health/Center for Communication Programs (CCP). Knowledge for health project. Family planning: a global handbook for providers (2011 update). Baltimore, MD; Geneva,Switzerland: CCP and WHO; 2011; and Trussell J. Contraceptive failure in the United States. Contraception 2011;83:397–404.

* The percentages indicate the number out of every 100 women who experienced an unintended pregnancy within the first year of typical use of each contraceptive method.

Table 2.1 Percentage of women experiencing an unintended pregnancy within the first year of typical use and the first year of perfect use and the percentage continuing use at the end of the first year: United States*

	% of Women Experiencing an Unintended Pregnancy within the First Year of Use		% of Women Continuing Use at One Year[1]
Method	**Typical Use[2]**	**Perfect Use[3]**	
Male Sterilization	0.15	0.10	100
Female Sterilization	0.5	0.5	100
Nexplanon	0.1	0.1	89
Intrauterine contraceptives			
Paragard (copper T)	0.8	0.6	78
Mirena / Liletta (LNG)	0.1	0.1	80
Depo-Provera	4	0.2	56
NuvaRing*	7	0.3	67
Evra patch*	7	0.3	67
Combined pill & Progestin-only pills	7	0.3	67
Diaphragm	17	16	57
Condom[8]			
Female (fc)	21	5	41
Male	13	2	43
Sponge			36
Parous women	27	20	
Nulliparous women	14	9	
Withdrawal	20	4	46
Fertility awareness-based methods	15		47
Standard Days method[6]	12	5	
TwoDay method[6]	14	4	
Ovulation method[6]	23	3	
Symptothermal method[6]	2	0.4	
Spermicides[5]	21	16	42
No Method[4]	85	85	

Emergency Contraceptive Pills: Treatment with COCs initiated within 120 hours after unprotected intercourse reduces the risk of pregnancy by at least 60-75%[9]. Pregnancy rates lower if initiated in first 12 hours. Progestin-only EC reduces pregnancy risk by 89%.

Lactational Amenorrhea Method: LAM is a highly effective, temporary method of contraception.[10]

Notes:

1 Among typical couples who initiate use of a method (not necessarily for the first time), the percentage who experience an accidental pregnancy during the first year if they do not stop use for any other reason. Estimates of the probability of pregnancy during the first year of typical use for spermicides, withdrawal, fertility awareness-based methods, the diaphragm, the male condom, the oral contraceptive pill, and Depo Provera are taken from the 1995 National Survey of Family Growth corrected for underreporting of abortion; see the text for the derivation of estimates for the other methods.

2 Among couples who initiate use of a method (not necessarily for the first time) and who use it perfectly (both consistently and correctly), the percentage who experience an accidental pregnancy during the first year if they do not stop use for any other reason. See the text for the derivation of the estimate for each method.

3 Among couples attempting to avoid pregnancy, the percentage who continue to use a method for 1 year.

4 The percentages becoming pregnant in columns (2) and (3) are based on data from populations where contraception is not used and from women who cease using contraception in order to become pregnant. Among such populations, about 89% become pregnant within 1 year. This estimate was lowered slightly (to 85%) to represent the percentage who would become pregnant within 1 year among women now relying on reversible methods of contraception if they abandoned contraception altogether.

5 Foams, creams, gels, vaginal suppositories, and vaginal film.

6 The Ovulation and TwoDay methods are based on evaluation of cervical mucus. The Standard Days method avoids intercourse on cycle days 8 through 19. The Symptothermal method is a double-check method based on evaluation of cervical mucus to determine the first fertile day and evaluation of cervical mucus and temperature to determine the last fertile day.

7 Without spermicides.

8 With spermicidal cream or jelly.

9 ella, Plan B One-Step and Next Choice are the only dedicated products specifically marketed for emergency contraception. The label for Plan B One-Step (one dose is 1 white pill) says to take the pill within 72 hours after unprotected intercourse. Research has shown that all of the brands listed here are effective when used within 120 hours after unprotected sex. The label for Next Choice (one dose is 1 peach pill) says to take 1 pill within 72 hours after unprotected intercourse and another pill 12 hours later. Research has shown that both pills can be taken at the same time with no decrease in efficacy or increase in side effects and that they are effective when used within 120 hours after unprotected sex. The Food and Drug Administration has in addition declared the following 19 brands of oral contraceptives to be safe and effective for emergency contraception: Ogestrel (1 dose is 2 white pills), Nordette (1 dose is 4 light-orange pills), Cryselle, Levora, Low-Ogestrel, Lo/Ovral, or Quasense (1 dose is 4 white pills), Jolessa, Portia, Seasonale or Trivora (1 dose is 4 pink pills), Seasonique (1 dose is 4 light-blue-green pills), Enpresse (one dose is 4 orange pills), Lessina (1 dose is 5 pink pills), Aviane or LoSeasonique (one dose is 5 orange pills), Lutera or Sronyx (one dose is 5 white pills), and Lybrel (one dose is 6 yellow pills).

10 However, to maintain effective protection against pregnancy, another method of contraception must be used as soon as menstruation resumes, the frequency or duration of breastfeeds is reduced, bottle feeds are introduced, or the baby reaches 6 months of age.

*Adapted from Trussell J, Kowal D. The essentials of contraception. In: Hatcher RA, et al. Contraceptive Technology, 21th ed., 2018 (page 100)

*Numbers for typical use failure of Ortho Evra and NuvaRing are not based on data. They are estimates based on pill data.

Thank you, James Trussell, for this remarkable table!

Table 2.2 Summary of major methods of contraception and some related safety concerns, side effects, and noncontraceptive benefits - may be useful for counseling

**Trussell 2018*

METHOD	NON-CONTRACEPTVE BENEFITS	SIDE EFFECTS / CAUTION	RISKS
Combined hormonal contraception (pill, patch and ring)	Decreases dysmenorrhea, menorrhagia, anemia and cyclic mood problems (PMS); protects against ectopic pregnancy, symptomatic PID, and ovarian, endometrial, and possibly colorectal cancer; reduces acne	Nausea, headaches, dizziness, spotting, weight gain, breast tenderness, chloasma	Cardiovascular complications (stroke, heart attack, blood clots, high blood pressure), depression, hepatic adenomas, increased risk of cervical and possibly liver cancers, earlier development of breast cancer in young women
Progestin-only pill	Lactation not disturbed Less nausea than with combined pills	Unscheduled spotting, breast tenderness	Efficacy dependant on daily adherence
IUD	LNG-IUDs decreases menstrual blood loss and menorrhagia and can provide progestin for hormone replacement therapy	Menstrual cramping, spotting, increased bleeding with non-progestin-releasing IUDs	Infection post insertion, uterine perforation, anemia (Copper IUD), expulsion
Male condom	Protects against STIs, including HIV; delays premature ejaculation	Decreased sensation, allergy to latex	Anaphylactic reaction to latex, slippage or breakage
Female condom	Protects against STIs	Aesthetically unappealing and awkward to use for some	None known
Implanon	Lactation not disturbed; decreases dysmenorrhea	Headache, acne, menstrual changes, weight gain, depression, emotional lability	Infection at implant site; difficult removal

METHOD	NON-CONTRACEPTVE BENEFITS	SIDE EFFECTS / CAUTION	RISKS
Depo-Provera	Lactation not disturbed; reduces risk of seizures; may protect against ovarian and endometrial cancers	Menstrual changes, weight gain, headache adverse effects on lipids	Depression, allergic reactions, pathologic weight gain, bone loss
Sterilization	Tubal sterilization reduces risk of ovarian cancer and may protect against PID	Pain at surgical site, psychological reactions, subsequent regret that the procedure was performed	Infection; possible anesthetic or surgical complications; if pregnancy occurs after tubal sterilization, risk that it will be ectopic
Abstinence	Prevents STIs, including HIV, if anal and oral intercourse are avoided as well		
Diaphragm, Sponge with spermicide		Pelvic discomfort, vaginal irritation, vaginal discharge if left in too long, allergy	Vaginal and urinary tract infections, toxic shock syndrome; possible increase in susceptibility to HIV/AIDS acquisition if exposed to positive partner
Spermicides		Vaginal irritation, allergy	Vaginal and urinary tract infections; possible increase in susceptibility to HIV/AIDS acquisition if exposed to positive partner
Lactational Amenorrhea Method (LAM)	Provides excellent nutrition for infants under 6 months old		

TIMING *(see table 2.3 page 14)*:

Traditionally, clients were counseled to start a new method on the first day of their upcoming menstrual cycle; however, some women become pregnant while they wait to begin their new method. We advocate for the use of the Quick Start method, which involves the patient starting the method on the day of the clinic visit in cases when you can be reasonably certain that the patient is not pregnant.

The QuickStart approach to starting the use of pills, intrauterine devices, implants, injections is now accepted as the proper way to start most contraceptives because it eliminates delay.

> **How to be reasonably certain a woman is not pregnant - no symptoms and signs of pregnancy AND she meets any of following criteria:**
>
> - no intercourse since last menses (period)
> - has been using a reliable method consistently and correctly
> - is 7 days or less after start of normal menses (period)
> - within 4 weeks postpartum
> - is 7 days or less post abortion or miscarriage
> - fully or near fully breastfeeding, amenorrheic and < 6 months postpartum (Some experts recommend relying on lactational amenorrhea only through 3 months because 20% of fully nursing mothers ovulate at 3 months)
>
> *CDC MMWR, June 21, 2013, Vol. 62, No.5*

Combined Hormonal Contraceptives (CHC):

- Healthy women who tolerate pills or CHC well and do not smoke can continue pills until menopause, *see page 125 (algorithm pills -> menopause)*
- No medical reason for periodic "breaks" from pils
- Extended use of combined pills with no pill free interval is an acceptable way for some women to take pills, with no increased risk of endometrial hyperplasia *[Anderson-2003]*.
- **QuickStart the method meaning**
    - Start pills, patch, or ring on day of office visit if you can be reasonably certain that she is not pregnant – *see box above [Westhoff-2002]*
    - If NOT within 5 days of the start of a period or miscarriage, recommend abstaining from sexual intercourse or back-up contraceptive for 7 days
    - If unprotected intercourse in preceeding 5 days offer EC.

Progestin Only Methods

- The first injection may be given at any time in the cycle if reasonably certain a woman is not pregnant *(see Box above)*.
- If NOT within 7 days of the start of a period or miscarriage, recommend to abstain or use back-up contraceptive for 7 days
- If unprotected intercourse in preceeding 5 days, offer EC. If QuickStart Depo-Provera with EC, repeat pregnancy test in 2-3 weeks
- Depo-Provera and progestin-only methods may be started postpartum:
    - At discharge from hospital up to 30 days: category 1 MEC non-breastfeeding, category 2 breastfeeding
    - >30 days: category 1 MEC for breastfeeding or not

IUDs

- May insert any time in a woman's menstrual cycle if reasonably certain she is not pregnant.
- If using an LNG-IUD, back-up recommended for 7 days if not inserted in the first 7 days of cycle.
- No back-up for Copper IUD because of its high efficacy as an emergency contraceptive.

Table 2.3 When to Start Using Specific Contraceptive Methods

U.S. Selected Practice Recommendations 2016

Contraceptive method	When to start (if the provider is reasonably certain that the woman is not pregnant)	Additional contraception (i.e., back up) needed	Examinations or tests needed before initiation[1]
Copper-containing IUD	Anytime	Not needed	Bimanual examination and cervical inspection[2]
Levonorgestrel-releasing IUD	Anytime	If >7 days after menses started, use back-up method or abstain for 7 days.	Bimanual examination and cervical inspection[2]
Implant	Anytime	If >5 days after menses started, use back-up method or abstain for 7 days.	None
Injectable	Anytime	If >7 days after menses started, use back-up method or abstain for 7 days.	None
Combined hormonal contraceptive	Anytime	If >5 days after menses started, use back-up method or abstain for 7 days.	Blood pressure measurement
Progestin-only pill	Anytime	If >5 days after menses started, use back-up method or abstain for 2 days.	None

Abbreviations: BMI = body mass index; IUD = intrauterine device; STD = sexually transmitted disease

[1]Weight (BMI) measurement is not needed to determine medical eligibility for any methods of contraception because all methods can be used or generally can be used among obese women. However, measuring weight and calculating BMI at baseline might be helpful for monitoring any changes and counseling women who might be concerned about weight change perceived to be associated with their contraceptive method.

[2]Most women do not require additional STD screening at the time of IUD insertion if they have already been screened according to CDC's STD Treatment Guidelines (available at http://www.cdc.gov/std/treatment). If a woman has not been screened according to guidelines, screening can be performed at the time of IUD insertion and insertion should not be delayed. Women with purulent cervicitis, current chlamydial infection, or gonorrhea should not undergo IUD insertion. Women who have a very high individual likelihood of STD exposure (e.g., those with a currently infected partner) generally should not undergo IUD insertion. For these women, IUD insertion should be delayed until appropriate testing and treatment occurs.

MMWR July 29, 2016, Vol. 65:No. 4

CHAPTER 3

SIMPLIFYING FAMILY PLANNING ACCESS DURING COVID-19 AND BEYOND

SIMPLIFYING ACCESS PER CDC GUIDANCE ISSUED DURING COVID APPLIES TO SERVICES AT ALL TIMES

https://www.cdc.gov/reproductivehealth/contraception/covid-19-family-planning-services.html

- Family Planning services are essential medical services
- Reduce barriers to accessing care
- Telehealth and other alternative practices such as curbside pick-up or mail delivery of contraception.
- Pharmacist-prescribed contraception: Many states allow access to some methods directly from a pharmacist, without a separate visit to a health care provider.
- Improving access during COVID applies to services at all times

FOR NEW CONTRACEPTIVE USERS OR THOSE WISHING TO SWITCH TO A NEW METHOD:

- ***Most contraceptive methods are safe for use by most patients.*** Consult the U.S. MEC *(see page 242)* to assess whether patients have any characteristics or medical conditions for which use of a specific contraceptive method should be restricted.
- ***Most contraceptive methods can be started with no physical examinations or laboratory tests.***

However, the following contraceptive methods* do *require physical examinations or laboratory tests:

- Intrauterine devices (IUDs): Bimanual exam and cervical inspection are necessary prior to IUD insertion. Most patients do not require additional STI screening at the time of IUD insertion, unless they have not been screened for gonorrhea and chlamydia according to CDC's STI Treatment Guidelines. Screening can be performed at the time of IUD insertion, and insertion should not be delayed.
- Combined hormonal contraception (CHC): Blood pressure should be evaluated before initiating CHCs. If blood pressure cannot be measured by a provider, blood pressure measured in other settings can be reported by the patient to the provider.
- Diaphragms and cervical caps: A bimanual examination (not cervical inspection) is needed for fitting some diaphragms that come in more than one size and could be considered to confirm fit for diaphragms that come in one size. Bimanual examination and cervical inspection are needed for cervical cap fitting.

All other methods: no exams or test are needed.

- ***All methods can be started on the day they are requested, if the provider is reasonably certain the patient is not pregnant.*** *see page 12*
  - Consider the need for emergency contraception at initiation.
  - Consider the need for a back-up depending on when method started.
- Immediate post-pregnancy contraception.
  - Combined hormonal methods can be started immediately after abortion.
  - Combined hormonal methods should not be initiated immediately postpartum due to concerns about increased risk of thrombosis.

- All other methods of contraception, including placement of IUDs and implants, can be started immediately post-pregnancy. IUDs should not be placed for women with sepsis.

FOR CURRENT CONTRACEPTIVE USERS WHO WANT TO INITIATE A NEW METHOD OR CONTINUE WITH THEIR CURRENT METHOD, LITTLE OR NO ONGOING FOLLOW UP IS NEEDED:

- No routine follow-up visit is required for any contraceptive method. Patients should be advised to contact a provider at any time to discuss side effects or other problems, to change or discontinue a method, and when it is time to remove or replace the method.
- A 1-year supply of CHC (COCs, patch, ring) can be provided or prescribed, depending on coverage allowances.
- Depot medroxyprogesterone acetate (DMPA), intramuscular (IM) or subcutaneous (SC) should be provided every 3 months (13 weeks); injections can be given up to 15 weeks from the last injection without requiring additional contraceptive protection. Consider self-administration of DMPA-SQ
  - Prefilled DMPA SQ syringe, 26-gauge needle, 0.65ml
  - Not labeled for self-administration
  - Several studies deem it safe and feasible

OTHER CONSIDERATIONS:

- An advance supply of emergency contraceptive pills can be provided or prescribed.
- Consider the need for STI / human immunodeficiency virus (HIV) prevention (including condom provision), diagnosis, testing and treatment, as well as need for HIV pre-exposure prophylaxis.
- Consider needs for other family planning services, such as pre-conception care, pregnancy testing and counseling, and basic infertility services.
- Consider the needs of different populations, including adolescents and others who may have more challenges overcoming barriers to accessing contraception at this time (e.g., issues around confidentiality, payment for services, and accessing new models of care).

CHAPTER 4

PROVIDING COMPREHENSIVE FAMILY PLANNING SERVICES

PROVIDING QUALITY FAMILY PLANNING (FP) SERVICES FROM CDC GUIDANCE*

Screening recommendations for women of reproductive age during FP visits

- What services should be offered during a FP visit?
  - Selected preventive health services tailored to FP visit
  - Does not include all preventive health services, such as screening for skin cancer or lipid disorders

Full recommendations at https://www.cdc.gov/mmwr/preview/mmwrhtml/rr6304a1.htm?s_cid=rr6304a1_w#Box2

DECIDE OR ASK:

- What is the purpose of this visit?
- What is the client's reproductive life plan?

Providers should discuss a reproductive life plan with clients receiving contraceptive, pregnancy testing and counseling, basic infertility, sexually transmitted disease, and preconception health services in accordance with CDC's recommendation that all persons capable of having a child should have a reproductive life plan.*

RECOMMENDED QUESTIONS TO ASK WHEN ASSESSING A CLIENT'S REPRODUCTIVE LIFE PLAN

- Do you have any children now?
- Do you want to have (more) children?
- How many (more) children would you like to have and when?

** Source: CDC. Recommendations to improve preconception health and health care—United States: a report of the CDC/ATSDR Preconception Care Work Group and the Select Panel on Preconception Care. MMWR 2006;55(No. RR-6).*

- If client is sexually active but not wanting pregnancy now, provide contraception and preconception health, *page 25*
- If client desires pregnancy testing, then test and counsel, *page 25*
- If client wants a child now, provide preconception health, *page 25*
- If client has difficulty conceiving, provide basic infertility services, *page 20*

** Providing Quality Family Planning Services (QFP) provides recommendations developed collaboratively by CDC and the Office of Population Affairs (OPA) of the U.S. Department of Health and Human Services (HHS).*

CONSIDER: WHAT OTHER PREVENTIVE SERVICES NEEDED?

Step 1: Establish rapport:

- Use open-ended questions
- Demonstrate expertise, trustworthiness, accessibility
- Ensure privacy and confidentiality
- Listen / observe client
- Encourage to ask questions
- Demonstrate empathy

Step 2: Obtain clinical and social information:

- Medical history
- Pregnancy intention or reproductive life plan
- Contraceptive experiences or preferences
- Ask method related questions *see page 5*

Sexual health assessment

TAKING SEXUAL HISTORIES

Initiating the Sexual History: Sample Questions

- Start with less direct questions and as trust builds, can ask more explicit questions
  - "Sexual information is necessary to provide complete care, you have the right to discuss only what you are comfortable with."
  - "These are routine questions I ask all patients."
  - "The information you share with me will be kept confidential but will be part of your medical record, unless you specifically request I do not include it."
  - "Some patients have shared concerns with me related to their risks of infections or concerns about particular sexual activities. If you have any concerns, please feel free to ask."

Sexual History Questions

Avoid assumptions: Making assumptions about a patient's sexual behavior and orientation can undermine patient trust and make the patient feel judged or alienated causing her to withhold information. This can result in diagnostic and treatment errors.

Do not assume that patients:

- ARE sexually active and need contraception
- Are NOT sexually active (e.g., older patients, young adolescents)
- Are heterosexual, homosexual or bisexual OR know if their partners have other partners
- Have power (within a relationship) to make or implement their own contraceptive decisions

The Five P's: Partners, Practices, Prevention of Pregnancy, Protection from STIs, and Past History of STIs

1. Partners

- "Do you have sex with men, women, or both?"
- "In the past 2 months, how many partners have you had sex with?"
- "Is it possible that any of your sex partners in the past 12 months had sex with someone else while they were still in a sexual relationship with you?"

2. Practices

- "To understand your risks for STIs, I need to understand the kind of sex you have had recently."
- "Have you had vaginal sex, meaning 'penis in vagina sex'?" If yes, "Do you use condoms: never, sometimes, or always?"
- "Have you had anal sex, meaning 'penis in rectum/anus sex'?" If yes, "Do you use condoms: never, sometimes, or always?"
- "Have you had oral sex, meaning 'mouth on penis/vagina'?"
- For condom answers:
  - If "never": "Why don't you use condoms?"
  - If "sometimes": "In what situations (or with whom) do you use or not use condoms?"

3. Prevention of pregnancy

- "What are you doing to prevent pregnancy?"

4. Protection from STIs

- "What do you do to protect yourself from STIs and HIV?"

5. Past history of STIs

- "Have you ever had an STI?"
- "Have any of your partners had an STI?"

Additional questions to identify HIV and viral hepatitis risk include:

- "Have you or any of your partners ever injected drugs?"
- "Have your or any of your partners exchanged money or drugs for sex?"
- "Is there anything else about your sexual practices that I need to know about?"

[MMWR/Vol 64/No.3 published June 5th, 2015]

Step 3: Work with client to select most effective / appropriate method. *see page 9*

Goals:

- Educate about safe methods for client
- Help to consider barriers to use
- Educate about typical effectiveness, correct use, noncontraceptive health benefits, side effects, protection from STIs

Potential barriers to successful use:

- Sociobehavioral including how partner may respond, or confidence in ability to use consistently like remembering daily pill
- Intimate partner violence
- Mental health and substance abuse

Step 4: Physical exam when warranted, *see page 25*

- Blood pressure before CHC
- BMI if indicated to note changes over time

Step 5: Provide method with instructions

- QuickStart, *page 12*, if reasonably certain not pregnant, *page 12*
- Provide or prescribe multiple cycles, e.g. one year supply short acting methods
- Make condoms easily available
- If method unavailable, provide bridge method
- Help client develop plan for successful use
- Discuss potential side effects and when to follow up
- Confirm understanding; may ask to "teach-back"

RETURNING CLIENTS

- Assess for satisfaction and concern with method and fertility goals
- Assess change in medical hx / eligibility
- Provide supplies and follow-up

BASIC INFERTILITY CARE FOR WOMEN IS A CORE FP SERVICE:

Infertility: failure to achieve pregnancy after 12 months

- Assess earlier at six months if: woman >35, h/o oligomenorrhea, possible tubal disease or endometriosis, partner known as subfertile
- Medical history assessing conditions that may impact fertility:
    - Past surgery, hospitalizations, injuries, endocrine disorders including thyroid, hirsutism, PCO, family h/o infertility
- Record time trying to conceive, coital frequency and timing, gravidity, parity, pregnancy outcomes
- Age of menarche, cycle length, dysmenorrhea, h/o STIs or PID
- Review of symptoms emphasizing Sx of thyroid Dz, pelvic or abdominal pain, dyspareunia, glactorrhea, hirsutism
- **Physical exam:** height, weight, BMI, thyroid, breast, R/O androgen excess
- **Pelvic exam:** assess tenderness and mobility, R/O enlargement, mass, nodularity and mobility
- Further Dx and Rx may include P levels, LH/FSH, TFTs, Prolactin, endometrial Bx, TVU, HSG, laparoscopy and clomiphene citrate

BASIC INFERTILITY CARE FOR MEN:

- Medical Hx including systemic illnesses e.g., diabetes, prior surgeries, infections, medications, lifestyle exposures.
- Reproductive history including coital frequency and timing, duration infertility, sexual history, gonadal toxin exposure including heat, sexual dysfunction
- Physical exam includes penis, location urethral meatus, palpation / size testes, presence / consistency vas deferens and epididymis, R/O varicocele, secondary sex characteristics, digital rectal
- Semen analysis. If abnormal, refer.

OTHER MEDICAL SCREENING SERVICES DURING FP VISIT:

Hypertension: Measure BP routinely

- May screen every 3-5 yrs. in 18-39 y/o without risk factors

Screen annually if high risk: Black clients, high normal BP, obese or overweight, age > 40

BP Category	Systolic mmHg		Diastolic mmHg
Normal	<120	and	<80
Elevated	120-129	and	<80
HTN stage 1	130-139	or	80-89
HTN stage 2	≥ 140	or	≥ 90
Hypertensive crisis	>180	and /or	>120

- ***Obesity:*** screen with height, weight, BMI, and if obese (BMI ≥ 30) refer for counseling and behavioral interventions

Diabetes: Screen adults 40-70 y/o overweight or obese

- **Screen younger if:** family hx, h/o gestational DM or PCO, or if Black, Asian American Pacific Islander, Latinx
- Diabetes tests normal results:
  - Fasting glucose < 5.6 mmol / L
  - HgA1C < 5.7%
  - Oral GTT done fasting in morning with 75g glucose load. 2-hr glucose < 140g/dl

Depression: screen if staff trained in a common depression screening tool and refer appropriately

Substance Use: Ask routinely about nicotine, alcohol and drugs including prescription opioids. Refer appropriately

Intimate Partner Violence: *(see ACOG CTE Opinion No. 518, Feb 2012)*

- Screen and refer to intervention if positive
- ***Sample screening framing statement:***
  - "We've started talking to all clients about safe and healthy relationships because they impact health."
- Statement of confidentiality
- ***Sample questions:***
  - "Has your current partner ever threatened you or made you afraid?"
  - "Has your partner ever hit, choked, or physically hurt you?"
  - "Has your partner ever forced you to do something sexually or refused to wear condoms?"

Immunization:

- Screen for influenza, Tdap, MMR, Varicella, Pneumococcal and meningococcal
- ACOG recommends Rubella titers in women unsure of status
- ***HPV vaccine:*** offer to ages 11-26 and counsel that the vaccine is indicated for both boys and girls (although can be started at age 9)
- ***Hepatitis B vaccine:*** offer to all unvaccinated under 19 years and all adults who are unvaccinated and do not have documented Hx of Hepatitis B infection

OTHER PREVENTIVE HEALTH SERVICES:

- ***Cervical cancer screening:*** *see page 28 for guidelines*
- ***Clinical Breast Exam*** recommendations for average risk women:
  - USPSTF says there is insufficient evidence to assess balance of benefits vs. harms.
  - ACOG recommends offering exam every 1-3 yrs for individuals ages 25-39 and yearly after 40.
  - American Cancer Society recommends Q3yrs ages 20-39 and yearly after 40
- ***Mammography:*** age < 50 screen based on individual risk and shared decision making
  - ***Age > 40:*** ACOG recommends yearly or biennial screening until age 75, then discuss.
  - ***Age 50-74:*** USPSTF recommends beginning screening at 50 and conducting bien-nialy until age 74

SEXUALLY TRANSMITTED INFECTIONS:

When counseling about and treating STIs, it is helpful to know comparative risks.

TABLE 3.1 Comparative risk of adverse consequences from vaginal or anal intercourse: Reproductive tract infection and unintended pregnancy

Unintended pregnancy (per coital act)	• 17%-30% midcycle • <1% during menses
HIV transmission (per coital act)	• 0.08% receptive vaginal sex • 0.04% insertive vaginal sex • 1.3% receptive anal sex • 0.11% insertive anal sex
Gonococcal transmission (per coital act)	• 50% receptive vaginal sex • 25% insertive vaginal sex
PID per woman infected with cervical gonorrhea	• 22% if not treated • 0% if promptly and adequately treated
Tubal infertility per PID episode	• 8% after first episode • 20% after second episode • 40% after three or more episodes

Marrazzo-2018

- ***Chlamydia:*** screen all sexually active women ≤ 25 annually and > 25 with risk factors

RISK FACTORS FOR CHLAMYDIA TRACHOMATIS	
• New partners • Partners with other partners	• >1 partner

  - If treating for CT, rescreen at 3 months for reinfection
  - Screen pregnant women at time of their pregnancy test if care may be delayed
- ***Gonorrhea:*** screen all sexually active women at risk annually

RISK FACTORS FOR GONORRHEA	
• Age <25 • Presence of other STIs • Inconsistent condom use	• Previous GC infection, • New or multiple partners • Commercial sex work, drug use

- If treating for GC, rescreen at 3 months for re-infection
- Screen pregnant women at time of their pregnancy test if care may be delayed

- ***Syphilis:*** screen those at risk:

RISK FACTORS FOR SYPHILIS	
• Men who have sex with men	• Sex workers
• Those who exchange sex for drugs	• In adult correctional facilities
• High prevalence areas	

- Screen pregnant women at time of pregnancy test if care may be delayed
- When prevalence high and woman high risk, testing should be repeated at 28-32 and at delivery

- ***HIV:*** screen ages 13-64 routinely and high risk annually

RISK FACTORS FOR HIV
• Injection drug users and their partners
• Those who exchange sex for money or drugs and their partners,
• Partners of HIV infected
• Men who have sex with men
• People with more than 1 partner since last HIV test

- CDC guidelines provide additional information about how to care for patients with HIV, which go beyond the level of care provided by most family planning service providers. *[clinicalinfo.hiv.gov/en/guidelines]*
- Providers should counsel the patient on **PrEP** (PO tenofovir/emtricitabine) if the patient has sex without consistent condom use with a partner living with HIV or if they are exposed to any other risk factors. *[Preexposure, 2014; CDC Clinical Practice Guidline]* Particularly if trying to conceive, pregnant, postpartum or breastfeeding *[clinicalinfo.hiv.gov/en/guidelines/perinatal/prep]*

- ***Hepatitis C:*** one time testing for people born between 1945-1965 (account for 75% of chronic HCV infections) as well as those at high risk.
  - HIV positive individuals should be screened annually for Hepatitis C

RISK FACTORS FOR HCV	
• Born between 1945-1965	• Ever injected illegal drugs
• Received clotting factors before 1987	• Ever on chronic hemodialysis
• Received organ transplant	• Blood transfusion before 1992
• Persistently abnormal alanine aminotransferase	
• Needlestick by someone HCV positive	
• Child born to HCV positive woman	

- ***Hepatitis B:*** screen high risk

RISK FACTORS FOR HBV	
• HIV-positive persons	• Injection drug users
• Injection drug users	
• Household contacts of persons with HBV infection	
• Persons from countries with a high prevalence of HBV infection	
• Men who have sex with men	

STI RECOMMENDATIONS:

- Provide high-intensity behavioral counseling for those at risk including: all sexually active adolescents, adults with current STI or in past year, adults with multiple partners, or those who live in high prevalence communities.
- When treating for an STI, counsel about need for partner treatment
  - partners in the past 60 days for CT and GC
  - partners in past 3 months for primary syphilis and 6 months for secondary syphilis PLUS the duration of lesions or signs
  - if partners cannot be examined, expedited partner therapy (giving prescription to treat partner for GC or CT) can be offered if permissible by state laws
- Advise to refrain from unprotected sexual intercourse during Rx.
- Return for retesting in 3 months.
- Encourage condom use.

Table 4.1 Footnotes

Abbreviations: BMI = body mass index; HBV = hepatitis B virus; HIV/AIDS = human immunodeficiency virus/acquired immunodeficiency syndrome; HPV = human papillomavirus; IUD = intrauterine device; STD = sexually transmitted disease.

* This table presents highlights from CDC's recommendations on contraceptive use. However, providers should consult appropriate guidelines when treating individual patients to obtain more detailed information about specific medical conditions and characteristics (Source: CDC. U.S. Medical Eligibility Criteria for Contraceptive Use. 2010. MMWR 2010;59(No. RR-4).

† STD services also promote preconception health but are listed separately here to highlight their importance in the context of all types of family planning visits. The services listed in this column are for women without symptoms suggestive of an STD.

§ CDC recommendation.

¶ U.S. Preventive Services Task Force recommendation.

** Professional medical association recommendation.

†† Weight (BMI) measurement is not needed to determine medical eligibility for any methods of contraception because all methods can be used (U.S. Medical Eligibility Criteria 1) or generally can be used (U.S. Medical Eligibility Criteria 2) among obese women (Source: CDC. U.S. Medical Eligibility Criteria for Contraceptive Use. 2010. MMWR 2010;59 Adobe PDF file [No. RR-4]). However, measuring weight and calculating BMI at baseline might be helpful for monitoring any changes and counseling women who might be concerned about weight change perceived to be associated with their contraceptive method.

§§ Indicates that screening is suggested only for those persons at highest risk or for a specific subpopulation with high prevalence of an infection or condition.

¶¶ Most women do not require additional STD screening at the time of IUD insertion if they have already been screened according to CDC's STD treatment guidelines (Sources: CDC. STD Treatment Guidelines: US Department of Health and Human Services, CDC; 2013. Available at http://www.cdc.gov/std/treatment. CDC. Sexually Transmitted Diseases Treatment Guidelines, 2010. MMWR 2010;59 Adobe PDF file [No. RR-12]). If a woman has not been screened according to guidelines, screening can be performed at the time of IUD insertion and insertion should not be delayed. Women with purulent cervicitis or current chlamydial infection or gonorrhea should not undergo IUD insertion (U.S. Medical Eligibility Criteria 4) Women, who have a very high individual likelihood of STD exposure (e.g. those with a currently infected partner) generally should not undergo IUD insertion (U.S. Medical Eligibility Criteria 3) (Source: CDC. US Medical Eligibility Criteria for Contraceptive Use. 2010. MMWR 2010;59 Adobe PDF file [No. RR-4]). For these women, IUD insertion should be delayed until appropriate testing and treatment occurs.

TABLE 4.1 CHECKLIST OF FAMILY PLANNING AND RELATED PREVENTIVE HEALTH SERVICES FOR WOMEN *(http://www.uspreventivetaskforce.org/uspstf/uspsstds.htm)*

Screening components	Family planning services (provide services in accordance with the appropriate clinical recommendation)					Related preventive health services
	Contraceptive services*	Pregnancy testing and counseling	Basic infertility services	Preconception health services	STI services†	
History						
Reproductive life plan§	Screen	Screen	Screen	Screen	Screen	
Medical history§,**	Screen	Screen	Screen	Screen	Screen	Screen
Current pregnancy status§	Screen					
Sexual health assessment§,**	Screen		Screen	Screen	Screen	
Intimate partner violence §,¶,**				Screen		
Alcohol and other drug use§,¶,**				Screen		
Tobacco use§,¶	Screen (combined hormonal methods for clients aged ≥35 years)			Screen		
Immunizations§				Screen	Screen for HPV & HBV§§	
Depression§,¶				Screen		
Folic acid§,¶				Screen		
Physical examamination						
Height, weight and BMI§,¶	Screen (hormonal methods)††		Screen	Screen		
Blood pressure§,¶	Screen (combined hormonal methods)			Screen§§		
Clinical breast exam**			Screen			Screen§§
Pelvic exam§,**	Screen (initiating diaphragm or IUD)	Screen (if clinically indicated)	Screen			
Signs of androgen excess**			Screen			
Thyroid exam**			Screen			
Laboratory testing						
Pregnancy test **	Screen (if clinically indicated)	Screen				
Chlamydia§, ¶	Screen¶¶				Screen§§	
Gonorrhea§, ¶	Screen¶¶				Screen§§	
Syphilis§,¶					Screen§§	
HIV/AIDS§,¶					Screen§§	
Hepatitis C§,¶					Screen§§	
Diabetes§,¶				Screen§§		
Cervical cytology¶						Screen§§
Mammography¶						Screen§§

CHAPTER 5

CERVICAL CANCER SCREENING AND HPV VACCINE

HPV & CERVICAL CANCER:

- Most HPV infections are transient, especially in young women (<30 y/o)
  - HPV detected in women >30 y/o is more likely to represent persistent infection, and increasing age has higher rates of high-grade squamous intraepithelial lesions (HSIL)
- **Oncogenic HPV accounts for 99% of cervical cancer**
  - Other risk factors: smoking, decreased immunity, HIV infection, number of sexual partners
  - HPV-16 accounts for 55-60% of cervical cancer worldwide, most oncogenic strain
  - HPV-18 accounts for 10-15% of cases worldwide
  - Only small fraction of women infected with HPV will develop dysplasia or cancer

Cervical CA incidence and mortality

- 12,820 new cases and 4,210 deaths from cervical CA in the US yearly (2017 estimates from the American Cancer Society)
- Worldwide in 2012 an estimated 530,000 new cases and 70,000 deaths *[WHO 2015]*.

PATIENT PREPARATION FOR PAP TESTING

- Preferred timing is mid-cycle, but may collect specimen during menses if using liquid based cytology
- Patient should abstain from vaginal medications, contraceptives, lubricants or douching 48 hours in advance, and sex the night before

PAP TESTING: RECOMMENDATIONS SAME IF WOMAN HAS RECEIVED HPV VACCINE

- May use conventional slide fixation or liquid based technique
  - Liquid allows for HPV co-testing as well as GC/CT and trichomonas testing
- Perform PAP test before bimanual exam, can use small amount water based lubricant on speculum. This does not interfere with PAP. Large amount of lubricant used for bimanual exam may interfere with PAP testing.

Table 5.1 Screening Recommendations based on the American Cancer Society *(updated 7/2020)*

Population	Recommended Screening Method	Comment
Women younger than 25	No screening	
Women aged 25-65 years	Preferred: Primary Human Papillomavirus testing alone every 5 years Acceptable: Cytology alone every 3 years or cotesting every 5 years	• 2 FDA approved Primary HPV tests • 5 FDA approved HPV tests for cotesting
Women older than 65 years	No screening is necessary after adequate negative prior screening results -no h/o CIN2 or more severe -2 consecutive negative primary HPV tests OR -2 neg co-tests OR 3 negative cytology within past 10 yrs with most recent within the past 3- 5 yrs	Women with a history of CIN 2, CIN 3 or adenocarcinoma in situ should continue surveillance for at least 25 years After 25 years surveillance at age 65 continue surveillance at 3 year intervals
Women who underwent total hysterectomy	No screening is necessary - no cervix - no h/o CIN2 or more in past 25 years	Applies to women without a cervix and without a history of CIN 2, CIN 3, adenocarcinoma in situ, or cancer in the past 20 years
Women vaccinated against HPV	Follow age-specific recommendations (same as unvaccinated women)	

Fontham ETH etal. CA Cancer, J Clin 2020; 70:321-346

FOR MANAGEMENT OF HPV TESTING AND CYTOLOGY:
consult ASCCP guidelines at *www.asccp.org/management-guidelines* or use the "ASCCP Management Guidelines" App

Table 5.2 Cervical Screening Recommendations endorsed by American College of Obstetricians and Gynecologists, American Society for Colposcopy and Cervical Pathology, Society of Gynecologic Oncology and United States Preventive Services Taskforce

asccp.org/screening-guidelines

Population*	Recommended Screening Method	Recommendation Grade±
Women aged less than 21 years	No screening	D
Women aged 21-29 years	Cytology every 3 years$	A
Women aged 30-65 years	Any one of the following: • Cytology alone every 3 years • FDA approved primary hrHPV testing alone every 5 years • Cotesting (hrHPV testing and cytology) every 5 years	A
Women aged greater than 65 years	No screening after adequate negative prior screening results §	D
Hysterectomy with removal of cervix	No screening in individuals who do not have a history of high-grade cervical precancerous lesions or cervical cancer	D

Abbreviations: FDA, U.S. Food and Drug Administration; hrHPV, high-risk human papillomavirus testing.

*These recommendations apply to individuals with a cervix who do not have any signs or symptoms of cervical cancer, regardless of their sexual history or HPV vaccination status. These recommendations do not apply to individuals who are at high risk of the disease, such as those who have previously received a diagnosis of a high-grade precancerous cervical lesion. These recommendations also do not apply to individuals with in utero exposure to diethylstilbestrol or those who have a compromised immune system (eg, individuals with human immunodeficiency virus).

±Grade A denotes that "The USPSTF recommends the service. There is high certainty that the net benefit is substantial." Grade D definition means that, "The USPSTF recommends against the service. There is moderate or high certainty that the service has no net benefit or that the harms outweigh the benefits." For more information on the USPSTF grades, see https://www. uspreventiveservicestaskf orce. org/Page/Name/ grade-definitions

$Primary hrHPV testing is FDA approved for use starting at age 25 years, and ACOG, ASCCP, and SGO advise that primary hrHPV testing every 5 years can be considered as an alternative to cytology-only screening in average-risk patients aged 25-29 years.

§Adequate negative prior screening test results are defined as three consecutive negative cytology results, two consecutive negative cotesting results, or two consecutive negative hrHPV test results within 10 years before stopping screening, with the most recent test occurring within the recommended screening interval for the test used (1, 5).

Data from Curry SJ, Krist AH, Owens DK, Barry MJ, Caughey AB, Davidson KW, et al. Screening for cervical cancer: U.S. Preventive Services Task Force recommendation statement. U.S. Preventive Services Task Force. JAMA 2018;320:674-86. Available at https:/ /jamanetwork.com/journals/jama/fullarticle/2697704. Retrieved April 12, 2021.

HPV VACCINE:

- Other cancers attributable to HPV are throat, larynx, anal and vulvar cancer.
- Vaccine is recommended and FDA approved (in U.S.) for both women and men 9-45.
- In the United States, just under 40% of women (39.7%) and 20% of men (21.6%) received all 3 doses of the vaccine in 2014. [CDC 2015]
- 3 HPV vaccines available but only 9-Valent is used in U.S.

Bivalent vaccine (Cervarix): protects against HPV types 16 and 18

Quadrivalent vaccine (Gardasil): protects against HPV types 16 and 18, and HPV types 6 and 11 which cause most genital warts

9-Valent vaccine (Gardasil 9): adds protection to 5 additional high-risk HPV types 31, 33, 45, 52, 58

- Gardasil 9 FDA approved for women and men ages 9-45.
- If administering to ages 9-15, two doses are given at time 0 and at 6-12 months.
- if administering at ≥ 15 y/o three doses are given at 0, 2, and 6 months
- Getting all 3 doses prior to onset of sexual activity reduces risk of certain HPV-related cervical cancer by 97%
- Less benefit as people get older because assumed prior exposure to HPV. If client has had limited sexual activity, may be greater benefit to vaccinating older people.
- Vaccine is not a substitution for cervical cancer screening.
- Women with previous HPV infection or abnormal cytology can still be vaccinated and may benefit from protection against strains they may not have yet acquired. Benefits in these women may be more limited and women should be informed it will have no effect on pre-existing HPV disease.
- Vaccination is not a treatment for genital warts
- Immunosuppression is not a contraindication to vaccination; efficacy may be affected

HAVING RECEIVED HPV VACCINE DOES NOT CHANGE CERVICAL CANCER SCREENING GUIDELINES

Contraindication: hypersensitivity to vaccine components. If sensitivity occurs after first dose, do not administer subsequent doses

Precaution: may not result in protection for all recipients

• Not intended to be given to pregnant women, pregnancy category B, although no known increase in adverse outcomes. Pregnancy registry: 1-800-986-8999

• Adverse events include pain, swelling, erythema, pruritis at injection site

CHAPTER 6

ADOLESCENT ISSUES

> To improve contraceptive effectiveness, prevent sexually transmitted infections, and prevent infertility due to tubal occlusion, CONDOMS should be used by most adolescents using ANY contraceptive, including LARC methods - IUDs and implants.

Talking to adolescent patients about the benefits of delaying sexual activity, the correct use of contraceptives, and the need for protection from STIs and HIV is important:

- Teen pregnancy has dramatically decreased in last decade. 2017 had the lowest recorded teen pregnancy rate in U.S. at 14 pregnancies per 1000 women ages 15-17 (down from 75 at peak in 1989). This is due to a decrease in sexual activity and an increase in contraception, including more effective methods
  - Between 1988-2015: girls who ever had sex decreased from 51% to 42%
  - Girls who used contraception at last sex increased from 80-90%
  - 50% US teens have had vaginal intercourse by 18
  - US teen birth rates still highest in developed world besides the Soviet Bloc

    [Guttmacher.org, Adolescent Pregnancy and Its Outcomes Across Countries]
- US teen birth rates have declined across several decades, and the 2017 birth rate of 18.8 births per 1,000 teens ages 15–19 years was the lowest recorded birth rate. *[Martin 2018]*
  - US teen pregnancy rate is still higher than other developed countries. Among 15-19 year olds 57 per 1000 females compared to lowest rate in Switzerland 8 per 1000 *[Adolese 2015]*

COUNSELING CHALLENGES POSED BY ADOLESCENTS

Teens are not "young adults." Developmentally appropriate approaches are needed.

- Age 11-14 – teens are concrete, egocentric (self-focused) and concerned with personal appearance and acceptance, with a short attention span. Sexual maturation and abstract thinking start.

> **LONG ACTING REVERSIBLE CONTRACEPTIVES,** also called LARC methods or forgettable methods (IUDs, implants), are the most effective methods for preventing teen pregnancy. Young teens (14-17) who chose a LARC method in St. Louis were more likely to choose an implant (63%), while most older teens who chose a LARC method chose an IUD (71%). *[Mestad Contraception 2011]*

Nonjudgmental, open-ended and reflective questions are better than direct yes-no inquiries. "What would you want to tell a friend who was thinking about having sex?" instead of "You're not having sex, are you?"

- Be sensitive to client's preferred gender identity, sexual orientation and pronouns

CONFIDENTIALITY: All teens should be entitled to confidential services and counseling, but billing systems and/or laws in some states affect confidentiality. Know your local laws and refer to sites that may be able to meet all the teen's needs if your practice can not.

ADOLESCENTS AND THE LAW: The Guttmacher Institute provides information on state laws regarding adolescent's right to consent to reproductive health, contraception, and abortion services. Visit *www.guttmacher.org/statecenter/spids/spib_OMCL.pdf* for current information.

TEENS AND CONTRACEPTION

- It is not necessary to perform a pelvic exam prior to prescribing any contraceptive other than an IUD or barrier method that requires fitting.
- Teens are eligible for all methods of contraception, regardless of pregnancy history.
- The CDC's U.S. Selected Practice Recommendations for Contraceptive Use provides clear guidance on best practices for contraceptive use, initiation, discontinuation, and problem management. https://www.cdc.gov/mmwr/volumes/65/rr/rr6504a1.htm *[CDC 2016 Selected Practice Recommendations]*

Over the counter (OTC) access to oral contraceptives would improve access for teens although contact with a provider is still encouraged. This approach is supported by the American College of Obstetricians and Gynecologists *[ACOG Committee Opinion #615 Jan 2015 Access to Contraception]*. It is generally predicted that progestin-only pills have a greater chance of being approved as OTC pills than combined pills.

ADOLESCENTS AS RISK TAKERS

- Ask each teen about Home, Education, Activities, Drugs, Sexuality (activity, orientation and abuse) and Suicide (HEADSS)
- Assess for the female athletic triad: eating disorders, amenorrhea and osteoporosis
- Discuss keeping EC at home and provide a prescription if needed or desired
- LARC are highly effective methods for this age group
- IUDs are safe and effective methods for nulliparous and parous adolescents *[US MEC]*
- As in adults, bone mineral density quickly recovers after discontinuation of DMPA use to levels as high as non-users by 12 months *[Curtis 2006]*. DEXA scans are NOT indicated in this age group as the scores cannot predict fracture risk in adolescents

HEALTH CARE SCREENING FOR ADOLESCENTS

- The initial visit for screening and provision of reproductive preventative health care services should take place between 13-15 years of age. *[ACOG CTE opinion 710, 2019]*
- Initiate cervical cancer screening beginning at age 21 (per ACOG) or age 25 (per ACS), unless immune deficiency or other special circumstances warrant earlier screening
- Teaching self-breast examination is not recommended in women younger than 19 years old as it leads to false positives and takes time from higher priority counseling issues

TEENS AND SEXUALLY TRANSMITTED INFECTIONS

Regardless of contraception chosen, discuss use of condoms to prevent STIs.

- 15-24 years olds account for 25% of the sexually active population, but experience almost half of STIs annually
- One study showed a decline in condom use after starting OCs. Subjects who were advised to ALWAYS use a condom, had a 50% increase in consistent condom use. *[Morroni 2014]*
- HPV infections account for half of the newly acquired STIs in this age group. *[see page 29 for vaccine information]*
- Screening for gonorrhea, chlamydia, and HIV is recommended for all sexually at-risk active teenagers. Treatment for gonorrhea and chlamydia should be followed by a rescreening test for reinfection in 3 months

SEX EDUCATION

Abstinence-only sex ed programs have been found ineffective in preventing or delaying teenagers from having sexual intercourse, and have no impact on the likelihood that if they do have sex, they will use a condom. Moreover, sex education, contraception and STI curricula offered in many schools are not medically correct. The information teens obtain from peers is also often inaccurate.

Common **MYTHS** are:

- *You cannot get pregnant the first time you have intercourse*
- *You cannot get pregnant if you douche after sex*
- *Having sex or having a baby makes you a woman and makes your boyfriend love you*
- *Making a girl pregnant means that you are a man*

Adolescents need concrete information and opportunities to role play and practice:

- How to open and place a condom and where to carry it
- How to negotiate NOT having sex and, in other cases, condom use
- How to punch out the pills, where to keep the pack, and how to remember them
- 7% is the typical-use failure rate of pills in a general population, but is higher in teens
- Dual protection: condoms and another contraceptive
- How to access and use emergency contraceptive pills and IUDs

Society for Adolescent Health and Medicine (SAHM) Position on Abstinence-Only-Until-Marriage (AOUM) programs

The goal of this revised position paper was to update the scientific and human rights evidence about AOUM programs and refine SAHM's recommendations regarding AOUM programs. Based on our review, SAHM believes:

- **Young people have a right to accurate and complete information to protect their lives and their health.**
- **Abstinence can be a healthy choice, but adolescents should decide for themselves when they are ready to initiate sex. An adolescent's choice of abstinence or sexual activity should never be coerced.**
- **Young people should be empowered to become full partners in the development and implementation of comprehensive sexuality education programs.**
- **Education for adolescents regarding abstinence is best provided within health education programs that provide adolescents with complete and accurate information about sexual and reproductive health.**
- **Sexuality education should be comprehensive, medically accurate, and culturally competent; promote healthy sexuality; and prepare young people to make healthy sexual decisions. Instruction in sexuality education should include essential concepts and issues such as sexual orientation, sexual health, gender identity and power dynamics, intimate partner violence and sexual exploitation, healthy relationships, social and structural determinants, personal responsibility, risks for HIV and other sexually transmitted infections (STIs) and unwanted pregnancy, access to sexual and reproductive health care, and the benefits and risks of condoms and other contraceptive methods.**
- **Health educators and health care providers should provide comprehensive information to young people.**
- **Governments and schools should eliminate censorship of information related to human sexuality, including sexual orientation and gender identity.**
- **Sexuality education curricula and programs should be based on scientific principles and evidence from research. Government policy regarding sexual and reproductive health education should be science based. The focus on evidence-based interventions in current U.S. federal programs to prevent adolescent pregnancy represents an important scientific advance over prior federal efforts which focused on abstinence only and ignored the evidence base. The USG and other governments should increase support for development and evaluation of programs to promote adolescent sexual and reproductive health, including school-based interventions, media efforts, and clinic-based interventions.**
- **United States government programs promoting abstinence-only-until-marriage are ethically flawed, are not evidence-based, and interfere with fundamental human rights to complete and accurate health information. U.S. federal funding for such programs should be eliminated and Title V, Section 510(b) of the Social Security Act, including subsections A–H, should be repealed. Current funding for abstinence-only-until-marriage programs should be replaced with funding for programs that offer comprehensive, medically accurate sexuality education.**
- **"Abstinence-only-until-marriage" as a basis for adolescent health policy and programs should be abandoned.**

https://www.jahonline.org/article/S1054-139X(17)30297-5/fulltext

CHAPTER 7

PRECONCEPTION AND PREGNANCY PLANNING

Preconception Health applies to any time a woman of reproductive potential is not pregnant but at risk of pregnancy, or a man is at risk of impregnating his partner.

GOALS

- Promote health before pregnancy to reduce adverse pregnancy outcomes
- Improve health regardless of pregnancy intentions
- Integrate into Family Planning visits

FOLIC ACID

- Women in the reproductive years should take 0.4 mg (400 micrograms) to 0.8 mg of synthetic folic acid daily to reduce the risk of neural tube defects in a developing fetus. All prenatal vitamins contain a minimum dose
- Women with a history of spina bifida, women on antiseizure medication and insulin dependent diabetics need 4.0 mg folic acid daily
- 0.45 mg per day is in Beyaz and Safyral oral contraceptive pills

Ask about Pregnancy Planning

- Would you like to become pregnant in the next year?
- How important is avoiding pregnancy in the next year?

PREGNANCY PLANNING

Reproductive history: Assess risk factors for preterm birth

RISK FACTORS FOR PRETERM BIRTH:

- non-white race
- age < 17 or > 35
- low socioeconomic status
- low prepregnancy weight
- maternal history of preterm birth especially in second trimester
- late or no health care during pregnancy
- using alcohol or illegal drugs
- vaginal bleeding in more than one trimester
- excessively physically stressful job (controversial)
- smoking
- being pregnant with twins, triplets or more
- pregnancy resulting from in vitro fertilization
- short time period between pregnancies
- diabetes and gestational diabetes

Reference: ACOG Practice Bulletin, 2001 and nichd.nih.gov

Assess Environmental Hazards:

- Chemical, radioactive and infectious exposures at workplace, home, hobbies
- Physical conditions, especially workplace

Assess Psychosocial Factors:

- Readiness of individual and partner for parenthood
- Mental health, anxiety, depression, domestic violence and history of PTSD
- Financial issues and support systems

Provide Genetic Counseling:

- For all individuals, may need additional specialized counseling if going to be > 35 y.o. when she delivers or has a significant personal or family history of genetic disorders, poor pregnancy outcome or partner of advanced paternal age
- Family history of developmental delays or genetic disorders such as sickle cell anemia, thalassemia, cystic fibrosis, Tay-Sachs, Canavan disease, neural tube defect
- High risk backgrounds: Ashkenazi Jews, French Canadian, etc.
- At risk of defects: seizure disorders, diabetes

Offer Screening and/or Counseling for:

- Infections (TB, gonorrhea, chlamydia, HIV, syphilis, hepatitis B & C, HSV as per CDC guidelines). Vaginal wet mount if discharge present
- Neoplasms (breast, cervical dysplasia, warts, etc.)
- Immunity (rubella, tetanus, varicella, HBV) HPV if applicable
- Alcohol use, tobacco use, substance abuse, obesity
- Advanced maternal and paternal age
- Intimate partner violence
- Depression
- Height, weight, BMI
- Blood pressure:
  - < 120/80, screen every 2 years
  - 120-139/80-89, prehypertension, screen yearly
- Diabetes: screen if BP > 135/80

Assess Medication Risks:

- Include OTC, prescription, herbal
- **For example:** Accutane and Tetracycline are teratogenic and require highly effective contraception and use of 2 methods
- Delay pregnancy at least 1 year after Accutane
- Hypertensive women on ACE inhibitors should switch to other meds
- Some antiepileptics are teratogenic
- Switch from Coumadin to Heparin or Lovenox

ACCUTANE SHOULD BE USED VERY CAUTIOUSLY IN REPRODUCTIVE AGE WOMEN

Accutane (isotretinoin) is a vitamin A isomer used in the treatment of severe cystic acne. If taken by a woman who is pregnant, it may cause a wide range of teratogenic effects:

CNS: hydrocephalus, facial nerve palsy, cortical blindness and retinal defects
Craniofacial: low-set ears, microcephaly, triangular skull and cleft palate
Cardiovascular: transposition of the great vessels, atrial and ventricular septal defects

Important contraceptive messages for women considering Accutane use:

- ***Use Two Methods:*** In addition to compulsive, careful and consistent use of a very effective hormonal contraceptive, also use condoms consistently and correctly.
- ***Repeated Pregnancy Tests:*** Pregnancy tests are essential prior to initiating and on a monthly basis thereafter.
- ***Consider Abortion if Contraceptive Failure:*** Many clinicians will not provide this drug unless the woman agrees to have an abortion should a pregnancy occur
- ***Use Accutane Sparingly:*** This drug is dangerous to a developing fetus and should not be used unless other approaches to managing acne have been used first AND unless the reproductive-age woman using it agrees to use contraception consistently and correctly.

Achieve Glucose Control

In DM, glucose control decreases adverse outcomes

Recommend:

- Ideally, planning a pregnancy should involve both an individual and partner
- Balanced diet
- Eat at least 8 oz and up to 12 oz (2 average meals) of fish lower in mercury, which can include up to 6 oz of albacore tuna per week. Non-albacore tuna has less mercury.
- No more than 1 serving of fish with moderate mercury levels and avoid all fish with high mercury levels (ACOG).
- Vitamin with folic acid 0.4 mg for all women planning pregnancy or at risk for unintended pregnancy (women with previous pregnancy with a neural tube defect, insulin dependent diabetic, alcoholic, malabsorption or on anticonvulsants need 4 mg folic acid daily)
- Minimize STI exposure risk
- Weight loss, if obese (gradual loss until conception)
- Moderate exercise
- Avoiding exposure to cat feces (toxoplasmosis) if no known immunity
- Encourage breastfeeding early in process of discussing pregnancy
- Early prenatal care when pregnancy occurs

CHAPTER 8

PREGNANCY TESTING

Early testing gives a woman time to pursue pregnancy options

- Prenatal care can be initiated promptly
- Unhealthy behaviors/exposures, such as smoking and alcohol intake, can be stopped sooner
- Ectopic pregnancies may be detected earlier
- Medical and surgical methods of abortion can be carried out more safely and less expensively

Timing of fertilization and production of hCG

- Sperm fertilizes ovum in fimbria of tube
- Fertilized ovum enters uterus at morula stage
- At 6 days after fertilization the embryo implants in the uterine decidua
- Embryo cells become placenta which produces hCG
- hCG can be detected 7-10 days after conception

PREGNANCY TESTS

Urine tests:

- Enzyme-linked immunosorbent assay (ELISA) test: Most tests positive at levels of 25 mIU/ml

BUT;

- Remind patients that no lab test is 100% accurate

AND THAT;

- False-negative tests (tests read as negative when a woman actually is pregnant) usually occur when done too early in the pregnancy and are far more common than false-positive tests, therefore pregnancy cannot be "ruled out" until test is 7 days after expected menses
- Any test can have false-negative results at low levels. If in doubt, repeat urine test in 1-2 days or obtain serum tests with a quantitative hCG

Serum tests (blood drawn):

- Radioimmunoassay:
    - Uses colorimetry, which detects hCG levels as low as 5 mIU/ml
    - Can quantify levels of hCG to monitor levels over time to assist in diagnosis of viability or ectopic pregnancy
    - For evaluation of early pregnancy, serial hCG testing should be done every 2 days until levels reach discriminatory levels of 1800-2000 mIU/ml, when a gestational sac can be visualized reliably by vaginal ultrasound. In normal gestations the levels of hCG doubles about every 2 days
    - Average time for hCG levels to become non-detectable after first trimester surgical abortion ranges from 31-38 days

PREGNANCY TEST NEGATIVE: WANTS TO AVOID PREGNANCY NOW

A negative pregnancy test for a woman not wanting to become pregnant provides the opportunity to offer effective contraception, and for discussion of a reproductive life plan. *(see page 17)*

1. If you haven't been using contraception, would you like to start now? What contraceptive method would work best for you? For maximal effectiveness you may want to consider using an IUD or an implant. You may be able to start your contraceptive today without a pelvic exam.
2. Don't try to become pregnant in order to see if you can become pregnant.
3. Unless you want to get pregnant, we can discuss protection against both infection and pregnancy.
4. Your negative pregnancy test today does not rule pregnancy from recent acts of intercourse (up to 2 weeks).
5. Provide information about emergency IUD insertion *(see page 81)* and emergency contraceptive pills *(see page 82)*.

PREGNANCY TEST POSITIVE: WANTS TO CONTINUE THIS PREGNANCY

Whether or not this pregnancy was planned and prepared for *(see page 34)*.

1. Start vitamins containing folic acid (0.4 mg) today.
2. Stop drinking alcohol or using any recreational drugs today.
3. Stop smoking today.
4. Are you on any medication? Are you taking any over-the-counter products? Assess for precautions with pregnancy
5. Use condoms if at any risk for HIV or other STIs.
6. Eat healthy foods. Gain 25-30 pounds during your pregnancy (if normal weight now).
7. Review current medical problems.
8. Provide appropriate prenatal care or make a referral.

CHAPTER 9

ELECTIVE ABORTION

OVERVIEW

- Nearly half of pregnancies in the United States are unintended
- Nearly one in 4 women in the U.S. will have an abortion by the age of 45
  - 59% of women having an abortion already have one or more children. *[Jerman 2016]*
  - Each year about 10-15,000 abortions occur as a result of rape or incest. The lack of availability of abortions for women who have been raped should be remedied.
  - Racial disparities in abortion rates: the rate per 1000 women was 38.7 for white / non-Hispanic, 33.6 for Black / non-Hispanic, 20.0 for Hispanic and 7.7 for other
- 92% of abortions are done at ≤ 13 weeks, 78% at <9 weeks, 27% are <7 weeks, 6.9% at 14-20 weeks and 1% at ≥ 21 weeks . *[Kurtsmut 2018]*
- **Abortion ratio** in 2017 was 19% (number of abortions per 100 pregnancies ending in either abortion or live birth)
- Abortion rate has been falling. In 2017 rate was 11.3 abortions / 1000 women ages 15-44
- Worldwide approximately 47,000 women die annually from unsafe abortions *[WHO 2015]*
  - Places where abortion is illegal have higher rates of morbidity and mortality from unsafe abortions.
  - In the U.S., serious complications from abortion and mortality are extremely rare
    - o Death related to pregnancy is 14 times higher than to abortion:
    - o Abortion related mortality: 0.6 per 100,000 abortions compared to pregnan cy-related mortality: 8-10 per 100,000 live births *[Grimes 2012]*
    - o Estimated mortality from medication abortion is 0.7 per 100,000
  - Some states require women considering abortion to hear information that is false and not evidence-based to present abortion as more risky than pregnancy & child birth
  - Women deserve accurate information *[Raymond and Grimes 2012]*

Many state laws impose mandatory restrictions, waiting periods, and consent requirements. For current information on your state's abortion laws: *www.naral.org/* or *www.guttmacher.org/state-policy/explore/overview-abortion-laws*

OPTIONS COUNSELING AND PREPARATION FOR ABORTION

- In a nondirective and compassionate way, discuss all pregnancy options, including continuing pregnancy, adoption and programs available for assistance with each option *(abortionfunds.org/need-abortion)*
- If patient chooses abortion, discuss available options when applicable (surgical versus medical)
- Offer emotional support, education, pre- and post-procedural instructions, and contraception

- Review protocol, risks, benefits, and visit schedule
- If choosing medication abortion, assess patient's access to provider if D&C is needed. Explain need for D&C if incomplete or if continuing pregnancy (clarify that it may not be possible to avoid surgery altogether)
- Obtain informed consent after all questions are answered
- Vaginal ultrasound to confirm dates if indicated and available

Features of Medical and Surgical Abortion	
Medical	***Surgical***
Generally avoids invasive procedure	Involves invasive procedure
Usually requires multiple visits	Usually requires one visit
Days to weeks until complete	Usually complete in a few minutes
Available during early pregnancy	Available early and later in pregnancy
High success rate (94% - 97%)	Higher success rate (99%)
Usually requires follow-up Telemedicine reduces this barrier	Does not require follow-up in most cases
May be more private in some circumstances; will vary for each individual patient	May be more private in some circumstances; will vary for each individual patient
Patient participation in multi-step process	Less patient participation in a single-step process
Analgesia available if desired	Allows use of sedation or anesthesia when available if desired
Does not require surgical training, but does require surgical back-up	Requires surgical training and sometimes a licensed facility

INDUCED SURGICAL ABORTION

DESCRIPTION

Voluntary termination of pregnancy using uterine aspiration in early intrauterine gestations. In later gestations (after 14-16 weeks) using instruments for tissue removal (standard dilation and evacuation [D & E].

EFFECTIVENESS

- 98-99% effective; failures are mostly incomplete abortions with small amounts of retained tissue

PROCEDURE

- After informed consent obtained according to local law, type of procedure is determined by gestational age and patient preference
- Perform careful bimanual exam to assess size and position of uterus
- Labs include pregnancy tests, Hgb / HCT and Rh status although some clinicians only test gestation > 8 weeks (56 days) since the risk of sensitization low in earlier gestation
- In second trimester, dilate the cervix with an osmotic dilator (laminaria, Dilapan AND /

OR with a prostaglandin analogue (misoprostol)
  - Same-day or 2-day procedures with dilator on day prior to procedure are options
  - Mifepristone may be used for cervical dilation the day prior to a second trimester procedure
  - The Society for Family Planning offers guidance for cervical preparation in the second trimester.
  - Some providers offer same day cervical preparation (more convenient for the patient) with Dilapan or misoprostol. It is associated with low complication rates and shorter operating time for gestations up to 21 weeks, 6 days. *[Lyons 2013], [Maurer 2013]*
- Peri-operative antibiotics reduce the risk of post-procedure infection. However, no studies demonstrate if a single regimen is better than others. First choice is single-dose doxycycline 200mg orally before the procedure.
  - For treatment of infections, e.g. presumtive chlamydia, a 7-day course of doxycycline, or a single dose of azithromycin 1 g may be given. If bacterial vaginosis (BV) is present, treat with appropriate antibiotics. Alternatives for preoperative prophylaxis are: metronidazole 500mg p.o or azithromycin 500mg p.o. before procedure
- Cleanse ectocervix and endocervix
- Administer cervical anesthesia; if desired, adjunctive analgesia and / or sedation can also be used.
- Place tenaculum and mechanically dilate cervix if not previously dilated adequately
- Pre-procedure dilation is typically in second trimester procedures or select individuals e.g. nulliparous, adolescents or uterine issues like prior surgery.
- Using sterile technique, insert a plastic cannula and apply suction to aspirate products of conception either with a machine, or manually with a manual vacuum aspiration (MVA) syringe
- Evaluate tissue to confirm presence of placental villi / gestational sac if early pregnancy. If more than 10 weeks should be able to visualize fetal parts. If no villi, consider immediate reaspiration, USG may be used, and consider the possibility of ectopic pregnancy
- Administer Rh immune globulin if woman is Rh negative
- Initiate contraceptive of choice prior to exit from the facility if desired.
- Placement of an IUD immediately after completion of an abortion is not associated with a significant increased risk of complications or expulsion, and may lead to increased use of the IUD at 6 months post-procedure *[Bednarek 2011]*

ADVANTAGES

- Fewer risks to maternal health than continuing pregnancy
- Can be provided as early as intrauterine pregnancy is diagnosed
- Provides individual complete control over her fertility
- Intervention for fetal or maternal health risks
- Safe and rapid; preoperative evaluation and procedure can usually be done in a single visit (notwithstanding local legal restrictions)

DISADVANTAGES

- Cramping and pain with procedure; the noise of the vacuum machine (if electrical vacuum used) may cause anxiety or distress.

COMPLICATIONS

- Infection < 1%, (may lead rarely to infertility)
- Incomplete abortion 0.5%-1.0%; Failed abortion 0.1%-0.5%
- Hemorrhage 0.03%-1.0%
- Perforation: < 0.6% overall and < 0.01% in first-trimester
- Retained products of conception: < 1%
- Hematometra (post-abortal syndrome) <1%
- Asherman's syndrome rare (more likely with septic abortion), with an uncommon complication of infertility
- Mortality: Induced surgical and medical abortion deaths <1 per 100,000

CANDIDATES FOR USE

- All women requesting abortion should be candidates. However some state laws include outright bans of abortion, affect access, and consent procedures. ***Adolescents:*** State laws vary regarding consent requirements *(See page 31)*
- Individuals with complex medical conditions or placental or uterine abnormalities may need hospital based procedures.

INSTRUCTIONS FOR PATIENT

- Most women have mild cramping and bleeding for a few days that decrease with time.
- While driving self home is not recommended, it can safely be done when procedures are done without sedation under local anesthesia
- Keep telephone number(s) nearby for any emergencies
- May resume usual activities same day if procedure done under local anesthesia
- One week pelvic rest (no tampons, douching or sexual intercourse) to reduce risk of infection
- Use NSAIDs or acetaminophen for cramping
- Showers are permitted immediately
- Call the clinic or seek medical care urgently if you are having heavy bleeding, specifically bleeding through more than 2 pads an hour for 2 hours in a row, fever, chills, increasing pain or malodorous discharge
- Contact clinic if pregnancy Sx unresolved at one week or if menses have not returned by 6-8 weeks.

FOLLOW-UP

- May choose to tell patient to follow up only if problem
- Or schedule routine follow-up at 1-2 weeks
- May be in person, by phone or telemedicine

PROBLEM MANAGEMENT

Infection

- Evaluate possibility of retained products and need for reaspiration
- Patients who develop endometritis can generally be treated using outpatient PID therapies
- Cases that are more complicated may require hospitalization and IV antibiotics (uncommon)

Persistent or excessive bleeding

- ***Possible causes***: uterine atony, retained products, uterine perforation, cervical laceration
- ***Treat likely cause(s):*** Use uterine-contracting agents for atony (methergine, hemabate, misoprostol). Reaspirate if retained products. If uterine perforation, give antibiotics, and evaluate surgically if there is concern for bowel or vascular injury. Suture external cervical lacerations; tamponade endocervical lacerations
- ***For significant hemorrhage (rare):*** transfuse if necessary. Provide blood factors to patients with coagulopathies. In extremely rare cases, uterine artery embolization, further surgery or hysterectomy may be necessary

INDUCED MEDICATION ABORTION

DESCRIPTION

- The first medication (mifepristone or methotrexate) is given to interrupt the further development of the pregnancy (the mifepristone/misoprostol regimen is the most common medical abortion regimen used currently)
- Misoprostol (MIS) is then given to induce expulsion of the products of conception *(see protocol, page 44)*
- Misoprostol is a prostaglandin analogue which causes the cervix to soften and the uterus to contract. May be taken orally, vaginally or by sublingual or buccal routes, either at home or in the office. (Not as effective when given alone as when given with either mifepristone or methotrexate) *[Goldberg 2001]*
- Increasingly chosen as method of abortion; accounts for 45% of abortions ≤ 9 weeks gestation when offered *[Jones 2017]*

Telehealth and Increasing Access to Medication Abortion

- In April 2021, FDA continued to temporarily lift the in-person dispersing requirement for mifepristone during COVID-19 permitting telehealth visits and mail order dispensing.
- FDA has agreed to review the current Risk Evaluation and Mitigation Strategy (REMS) for mifepristone
- State laws that require the drug be dispensed in person remain in effect
- Research has demonstrated that the medication abortion via telehealth is a safe option that increases access to time-sensitive care.
- There is no scientific justification for an in-person visit to pick up medication
- Like other abortion restrictions, this affects people of color the most as well as rural and low income people.
- ACOG and the National Abortion Federation support alternatives to in-person visits

MIFEPRISTONE (RU-486) AND MISOPROSTOL (MIS)

Most medical abortions in the U.S. and abroad now use mifepristone rather than methotrexate. Mifepristone used as an abortifacient in France since 1988

Mechanism - Mifepristone acts as an antiprogesterone to block continued support of the pregnancy. This causes decidual necrosis and detachment of products of conception. Also causes cervical softening

Dose of mifepristone - 200 mg p.o.

Effectiveness - 95-98% effective depending on gestational age and MIS doses used. Mifeprex FDA approved for use up to 70 days but data suggest safe and effective use through 77 days.

Contraindications - Suspected ectopic pregnancy, chronic corticosteroid users, chronic adrenal failures, porphyrias, history of allergy to mifepristone or prostaglandins, known anemia (Hgb < 9.0 g/dl) due to potential for heavy bleeding or hemorrhagic disorder. If an IUD in place, must be removed. Client must be willing to have access to care should complications occur.

Protocol - (evidence-based regimens)

- ***Initial visit:*** Confirm pregnancy by hCG or USG if available. Gestational age assessment (by LMP, bimanual exam, hCG, USG of any combination of these), baseline labs including Rh, hemoglobin, blood typing
- FDA approved for pregnancies up to 70 days (10 weeks)
- Planned Parenthood has extended use up to 11 weeks along with using a second dose of MIS for clients at 9-11 weeks to be given 3-6 hours after first dose.
- ***Mifepristone:*** administer 200 mg orally. Give Rh immune globulin if Rh negative at this time.
- ***Misoprostol (MIS):*** 800mcg given to client at initial visit to be self administered at home either vaginally or buccally 24-48 hours after taking mifepristone
  - Oral may be less effective at later gestations and associated with more side effects.
  - Recent evidence suggests a second dose of MIS may increase effectiveness at later gestations
- The Society of Family Planning, NAF, ACOG and WHO do not recommend prohylactic antibiotics for medication abortion, although practitioners may choose to administer.
- ***Follow-up:*** most visits are at 5-14 days after mifepristone use.
  - Follow-up may be an ultrasound or serial hCG tests along with a phone or video visit
  - Perform D&C for heavy bleeding, signs of infection or continuing pregnancy. If ≤ 11 weeks, can perform D&C or repeat misoprostol 800mcg vaginally or buccally with return evaluation in 1-2 weeks.
  - At-home over-the-counter pregnancy tests may be used for follow-up. This can be done in combination with phone-support from facility staff to provide women with an alternative to the usual in-clinic follow up, although the ideal protocol for an alternative follow up strategy has not been determined.
- Pregnancy tests may be positive for up to 1 month after the completed procedure
- ***Goal:*** confirm complete abortion, assess for complications, address contraceptive needs
  - Ask about ongoing pain, bleeding or Sx infection

ALTERNATIVE REGIMENS:

Medical Abortion with Methotrexate (MTX) and Misoprostol (MIS)

Regimens with MTX were developed before availability of MIF. MTX is widely available and cheap. MTX prevents reduction of folic acid to tetrahydrofolate by binding to dihydrofolate reductase, which interferes with DNA synthesis. This action, in early pregnancy, prevents continued implantation (inhibits syncytialization of the cytotrophoblast). MTX 50 mg/m^2 IM or 50 mg PO is combined with MIS 800 mcg vaginally 3-7 days later in women up to 49 days gestation. Efficacy within 1 week is typically 70-80%. The MIS dose can be repeated if no bleeding after 24 hours or if no abortion by 1-week visit. If the remaining non-continuing pregnancies are managed expectantly, the overall success rate is as high as 95%. Because of the significant delay in abortion for many women and the limit of efficacy to gestations only up to 49 days, the combination of MTX and MIS is generally not recommended for medical abortion.

MEDICAL ABORTION WITH MISOPROSTOL ALONE

Misoprostol, when used without mifepristone or MTX, can cause abortion after 1-3 doses. Treatment regimens in the first trimester typically include MIS 800 mcg vaginally or sublingually or buccally at intervals ranging from every 3 hours to every 12 hours. Efficacy rates are generally around 70-80% with one dose of misoprostol in the first trimester and 80-90% effective with repeat doses after 13 weeks. Given the existence and availability of safe alternative regimens, MIS alone is generally not recommended for medical abortion. However, in situations where mifepristone is unavailable (or illegal e.g. international or due to poor abortion access), MIS alone is an option. At ≥ 12 weeks, 400mcg MIS is typically given every 3 hours.

CONTRACEPTION AFTER ABORTION

- ***Surgical abortions:*** all methods may be started on the day of procedure
  - Advantages of starting immediately: know patient is not pregnant, immediate contraceptive protection
  - If inserting IUD after second-trimester abortion procedure, may have slightly higher expulsion rate. However if placed immediately, may be associated with higher use of an IUD at 6 months post-abortion.
- ***Medication abortions:*** start contraceptives on day mifepristone is ingested.
  - This includes the implant, DMPA and CHC. CHC should be started within 7 days of mifepristone.
- IUD can be inserted when the abortion is deemed complete by USG or history.

CHAPTER 10

POSTPARTUM CONTRACEPTION

Planning for postpartum (PP) contraception should begin during pregnancy and contraceptive use should be initiated as early as possible postpartum.

- Spacing of pregnancies at least 18-23 months apart reduces risk of: preterm delivery, low birth weight, and small for gestational age infants *[Zhv 2005]*
- Between 40 and 57 percent of women report engaging in unprotected intercourse before their 6-week postpartum visit *[BRITO 2009][Connolly 2005]*.
- Ovulation may resume before a woman realizes she is at risk, because she has not had her first period
- 70% of pregnancies in the first year postpartum are unintended. *[White 2015]*
- The PP visit should be at 2-4 weeks.
  - Waiting 6 weeks may miss postpartum depression, postpartum pain and bleeding, resumption of sex, breastfeeding problems, and adaptation to having a baby
- Contraception should be discussed with a breastfeeding woman before she leaves the hospital. Breastfeeding delays return to fertility, but the duration of this contraceptive effect is difficult to predict. Many women stop breastfeeding completely or supplement breastfeeding with other nutrition by the time of their six week exam. *[Ford 1998]*

AT DELIVERY

- Tubal sterilization at C-section or after vaginal delivery
- May be required to sign consent 30 days prior
- IUDs may be inserted within 10 minutes of placental delivery but expulsion risk higher *(see page 98)*
  - 40-75% of women who plan to use an IUD do not return to have it inserted PP exam. *[Trussell 2016]*

ACOG RESOURCES ON POST-PLACENTAL IUDS

- Committee Opinion No. 670, *Immediate Postpartum LARC*
- Practice Bulletin No. 186, LARC
- eModule: Coding for LARC: Billing quiz series
- Committee Opinion No. 672, *Clinical Challenges of LARC*
- Webinar, *Role of Nursing in Immediate Postpartum LARC*

PRIOR TO LEAVING HOSPITAL

- Discuss vaccination for COVID-19 if unvaccinated
- Encourage breastfeeding. Reinforce education about lactational amenorrhea *(see page 54)*
- Schedule PP visit at 2-4 weeks
- May start IUC, DMPA, POPs or implant prior to discharge from hospital
- A review of observational studies of progestin-only contraceptives, including progestin-only pills, injectables, implants, and hormonal intrauterine devices, indicates they have no effect on the successful start and continuation of breastfeeding or on infant growth and development.

- Male or female condoms to reduce risk of sexually transmitted infections
- Estrogen-containing contraceptives may be prescribed for nonlactating women to start 3 weeks postpartum (increased risk of thrombosis associated with pregnancy is reduced by that time)
  - Recommend to start after the 21st day PP. Give a prescription when she leaves the hospital
  - If lactating, start CHCs at 1 month PP, US MEC category 2. Provide backup method as needed

AT POSTPARTUM VISIT (2-4 WEEKS) *(see CDC MEC page 242)*

- Discuss COVID-19 vaccination if unvaccinnated
- Ask if woman has resumed sexual intercourse
- Pregnancy is possible 6 weeks to 2 months after delivery even if fully breastfeeding
- Support continued breastfeeding if applicable
- Lactational amenorrhea follow-up. Provide condoms as transitional method and discuss other methods before transition to decreased breastfeeding
- Emergency contraception may be given if needed
- Progestin-only methods may be provided. Provide back-up method as needed
- Condoms (male or female) may be given as primary or backup to provide STI risk reduction; withdrawal can be used at any time
- Tubal sterilization via laparoscopy may be provided after uterine involution, usually later than 4 weeks. Vasectomy may be provided anytime.
- ***Fertility Awareness Methods:*** should await resumption of 3 consecutive normal cycles
- Acknowledge that having a newborn can be challenging – where sleep schedules may be inconsistent and it is common to feel overwhelmed. Discuss support network and need for self-care. For contraception, discuss that daily adherence to contraception may be more difficult during this time, increasing one's risk for repeat pregnancy.
- Screen for postpartum depression

All breastfeeding women should be provided contraception because:

- Duration of breastfeeding in the U.S. is brief (median: about 3 months)
- Most couples resume intercourse a few weeks after delivery
- Postpartum visit should be no later than 3 weeks to ensure contraceptive coverage
- Ovulation may precede first menses
- LAM is an appropriate choice only when fully breastfeeding (90% of baby's nutrition)

Table 9.1 ***When to initiate contraception in lactating women:***

METHOD	WHEN TO START IN LACTATING WOMEN	EFFECT ON BREAST MILK
Condoms (Male & Female), Sponge	• Immediately	No effect
Cervical Cap, Diaphragm	• 4-6 weeks postpartum, after cervix and vagina normalized (need to be refitted for postpartum women unless the Caya diaphragm)	No effect
Progestin-Only Methods • Depo-Provera • Progestin - Only Pills • Implanon/Nexplanon	• US Medical Eligibility Criteria *(see page 242)*. Category 2 for initiation before discharge from hospital through first 30 days. Category 1 after 30 days.	• No significant impact on milk quality or production • Breast fed children of DMPA users grow at normal rate
Combined Pills Patch Vaginal Ring	• American Academy of Pediatrics recommends use of low-dose combined hormonal contraceptives when infant is not relying solely on breastmilk. No sooner than 3-6 weeks postpartum. • CDC Medical Eligibility Criteria *(see page 242)* ◆ <21 days: U.S. MEC:4 ◆ 21-30 days: U.S. MEC: 3 ◆ 30-42 days: U.S. MEC: 3 (if has other risk factors for VTE); U.S. MEC: 2 (no other risk factors for VTE) ◆ >42 days: U.S. MEC: 1	Quality and quantity of breast milk may be diminished if used prior to establishment of lactation. After lactation establishment, low-dose COCs have no significant impact
IUD: • Copper • Levonorgestrel	• May insert Copper or Levonorgestrel IUD within first 10 minutes after delivery of placenta with special technique	No effect with Paragard. Mirena - same as other progestin-only methods
Tubal Sterilization	Usually done in first 24-48 hours postpartum, or await complete uterine involution for interval tubal sterilization (laparoscopy) (> 6 weeks postpartum)	No effect

CHAPTER 11

PERIMENOPAUSE

PERIMENOPAUSE

- Changes in hormonal status and menstrual cycle that start before, and last through, menopause.
- Fluctuations in ovarian hormones resulting in intermittent vasomotor symptoms, menstrual changes and reduced fertility.
- Average age of onset: 47
- Average duration: 3-5 years
- Contraception should be used until menopause confirmed (amenorrheic for one year), although spontaneous pregnancy after 50 is rare
- Women over 40 have second highest abortion ratio due to unintended pregnancy (# abortions/1000 live births), second to women under 15
    - Pregnancies in older individuals are associated with higher risks of poor fetal and maternal outcomes
- All methods of birth control are available to most healthy, nonsmoking women until menopause, although medical conditions become more prevalent with age
    - Sterilization popular: 50% contraceptors > 40 use tubal occlusion plus 20% vasectomy
    - Fertility awareness methods that rely on timing of ovulation are less accurate due to increasing anovulatory cycles during perimenopause
    - Combined hormonal contraceptives have specific benefits for perimenopausal women: May regulate cycles, prevent osteoporosis, treat hot flashes. Usually should not be used for women > 35 who smoke, have migraines or have significant cardiac risk factors
    - Smokers > 35 or women with hypertension may use any non-estrogen containing methods, POPs, DMPA, IUDs or barriers unless they have other risk factors

MENOPAUSE:

- Average age: 51.1-51.4
- Determined retrospectively after one year of amenorrhea without another cause
- Some diagnose with FSH > 30 IU/L on 2 separate occasions, 6-8 weeks apart
- At age 55, 95% are menopausal so can assume sterility

See page 125 for transitioning woman on combination hormonal contraceptives to menopause with or without transitioning to menopausal hormone therapy

CHAPTER 12

MALE REPRODUCTIVE HEALTH

Reproductive health is a term generally associated with women. Efforts have increased to include males in health education and outreach programs, acknowledging that men have important reproductive and sexual health needs.

MEN AND SEXUAL EXPERIENCE

- Most adult men and almost half of adolescent men (44%) have had sexual intercourse *[Guttmacher 2008]*
- Survey data from 2011-2017 suggest 7.6% of men were sexually active before age 13
- 6.2% of males aged 18-49 have had sexual contact with another male

WHERE MEN GET THEIR REPRODUCTIVE HEALTH INFORMATION

- A study of adolescent primary care appointments found that 35% of interactions did not involve a discussion about sexuality and men are less likely to be counseled on sexual health than women. When those conversations do happen, the average time of sexuality talk was 36 seconds *[Alexander 2014]*
- Although most men get some sexuality education in high school, for 3 out of 10 men this instruction comes too late – after they have begun having sexual intercourse *[Sonfield 2002]*

What can healthcare providers do?

- Discussion should start with boys before puberty starts. The HPV vaccine is approved for males starting at age 9 and can be a useful entrypoint for discussion of sexuality
- The yearly physical is an appropriate place to discuss concepts such as the changing body in puberty, healthy relationships, consent, and the importance of consistent condom use for STI and pregnancy prevention

MEN AND CONTRACEPTION

When you come into contact with a man who is playing an active role in safely, effectively and carefully using contraceptives, go out of your way to give him positive reinforcement.

- As men get older, condom use declines. 7 out of 10 men age 15-17 use condoms, compared to 4 out of 10 men in their 20s, and 2 out of 10 men in their 30s. *[Sonfield 2002]*
- Vasectomy is a very effective male option for permanent birth control that is safer than female sterilization. However, it is estimated that approximately 500,000 men receive a vasectomy in the U.S. each year, in contrast to 700,000 women who have a female sterilization procedure. *[Hawes 1998]* In only 4 countries throughout the world, Great Britain, Netherlands, New Zealand and Bhutan, do vasectomies exceed tubal sterilization as a method of birth control. Vasectomy has not been found to cause any long-term adverse effects except chronic pain in approximately 2% of men which is usually relieved by anti-inflammatory agents. *[1997-IPPF Handbook]*

Men's support of women's birth control methods matters

- Education of adolescent males about birth control (including female methods) leads to improvement in use of the method by their partner(s) *[Edwards 1994]*

MEN AND SEXUALLY TRANSMITTED INFECTIONS

How many men acquire sexually transmitted infections?

- 17% of men aged 15-49 have genital herpes
- Among men in their 20s, there are 500-600 new cases of gonorrhea and chlamydia per year for every 100,000 men *[Sonfield 2002]*
- 8 out of 10 Americans living with HIV are men *[Sonfield 2002]*
- Rates of STIs are higher among young, poor, and minority men

Decreasing STI rates in men helps their female partner(s)

- Treating men decreases initial infection rate and reinfection rate in women, which could decrease female complications such as pelvic inflammatory disease, ectopic pregnancy, and infertility.

Decreasing STI rates in men helps themselves

- While the link between gonorrhea and chlamydia infection and infertility in men has not been proven, there is some clinical evidence that it does have some effect:
  gonorrhea/chlamydia infection → urethritis → epidymo-orchitis → infertility
  - If urethritis is treated promptly, there is less likelihood it will proceed to epidymo-orchitis *[Ness 1997]*
  - The most common cause of epidymo-orchitis in men younger than 35 years old is gonorrhea and chlamydia infections *[Weidner 1999]*

MEN AND REPRODUCTIVE CANCERS

Testicular cancer

- "Testicular cancer is the most common solid malignancy affecting males between the ages of 15 and 35. It accounts for 1% of all cancers in men." *[Michaelson 2004]*
- The number of deaths from testicular has dropped due to advances in therapy.
- Some signs or symptoms of testicular cancer are testicular enlargement, a dull ache in the abdomen or groin, scrotal pain, and fluid in the scrotum.
- The American Urological Association says that monthly testicular self exams are the most important way to detect a tumor early. A fact sheet with instructions available at *www.urologyhealth.org/resources/testicular-self-exams*.
- The treatment for testicular cancer may be removal of the affected testicle.

Prostate cancer

- The most important risk factor for prostate cancer is age.
- Screening includes digital rectal exam and prostate-specific antigen level.
- Some of the treatments for prostate cancer can affect male fertility. For instance, surgery to remove the prostate causes the male ejaculate to become "dry" so the ability to have children is usually lost. Prostate surgery can also cause erectile dysfunction.

CHAPTER 13

ABSTINENCE OR DELAYING SEXUAL INTERCOURSE

DESCRIPTION

Avoidance of genital contact that could result in a pregnancy (i.e. penile penetration into the vagina).

WAYS TO THINK ABOUT ABSTINENCE

- ***Primary Abstinence:*** delaying first sexual intercourse
- ***Return to Abstinence:*** after being sexually active
- ***Abstinence "for a while" - for example, until***
  - Effective contraception has been achieved
  - STI tests are negative and prevention of STIs discussed and agreed upon by both partners
  - Until 2, 4, or 6 week postpartum visit
  - Trust and communication (and monogamy) well-established in relationship and consequences of sex including unplanned pregnancy are discussed

EFFECTIVENESS

When abstinence is adhered to, there is no pregnancy.

HOW ABSTINENCE WORKS

Sperm does enter into the female reproductive tract, preventing fertilization

COST: None

ADVANTAGES: Can be used as an interval method

Menstrual: none

Sexual / psychological: May contribute to positive self-image if consistent with personal values

Cancers, tumors, and masses: Risk of cervical cancer far less if no vaginal intercourse has ever occurred.

Other:

- Reduces risk of STIs (unless vaginal intercourse replaced with oral or anal sex)
- Many religions and cultures endorse
- May encourage people to build relationships in other ways

DISADVANTAGES

Menstrual: None

Sexual / psychological: Frustration if abstinence is not adhered to

Substance abuse may lead to failed adherence to abstinence

Cancers, tumors, and masses: None

Other:

- Requires commitment and self control; nonunderstanding partner may seek other partner(s)
- Patient and her partner may not be prepared to contracept if they stop abstaining

COMPLICATIONS

- No medical complications
- Both partners do not agree to abstain

CANDIDATES FOR USE

- Individuals or couples who feel they have the ability to refrain from sexual intercourse
  - ***Adolescents:*** requires maturity. Provide information about contraceptive methods for future
  - Counseling may include discussions on masturbation (solo or mutual)

MAINTAINING ABSTINENCE USUALLY REQUIRES OPEN COMMUNICATION

- Teach negotiating skills, how to say "no" or "not now", and how to resist peer (societal) pressures
- Stress that abstinence may just be a decision to delay intercourse. It may mean "not now" instead of "never." Remind her she may use or return to abstinence at any time
- Prepare for time when (or if) decision to stop abstaining arises, contraceptive education
- Advise to consider having condoms and emergency contraception in case of need

PROBLEM MANAGEMENT

Partner does not want to abstain:

- Recommend continued communication and be available to discuss options
- Provide counseling on other forms of sexual pleasuring if patient is interested
- Consider birth control method or end the relationship

FERTILITY ISSUE

- Protects against upper reproductive tract infection preserving a woman's fertility

CHAPTER 14

BREASTFEEDING: LACTATIONAL AMENORRHEA METHOD (LAM)

DESCRIPTION: The lactational amenorrhea method (LAM) is contingent upon nearly exclusive, frequent breastfeeding.

- Both day and night feedings and at least 90% of baby's nutrition derived from breastfeeding
- The individual is amenorrheic (spotting which occurs in the first 56 days postpartum is not regarded as menses)
- The infant is less than 6 months old.
- It is important to provide a woman with another method in advance to use when she no longer fulfills all the above conditions for effective use of LAM. Half of women in the U.S. who start breastfeeding stop within 3 months.

EFFECTIVENESS: Controlled Studies

Life table pregnancy rate at 6 months: 0.45 and 2.45% in 2 published studies

Uncontrolled studies: range from 0 - 7.5%. Cochrane review found no difference between a woman using LAM and women who were fully breastfeeding and amenorrheic but not using any method (not using "LAM") *[Cochrane Review]*

Any time of concern about a user's contraception protection, emergency contraception may be used while nursing. When taking EC with UPA, breastfeeding is not recommended for first 24 hours. Breast milk can be expressed and discarded during this time period.

MECHANISM

- Suckling causes a surge in prolactin, which inhibits ovulation.
- If ovulation occurs and fertilization occurs, hypoestrogenic thin uterine lining may prevent implantation

ADVANTAGES OF BREASTFEEDING

Menstrual: Involution of the uterus occurs more rapidly; and breastfeeding suppresses menses

Sexual / psychological: Breastfeeding pleasurable to many women

- Facilitates bonding between mother and child (if not stressful)

Cancers, tumors, and masses: Reduces risk of breast, ovarian and endometrial cancer

Other:

- Provides the healthiest, most "natural" food for baby
- Protects baby against gastrointestinal and respiratory infections, otitis media
- Facilitates postpartum weight loss
- Ranges from no cost and less time preparing bottles and feedings to several fairly high expenses for pumps, bottles to store breast milk and even medical visits for pain or failure of infant to nurse adequately.
- Provision of COVID-19 vaccine to pregnant women protects both the woman and infant. Antibodies are passed in breastmilk and studies are underway to see if this protects the infants.

DISADVANTAGES

Menstrual: Return to menses unpredictable

Sexual / psychological:

- Breastfeeding mother may be self-conscious in public or during intercourse
- Hypoestrogenism of breastfeeding may cause temporary atrophic vaginal changes
- Tender breasts may decrease sexual pleasure
- No protection against STIs, HIV, AIDS
- Half of U.S. women who start breastfeeding stop within 3 months.

Cancers / tumors / masses: None

Other:

- Working women need support to find time/place/resources to pump
- Effectiveness after 6 months is markedly reduced; return to fertility often precedes menses
    - Here is why: the probability that ovulation will precede the first menstrual period in a lactating woman increases from 33-45% during the first 3 months to 64-71% during months 4 to 12 and 87% after 12 months. Among lactating women, 66% are sexually active in the first month postpartum and 88% are sexually active in the second month postpartum *[Ford 1998]*
- Frequent breastfeeding may be inconvenient or perceived as inconvenient, particularly if a woman is working outside of the home.
- If the mother is HIV+, there is a 14%-29% chance that HIV will be passed to infant via breast milk. Antiretroviral therapy decreases risk of transmission. Breastfeeding is not recommended for HIV+ women in the U.S.
- Sore nipples and breasts; risk of mastitis associated with breastfeeding

COMPLICATIONS: Risk of mastitis

CANDIDATES FOR USE

- Amenorrheic women less than 6 months postpartum who exclusively breastfeed their babies may consider breastfeeding as a contraceptive
- Women free of a blood-borne infection which could be passed to the newborn
- Women not on drugs which can adversely affect their babies

INITIATING METHOD

- Immediately or as soon as possible after delivery
- Breastfeeding fully or almost fully (>90% of baby's feedings); feedings around the clock
- Access to baby or pump
- Can supplement with a second method of contraception

INSTRUCTIONS FOR PATIENT

- Support/resources *(www.lalecheleague.org)*
- Breastfeed consistently (2-3 hours), exclusively and correctly for maximum effectiveness
- Breastfeed often (8-10 times daily), eat well, get additional rest, drink lots of fluids and take prenatal vitamins and iron supplements
- Breast milk should constitute at least 90% of baby's feedings
- Consider future methods for when menses return or at 6 months

PROBLEM MANAGEMENT

Deficient milk supply:

- The more frequently a breast is emptied, the more milk is produced,
- Use of artificial nipple (e.g. pacifier), fatigue or maternal stress
- Consult lactation specialist

Sore nipples:

- Commonly caused by incorrect application of the baby's mouth to the breast. Uncommonly caused by infection
- Check for correct ways of latching and suckling; be sure to break the suction before removing the baby from the breast
- Improve with practice; change the pressure points on the nipple by changing the baby's position for feeding
- Allow nipples to air dry with breast milk on the areola to reduce infection and nipple soreness. Apply lanolin to nipples after each feeding
- Do not cleanse breasts other than with water
- Apply cool gel packs to decrease soreness

Sore breasts:

- Wear a well-fitted, supportive nursing bra; avoid underwire
- Apply heat, or teabag
- Nurse frequently or use pump to empty sore breast
- Use of an anti-inflammatory agent and a complex of bromelain/trypsin both significantly improved symptoms of engorgement. *[Cochrane Database 2008]*
- Encourage additional rest
- Seek medical evaluation if any erythema, fever or signs or symptoms of infection

Other:

- Stress, fear, lack of confidence, lack of strong motivation to succeed at breastfeeding, lack of partner and/or societal support, and/or poor nutrition can cause problems

FERTILITY AFTER USE: Patient's baseline fertility (ability to become pregnant) is not altered once she discontinues breastfeeding

TEN STEPS TO SUCCESSFUL BREASTFEEDING IN YOUR FACILITY

From: Protecting, Promoting and Supporting Breastfeeding: The Special Role of Maternity Services. *(A Joint WHO/UNICEF Statement. Geneva, WHO, 1989)*

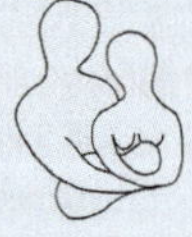

1. Written breastfeeding policy routinely communicated to all staff.
2. Train all staff in skills necessary to implement this policy.
3. Inform all pregnant women about the benefits and management of breastfeeding.
4. Help mothers initiate breastfeeding within the first 30 minutes after birth.
5. Maintain lactation even if mothers separated from infants due to medical reason.
6. Give infants only breast milk; no water or formula unless medical reason.
7. Allow mothers and infants to remain together 24 hours a day from birth.
8. Encourage natural breastfeeding on demand.
9. Do not give or encourage the use of artificial nipples to breastfeed infants.
10. Promote and refer to breastfeeding support groups .

CHAPTER 15

FERTILITY AWARENESS METHODS (FAM)

Description: FAMs should generally be limited to use by women with regular menstrual cycles. They involve monitoring the cycle and having intercourse only during infertile phases or using another method, e.g. condoms, during fertile phases. A woman cannot identify the exact day of ovulation using FAM methods; rather she estimates when the fertile phase of her cycle begins and ends. A woman's fertile phase may begin 3-6 days before ovulation (because sperm can live in cervical mucus for 3-6 days) and ends 24 hours after ovulation

For purposes of FAM, a woman's menstrual cycle has 3 phases:
1. ***Infertile phase:*** Before ovulation
2. ***Fertile phase:*** Approximately 5-7 days in the mid-portion of the cycle, including several days before and the day after ovulation;
3. ***Infertile phase:*** after the fertile phase

- During the fertile phase, a couple should be abstinent or use a barrier method to avoid pregnancy.

EFFECTIVENESS *(also see Table 2.1, page 9)*

First-year failure rate (100 women-years of use)

Method	Typical use	Perfect use
Calendar	24	9
Standard Days Method	24	5
Ovulation Method	24	3
Symptothermal	24	0.4
Post-ovulation	24	1
TwoDay Method	24	4

[Trussell 2018]

MECHANISM OF ACTION: Abstinence or barrier methods used during fertile period

- As couples using either the Calendar or the Cervical Mucus Methods can theoretically identify the beginning and the end of the fertile period, they may have unprotected intercourse during the pre-ovulatory infertile phase and the post-ovulatory infertile phase. However, in order to minimize the chance of an unintended pregnancy, some advocate that couples only have unprotected intercourse during the post-ovulatory infertile phase regardless of the method of FAM they are using.
- Apps may be useful to track cycle and assess fertile phase
- FDA approved App: "Natural Cycles"

Cost: Training, supplies (special digital basal body thermometer, Cycle Beads, charts)

ADVANTAGES

Menstrual: No change. Helps woman learn more about her menstrual physiology
Sexual / psychological: Men and women can work together in using this method. Men must be aware that abstinence or use of second method is essential during the fertile phase

Other:

- May be only method acceptable to couples for cultural or religious reasons
- Helps couples achieve pregnancy when practiced in reverse

Comparative efficacy of FAM methods is unknown due to poor subject retention in efficacy trials *[Grimes 2005]*

METHODS

1. Calendar Method: To calculate the fertile days:

- Record days of menses prospectively for 6-12 cycles
- Most estimates assume that sperm can survive 2-3 days and ovulation occurs 14 days before menses (motile sperm have been found as long as 7 days after intercourse and the extreme interval following a single act of coitus leading to an achieved pregnancy is 6 days *[Speroff 1999]*
- Earliest day of fertile period = day # in a cycle corresponding to **shortest cycle length minus 18**
- Latest day of fertile period = day # in a cycle corresponding to **longest cycle length minus 11**

2. Standard Days Method Utilizing Color-Coded Beads; CycleBeads™

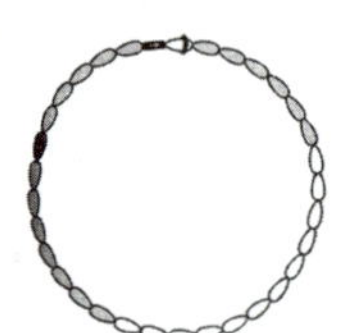

- For women with most cycles 26-32 days long, avoid unprotected intercourse on days 8-19 (white beads CycleBead necklace). No need for months of extensive cycle calculations
- 4.75% failure over 1 year with perfect use; 11.96% with typical use *[Arevalo 2002]*
- Resources available from the Institute for Reproductive Health, *www.irh.org* (CD, training manual, patient brochure, sample beads). Beads can also be ordered from *www.cyclebeads.com*

3. Cervical Mucus Ovulation Detection Method

- Requires avoiding unprotected intercourse approx. 15-17 days per month
- Women check quantity and character of mucus on the vulva or introitus with fingers or tissue paper each day for several months to learn cycle:
  - Post-menstrual mucus: scant or undetectable
  - Pre-ovulation mucus: cloudy, yellow or white, sticky
  - Ovulation mucus: clear, wet, stretches, more slippery
  - Post-ovulation fertile mucus: thick, cloudy; sticky
  - Post-ovulation post-fertile mucus: scant or undetectable
- When using method during preovulatory period, must abstain 24 hours after intercourse to make test interpretable as semen and vaginal fluids can obscure character of cervical mucus
  - Abstinence or barrier method through fertile period (i.e. abstinence for a given cycle begins as soon as the woman notices any cervical secretions)
  - Intercourse without restriction beginning 4th day after the last day of wet, clear, slippery mucus (post-ovulation)

4. TwoDay Method

- Uses cervical secretions, but is much simpler
- Each day woman asks herself 1) "Did I notice secretions today?" and 2) "Did I notice secretions yesterday?"
- If no secretions two consecutive days, OK to have intercourse
- Users typically avoid unprotected intercourse for 13 days per cycle (range 10-14)

5. Basal Body Temperature Method (BBT)

- BBT Method can only be used to identify the end of the fertile period.
- Couples using the BBT Method could only safely have unprotected intercourse during the post-ovulatory period, as the method cannot be used to define the pre-ovulatory infertile phase.

Figure 15.1 Basal body temperature variations during a menstrual cycle

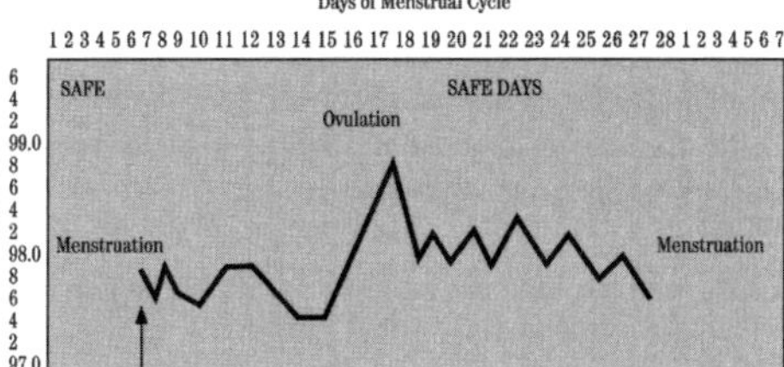

- Assumes early morning temperature measured before arising will increase noticeably (0.4-0.8° F) with ovulation; fertile period is defined as the day of first temperature drop or first elevation through 3 consecutive days of elevated temperature. Temperature drop does NOT always occur
- Abstinence begins first day of menstrual bleeding and lasts through 3 consecutive days of sustained temperature rise (at least 0.20 C or 0.40 F). Using this regimen means a couple must avoid unprotected vaginal intercourse about 17 days out of each 28 day cycle.

Natural Cycles is an FDA-approved contraceptive App where a user enters her BBT each morning to determine her fertile window. The company reports 93% effective with typical use and 98% with perfect use.

6. Post-ovulation Method

- Permits unprotected intercourse only after signs of ovulation (BBT, cervical mucus, etc.) have subsided

7. Symptothermal Method

- Combines at least two methods — usually cervical mucus changes with BBT
- May also include mittelschmerz, change in libido, and changes in cervical texture, position and dilation to detect ovulation:
  - During preovulatory and ovulatory periods, cervix softens, opens and is moister
  - During postovulatory period, cervix drops, becomes firm and closes

8. The Marquette Method (MM) of FAM

- An online site that aids users who choose either electronic hormonal fertility monitor (EHFM), cervical mucus monitoring (CMM) or both.
- RCT comparing the EHFM plus fertility algorithm vs. CMM plus algorithm found that over 12 months, EHFM (N=197) had 7 per 100 pregnant and CMM (N=164) had 18.5 per 100. *[Fehring 2013]*

DISADVANTAGES

Menstrual: No effect on menses

Sexual / psychological:

- Requires abstinence at time of ovulation, which typically is the time of peak libido
- Requires rigorous discipline, good communication and full commitment of both partners
- Requires abstinence, barrier method, or another contraceptive that does not change pattern of ovulation during 6-12 month learning / data-gathering period (unless CycleBead method is used)
- Complete abstinence in an anovulatory cycle, if using post-ovulation techniques. This method demands great self-control: either abstinence or use of another method must be used during long periods of time when woman is or may become fertile

Cancers, tumors, and masses: None

Other:

- Difficult to use in early adolescence, when approaching menopause, and in postpartum when cycles are irregular (or absent)
- Even women with "regular" periods can vary as much as ±7 days in any given cycle
- Cervical mucus techniques may be complicated by vaginal infections
- May be more challenging during time of stress, depression or major life changes
- Method very unforgiving of improper use
- Does not protect against STIs
- High failure rates with typical use
- Less reliable if woman has a fever, vaginal infection, or is in the practice of douching

Complications: None

CANDIDATES FOR USE

- Women with regular menstrual cycles at minimal risk for STIs
- Women wanting to avoid hormones and devices
- Couples with religious / cultural proscriptions against using other methods.
- Highly-motivated couples willing to commit to extensive abstinence or to use barriers during vulnerable periods or on demand methods such as condoms and spermicides.

Adolescents: Not appropriate until regular menstrual cycles established

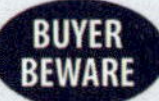

A woman considering use of the fertility awareness methods must be aware of **the five "R's"**:

- Restrictions on sexual spontaneity (method requires periodic abstinence or the use of backup method)
- Rigorous daily monitoring
- Required training
- Risk of pregnancy during prolonged training period
- Risk of pregnancy on unsafe days

INSTRUCTIONS FOR PATIENT

- Requires discipline, communication, listening skills, full commitment of both partners. Mistakes using this method are particularly likely to lead to unintended pregnancies as intercourse is then occurring at the time in the cycle when a woman is most likely to become pregnant
- If using FAM and decide to have sex during fertile days, use contraception
- Discuss other forms of sexual satisfaction for fertile phase

FOLLOW UP

- Have you had sexual intercourse during "unsafe" times during your cycle?
- Discuss use of emergency contraception if having sex during "unsafe" times during cycle
- Provide emergency contraceptive pills for use if needed

PROBLEM MANAGEMENT

Inconsistent use and risk taking: Educate about emergency contraception when women start using method

Fertility after discontinuation of method: No effect

CHAPTER 16

CONDOMS FOR MEN

DESCRIPTION: Condoms for men are sheaths made of latex, polyurethane or natural membranes, placed over the penis prior to sexual contact and worn until after ejaculation when the penis is removed from the orifice (vagina, mouth, or anus).

- Used correctly and consistently, male latex condoms are highly effective in preventing sexual transmission of HIV and can reduce the risk for other STIs.
- May be used as a primary contraceptive method or with another method to provide STI risk reduction.
- **As a primary contraceptive method, it is important that condoms be coupled with advice to buy OTC emergency contraceptive pills (ECPs) since couples experience a condom break or slippage during approximately 3-5% of acts of intercourse.**

EFFECTIVENESS

Typical use failure rate in the first year of use: 13% *[Trussell 2018]*
Perfect use failure rate in the first year of use: 2%

- The most common reason for condom failure is not using a condom with every act of intercourse *[Werner 2004] [Steiner 1999]*. Condoms are not used when:
  - *no condom is available*
  - *a couple thinks they are not at risk of either pregnancy or risk of infections*
- Dual use of a condom plus another contraceptive may dramatically reduce the risk of both pregnancy and an STI. *[Warner 2004][Cates 2002]*.
- Although they provide the same pregnancy protection, polyurethane condoms are more likely to slip or break (2.6 to 5 times more likely *[Gallo 2008]*) than latex condoms (1.6-1.7%).

MECHANISM OF ACTION

- Condoms act as a barrier; they prevent the passage of sperm into the vagina. Sheathing the penis also reduces transmission and acquisition of STIs, including HIV. **Spermicidal condoms are no longer recommended as they provide no additional protection against pregnancy or STIs and have more adverse effects.**

COST

- Average retail cost for latex condoms is $0.50, but some designer condoms cost several dollars. Polyurethane condoms cost $0.80-$2.00 each
- Some public health agencies and some college health services offer large numbers of free condoms

ADVANTAGES

Menstrual: No direct impact on menses.
Sexual / psychological:

- Some men may maintain erection longer with condoms, making sex more enjoyable for him, or for both partners.
- Individuals interested in using Multipurpose Prevention Technologies (MPTs), which act both to prevent pregnancy and STIs. *[Hynes 2018]*.

- Lubricated condoms are a particularly good contraceptive option during breast-feeding and for post-menopausal women when vaginal atrophy may occur.
- Availability of wide selection of condoms and designs can add variety and comfort
- Makes sex less messy by catching the ejaculate
- Intercourse may be more pleasurable because fear of pregnancy and STIs is decreased

Cancers / tumors / masses: Decrease in HIV and HPV transmission reduces risks of AIDS and HPV-related malignancies

Other:

- Consistent condom use reduces risks of HIV transmission by approximately 80% *[Welles 2001]*
- Consistent condom use reduces risk of cervical and vulvovaginal HPV infection among newly sexually active women *[Winer 2006]*
- Readily available over the counter; no medical visit required
- Usually inexpensive for single use
- Easily transportable.

DISADVANTAGES: May break or fall off. *Options:* *see Fig. 16.2, page 68*

Menstrual: None

Sexual / psychological:

- Condom use may interrupt sex
  - Interruption of sex may cause man to lose erection
- Blunting of sensation or "unnatural" feeling with intercourse
- Plain condoms may decrease lubrication and provide less stimulation for woman
- Requires prompt withdrawal after ejaculation, which may decrease pleasure

Other:

- Requires education / experience for successful use
- Either member of couple may have latex allergy or reaction to spermicide; polyurethane condom is an appropriate alternative
- Users must avoid petroleum-based lubricants and vaginal products when using latex condoms as can increase breakage
- Users should check the condom after ejaculation for any holes or tears that represent a compromised barrier. EC should be considered if there is a tear.

COMPLICATIONS

- Allergic reactions to latex are rarely life threatening; 2-3% of Americans (men and women) have a latex allergy; up to 14% of individuals working with latex are latex sensitive. Polyurethane condoms do not cause allergic reactions.
- Condom retained in vagina (uncommon) exposes woman to risk of infection as well as pregnancy. If this occurs: attempt to remove the condom with the help of the partner; if unable, go to a clinician. Use emergency contraception ASAP ro prevent pregnancy.

PRECAUTIONS

- Women who require high contraceptive efficacy should not be using condoms as their primary contraceptive method. They should, add another more effective method.
- Couples in which either partner has latex allergy should avoid latex condoms; can use male polyurethane or female nitrile condoms (female is FC2 condom).

- Couples in which either partner has spermicide allergy or is at high risk for HIV should avoid spermicide-coated condoms

CANDIDATES FOR CONDOM USE

- Anyone at risk for an STI
- Those looking for both STI and pregnancy prevention

Special applications for infection control:

- Non-monogamous couples (i.e. if either partner has multiple partners)
- During pregnancy
- After delivery or pregnancy loss to reduce risk of endometritis
- Couples with known viral infections (HIV, HPV, HSV-2)

Adolescents: Excellent option, especially when combined with another method

INITIATING METHOD

Couples desiring to use condoms often benefit from concrete instructions. Can demonstrate on a banana or finger. Encourage couple to practice. Counsel new users about:

- Options among condom types
- Storage for safety and ready access (limit storage in wallet to a month).
- How to open package and place correct side of condom over penis
- How to unroll and allow space for ejaculate (depending on condom design)
- Provide ECPs to all couples relying on condoms for birth control to ensure immediate use in the event of condom mishap or problem

INSTRUCTIONS FOR PATIENTS *(See Figure 16.1, page 67)*

- Learn how to use a condom long before you need it. Both women and men need to know how. Practice with models: fingers or banana. Individuals may enjoy when their partner places the condom.
- Buy condoms in advance, carry with you; Keep extra condoms out of sunlight and heat
- Check expiration date, and do not use if expired. If only a production date is given, condoms are good for 5 years (nonspermicidal) or 2 years (spermicidal).
- Open package carefully, squeeze condom out, avoid tearing with fingernails, teeth, scissors, etc.
- Routinely use appropriate water-based or silicone-based lubricant with latex condoms. Never put lubricant inside the condom
- Place condom over penis before any genital contact. Either partner can put it on.
- If condom used for oral or rectal intercourse before vaginal sex, replace first condom with a new condom prior to entry into vagina
- Vigorous sex can break the condom
- Immediately after ejaculation (before loss of erection) hold rim of condom against shaft of penis and remove penis from vagina
- Remove condom from the penis and visually inspect carefully for any breaks
- Dispose of used condom with waste. Do not flush into toilet. Do not reuse.
- If a condom falls off, slips, tears or breaks, start ECPs as soon as possible. Plan B is available OTC.

FOLLOW-UP QUESTIONS FOR THE PATIENT

- Are you and your partner comfortable using condoms?
- Have you had any problems with using the condom? Breaking? Slipping off? Decreased sensation? Vaginal soreness with use? Skin irritation or redness during the day after using it?
- Have you had any post-coital "yeast infection" symptoms? (May confuse an allergic reaction to the condom and/or spermicide with an infection)
- Have you had intercourse without a condom—even once in the past year?
- Did you have any questions about emergency contraceptive pills (ECPs)?
- Do you have ECPs at home?

PROBLEM MANAGEMENT

Allergic reaction: *[See Warner 2004]*

- Beware that latex can induce anaphylaxis and that the severity of allergic reaction increases with continued exposure. More often a person who says he (or she) is "allergic" to condoms means:
  - condoms are difficult to put on
  - condoms lead to loss of erection
  - the couple simply doesn't like condoms
  - is being irritated by a spermicide or lubricant
  - an ongoing infection may be causing irritation. Irritation can also be caused by thrusting during sex. Couple may try another brand of latex condoms
- If either partner is allergic to latex, switch to polyurethane condoms or the female condom

Condom breakage: *(Figure 16.2, page 68)* (1-2% for latex condoms)

- Ensure correct technique. Common problems: pre-placement manipulations (stretching, etc), use of inappropriate lubricant, and prolonged or extremely vigorous sex
- May need to recommend larger condom.
- May need to switch method if condoms repeatedly break
- Confirm that woman is using ECPs and has supply available at home
- The risk of HIV transmission following a condom break is quite low, but treatment lowers it still further. Consult an HIV clinic immediately if this is a concern.

Condom slippage: *(Figure 16.1, page 67)*

- Ensure correct technique. Common problems: condom not fully unrolled, lubricant placed incorrectly, and excessive delay in removing penis from vagina after ejaculation. Use of proper-sized condom is important (if condom is too large it may slip off). "Snugger fit" condoms are available
- Rule out erectile dysfunction. Condoms may not be appropriate if man loses erection with condom placement or use
- Confirm that woman has supply of ECPs at home

Decreased sensation:

- Common causes: condom too small, too thick or too tightly applied; inadequate lubrication
- Suggest experimentation with different textured or thinner condoms
- Integrate condom placement into lovemaking

Condoms that are the wrong size are a problem. Usually they are too long or too tight.

- Most U.S. condoms are longer by 1-2 inches than men's mean erect penile length. *[Warner 2017]*
- Most U.S. condoms have a circumference that is smaller than a man's penis. 32% of men describe their condoms as too tight. *[Reese 2009]*
- 45% of men report that their condoms do not fit.
- For information on ordering the right sized condom for you, go to https://www.onecondoms.com/pages/myone

Figure 16.1

HOW TO USE A LATEX CONDOM

(...Or rubber, sheath, prophylactic, safe, french letter, raincoat, glove, sock)

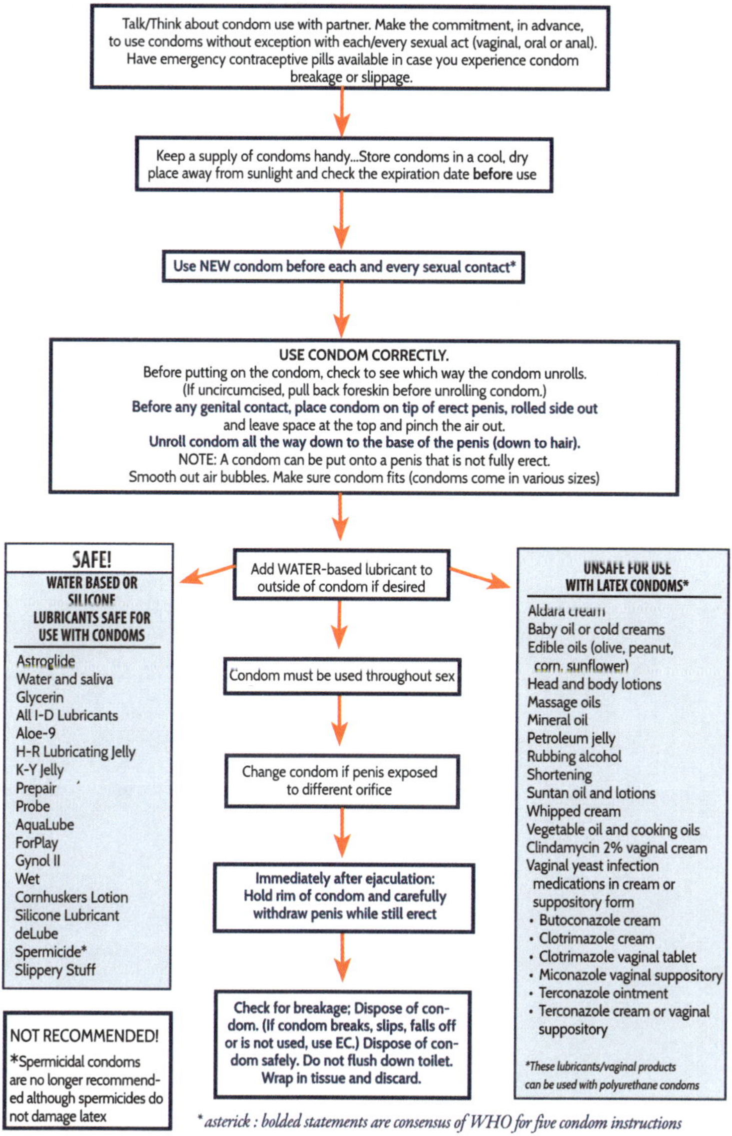

Talk/Think about condom use with partner. Make the commitment, in advance, to use condoms without exception with each/every sexual act (vaginal, oral or anal). Have emergency contraceptive pills available in case you experience condom breakage or slippage.

↓

Keep a supply of condoms handy...Store condoms in a cool, dry place away from sunlight and check the expiration date **before** use

↓

Use NEW condom before each and every sexual contact*

↓

USE CONDOM CORRECTLY.
Before putting on the condom, check to see which way the condom unrolls.
(If uncircumcised, pull back foreskin before unrolling condom.)
Before any genital contact, place condom on tip of erect penis, rolled side out and leave space at the top and pinch the air out.
Unroll condom all the way down to the base of the penis (down to hair).
NOTE: A condom can be put onto a penis that is not fully erect.
Smooth out air bubbles. Make sure condom fits (condoms come in various sizes)

↓

Add WATER-based lubricant to outside of condom if desired

↓

Condom must be used throughout sex

↓

Change condom if penis exposed to different orifice

↓

Immediately after ejaculation: Hold rim of condom and carefully withdraw penis while still erect

↓

Check for breakage; Dispose of condom. (If condom breaks, slips, falls off or is not used, use EC.) Dispose of condom safely. Do not flush down toilet. Wrap in tissue and discard.

SAFE!

WATER BASED OR SILICONE LUBRICANTS SAFE FOR USE WITH CONDOMS

- Astroglide
- Water and saliva
- Glycerin
- All I-D Lubricants
- Aloe-9
- H-R Lubricating Jelly
- K-Y Jelly
- Prepair
- Probe
- AquaLube
- ForPlay
- Gynol II
- Wet
- Cornhuskers Lotion
- Silicone Lubricant
- deLube
- Spermicide*
- Slippery Stuff

UNSAFE FOR USE WITH LATEX CONDOMS*

- Aldara cream
- Baby oil or cold creams
- Edible oils (olive, peanut, corn, sunflower)
- Head and body lotions
- Massage oils
- Mineral oil
- Petroleum jelly
- Rubbing alcohol
- Shortening
- Suntan oil and lotions
- Whipped cream
- Vegetable oil and cooking oils
- Clindamycin 2% vaginal cream
- Vaginal yeast infection medications in cream or suppository form
  - Butoconazole cream
  - Clotrimazole cream
  - Clotrimazole vaginal tablet
  - Miconazole vaginal suppository
  - Terconazole ointment
  - Terconazole cream or vaginal suppository

**These lubricants/vaginal products can be used with polyurethane condoms*

NOT RECOMMENDED!
*Spermicidal condoms are no longer recommended although spermicides do not damage latex

** asterick : bolded statements are consensus of WHO for five condom instructions*

Figure 16.2

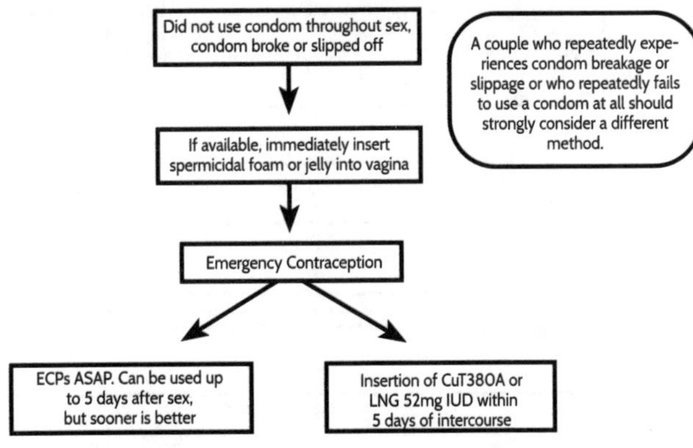

To purchase the 21st edition of ***Contraceptive Technology****, with an excellent chapter on condoms by David Lee Warner (CDC) and Markus Steiner (FHI), call (404) 875-5001 or go to www.managingcontraception.com*

CHAPTER 17

FEMALE-CONTROLLED BARRIER METHODS

DESCRIPTION

- Female-Controlled Barrier Methods: cervical cap, diaphragm, sponge and female condom
- One cervical cap is FDA approved and currently available in the US: FemCap. It is made of silicone rubber (latex-free), covers the cervix completely, and creates suction between the cervix and the cap.
- Diaphragms available in the U.S. are made of silicone; a dome-shaped device placed to cover the cervix, and held in place by the vagina.
  - available in single size (one size fits all) or multi-size that require fitting
- Both caps and the diaphragm are reusable, but should be replaced if they have any signs of damage.
- The female condom: a disposable, single use, polyurethane (FC) or nitrile (the FC2) sheath placed in the vagina.
- When used as a primary method, women should have ECP on hand at home.

EFFECTIVENESS

- The typical use failure rate for the FemCap is 13-16% for nulliparous women and 23-32 % for multiparous.
- A Cochrane Review found pregnancy rates during one year of use to be 11% to 13% for the diaphragm

Diaphragm:	Typical use failure rate in first year:	17% *[Trussell 2018]*
	Perfect use failure rate in first year:	6%
Female Condom:	Typical use failure rate in first year:	21% *[Trussell 2018]*
	Perfect use failure rate in first year:	5%

MECHANISM OF ACTION: Act both as a mechanical barrier to sperm migration into the cervical canal and as a chemical agent by applying spermicide directly to the cervix

ADVANTAGES

Menstrual: none

Sexual / psychological:

- Female controlled
- Intercourse may be more pleasurable because fear of pregnancy is reduced
- Can be inserted several hours before sexual intercourse to permit spontaneity
- Can remain in place for multiple acts of intercourse up to 24 hours (diaphragm) to 48 hours (cervical cap) total from time of placement (except for female condom)

Cancers / tumors / masses

- Follow-up studies of earlier cervical caps show no associated increase in cervical dysplasia with use. Labeling of current cervical caps or diaphragms does not require additional pap smears

Other:

- May reduce risk of cervical infections, including gonorrhea, chlamydia, and PID, but offers no protection against HIV infection
- Immediately active after placement
- May be used during lactation
- Used only when needed
- May be reusable (diaphragm and cap)
- Relatively low cost
- Immediately effective and immediately reversible
- May be part of "dual-method" use

DISADVANTAGES

Menstrual: none

Sexual / psychological:

- Requires placement prior to genital contact, which may reduce spontaneity of sex
- Some women do not like placing fingers or a foreign body into their vagina
- Requires motivation to use at time of sex
- Requires some skill
- Devices that require spermicide must be left in place for 6 hours after sex

Other:

- Lack of protection against HIV and some STIs. Must use condoms if at risk
- Higher failure rates than with hormonal contraception or LARC
- Odor may develop if left in place too long or if not appropriately cleaned (if reusable)
- Severe obesity or arthritis may make insertion/removal difficult
- Devices that require fitting need to be refitted after pregnancy

COMPLICATIONS

- UTIs may increase
- Superficial cervical erosion may occur causing vaginal spotting and/or cervical discomfort and discontinuation
- Rare cases of toxic shock syndrome with diaphragm and sponge have been reported. The risk may be increased if these methods are left in too long or used during menses

CANDIDATES: Women NOT at high risk of HIV

- Women willing and able to insert device prior to coitus and remove it later
- Motivated women willing to use with every coital act
- Women with pelvic relaxation are better candidates for cap than for diaphragm
- Women who are sensitive to use of hormones
- Women and partner(s) who have no sensitivity to spermicides

Adolescents: Appropriate, but requires discipline and preparedness to use consistently and correctly. If at risk for STIs use condoms in addition.

INITIATING METHOD

- Given the high failure rates for these methods, it is important to provide ECPs in advance for use if needed or recommend purchase OTC for adults
- A speculum and bimanual exam is recommended before initiating use. Should not be used in the presence of vaginal infections, or vaginal or cervical abrasions

- Encourage use of a back-up method for the first few uses until she is confident with correct use. Continual use of male condoms with these methods will reduce pregnancy and STI risk
- If device dislodges during use, EC should be used ASAP.
- For reusable devices, instruct the woman to wash with mild soap and water after each use, dry, and store in container until next use. The sponge and female condom should be disposed of after removal

FOLLOW-UP

- Are you or your partner noticing any discomfort during sex?
- Do you notice an odor when you remove the device?
- Have you had any burning with urination, vaginal irritation or itching?
- Do you use the device every single time you have sexual intercourse?
- For the cap or diaphragm, do you always apply spermicide before insertion?
- Do you have ECPs at home?

PROBLEM MANAGEMENT

- Spotting/cervical or vaginal discomfort/erosion: Rule out infection; stop use to allow healing; consider different size or alternative method
- Urinary tract infections: Urinate postcoitally to reduce bladder contamination with vaginal bacteria. Check fit to be sure there is not excessive urethral pressure
- Odor upon removal: Rule out infection. Try Listerine soaks if reusable, shorten time left in place, or replace
- Dislodged during sex (ensure proper fit) or other failure to use correctly: Use EC. Provide ECPs to have on hand. Consider alternative method

FERTILITY AFTER DISCONTINUATION

- Immediate return to baseline fertility

THE FC2 - FEMALE CONDOM

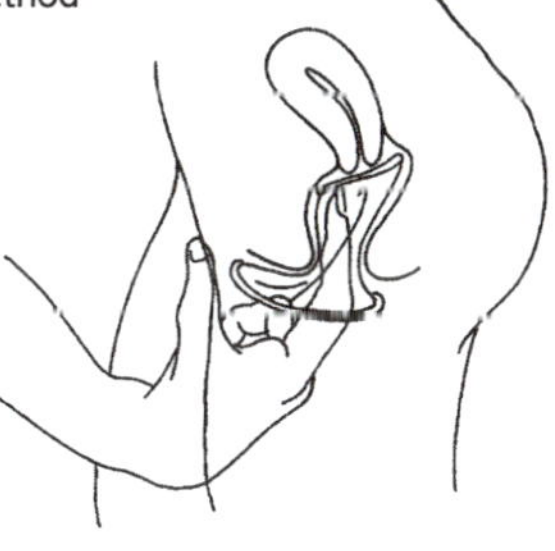

- The "FC1" (no longer available) is a polyurethane sheath. The FC2 is a nitrile sheath that is cheaper to produce and buy
- Sold over-the-counter, without need for prescription ($3.30 - $6.00; $1.50 in public clinic)

Instructions for Use:

- Can be inserted up to 8 hours before sex to allow for spontaneity
- In squatting, leg-up, reclining or lithotomy position, compress inner ring and introduce into vagina guiding sheath high into vagina until outer ring rests against vulva. Rotate inner ring to stabilize device in vault
- Manually place penis in sheath
- Excessive friction between penis and device can cause breakage or device inversion
- Remove condom immediately after intercourse. Twist outer ring to seal off contents and then pull out of vagina. Inspect condom for patency, then discard
- If condom dislodges or breaks, or if any spillage of ejaculate occurs, use EC ASAP
- If a male latex condom is used with a FC2, theoretically, there can be increased risk of breakage of either or both condoms

CERVICAL CAP

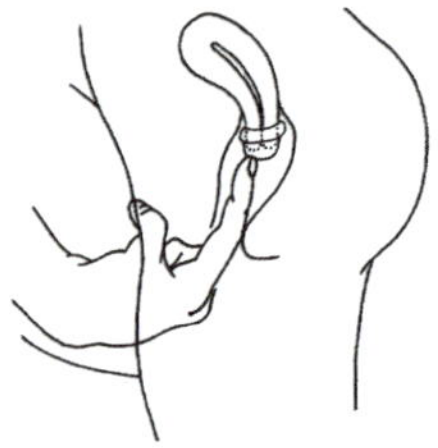

FemCap:

- Only cap available in U.S.
- Silicone
- Three sizes available. Approximately 85% of women can be assigned the correct size of FemCap based on their obstetrical history: nulligravid women using the small (22mm) size, parous women who have not delivered vaginally using the medium (26 mm) size, and women who have delivered vaginally using the largest (30 mm) size
- Proper fit can be confirmed in the office or clinic by checking that: insertion instructions have been followed, the cervix is covered entirely, and the device is comfortable for the woman
- FemCap may be bought over the internet at www.femcap.com with recommendation for fit to be checked by clinician

Instructions for Use:

- Can be placed up to 6 hours before sex
- Coat the inside of the bowl and the rim with spermicide. Place a small amount of spermicide along the outer part of the cap.
- In the squatting, leg-up or reclining position, press the rims on each side of the bowl together and hold with the dome strap side of the bowl pointing downward.
- Insert long/thick side first as far into the vagina as possible. Push the device over your cervix so that it covers the cervix completely so wider part of the cap brim is posterior and narrower part is anterior. Then press upwards to create suction between the cap and your cervix. You might feel air venting out as the suction is created between the cap and the cervix.
- The device should be left in place for at least 6-8 hours after the last act of intercourse, up to 48 hours total.
- Insert dose of spermicide in vagina for additional acts of intercourse
- To remove, use fingers to grasp loop, twist or push on cap to break the suction (hearing a "pop"), and remove device from the vagina

DIAPHRAGM

- Caya (aka SILCS):
  - single-size silicone diaphragm
  - no pelvic exam required but prescription required
- Milex: wide-seal omniflex style, made of silicone
  - order from Cooper Surgical
  - formerly the Ortho All-Flex
  - sizes 60, 70 ,75, 80, 85, 90 and 95mm
  - fits 98% of individuals
  - on bimanual exam, determine degree of version of uterus; not a good method for extremely anteverted or retroverted uterus. Introduce your third finger into the posterior fornix and and tilt your wrist upward to mark where your index finger/

hand contacts the symphysis. Use that measurement as a guide and place a fitting diaphragm in the vagina

- have woman walk around in your office to test its comfort
- alternatively, try a 70mm sample size and see if it covers the cervix from posterior vaginal fornix to just above the posterior of the symphysis
- recheck the fit of the diaphragm whenever there is a 20% weight change and/or pregnancy

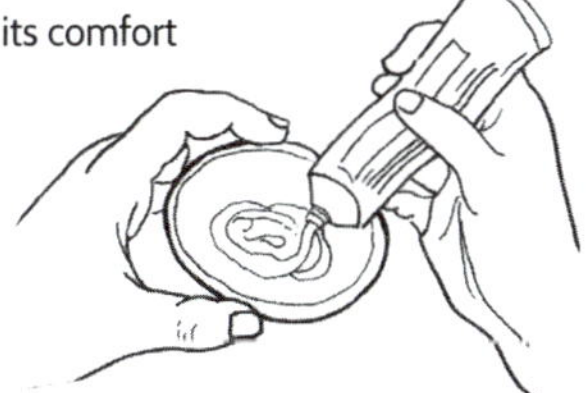

Figure 18.1
Risk of pregnancy increases when a spermicide is not used. Put spermicide on outside and on inside

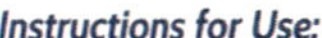

Instructions for Use:

- Can be placed up to 6 hours before sex
- Place about one tablespoon of spermicide in the dome and along rim
- In the squatting, leg-up or reclining position, press the rims on each side of the diaphragm together and hold with the dome of the bowl pointing downward.
- Insert with the dome side down as far into the vagina as possible. Push the diaphragm over your cervix so that it covers the cervix completely. Prior to each act of coitus, reconfirm correct placement and place additional spermicide

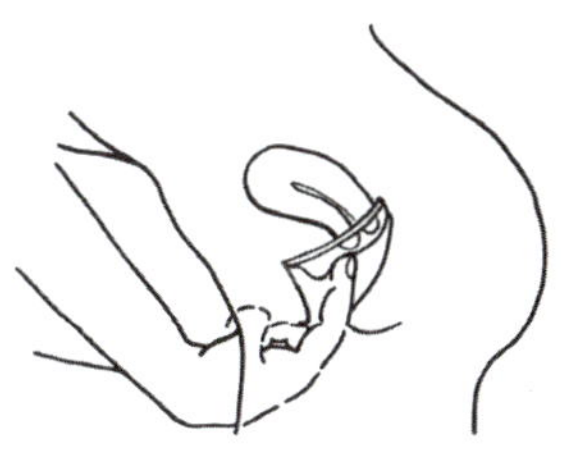

- Check to ensure diaphragm is lodged behind symphysis and completely covers the cervix. Bear down and digitally check to ensure that diaphragm does not move from behind pubic arch
- Insert another application of spermicide in vagina after insertion and before additional act of intercourse
- The diaphragm should be left in place for at least 6 hours after the last act of intercourse, up to 24 hours total from the time it was placed

TODAY™ CONTRACEPTIVE SPONGE

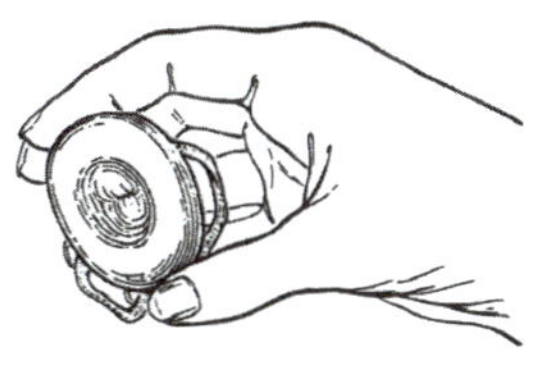

- The sponge is pre-filled with spermicide that is continuously released into the vagina during use

Instructions for Use:

- Hold the sponge "dimple" side up and thoroughly wet sponge with tap water before insertion. Squeeze the sponge to produce suds
- In the squatting, leg-up or reclining position, press the rims on each side of the sponge together with the dimple still pointing upward
- Insert with the dimple first and loop last as far into the vagina as possible. Push the sponge over your cervix so that the dimple covers the cervix completely. To check positioning, squat or bear down to be sure it does not move

- May be inserted up to 24 hours before sex but should not be in place >30 hours
- Should be left in place for at least 6 hours after the last act of intercourse, up to 24 hours total
- May have multiple acts of intercourse
- To remove, use fingers to grasp loop and remove device from the vagina. Dispose of sponge after use
- In France, the perfect use failure rate is 20% while the typical use failure rate is 27%
- In nulliparous women, the perfect use failure rate is 9% while the typical use failure rate is 14%. For multiparous woman the perfect use is 20% and typical use 27%.

CHAPTER 18

SPERMICIDES

DESCRIPTION: The search for an effective vaginal microbicide that would also kill sperm remains an important research priority. In the U.S., nonoxynol-9 (N-9) is available over the counter. In addition to N-9, patients around the world use menfegol, benzalkonium chloride, sodium docusate, and chlorhexidine. Spermicides are available as vaginal creams, films, foams, gels, suppositories, sponges and tablets.

> **Women at high risk of HIV** should not use spermicides (U.S. MEC:4). Nor should women who are HIV-infected (U.S. MEC:4) Condoms without nonoxynol-9 lubrication are effective and widely available. Women at high risk of HIV infection should also avoid using diaphragms and cervical caps to which nonoxynol-9 is added (U.S. MEC:3). There is good evidence that N-9 does not protect against STIs and some evidence that it may be harmful by increasing genital irritation *[Cochrane Review 2008]*.

- **A new product administered like a spermicide called a "pH vaginal modulator" was approved in 2020 called Phexxi, which makes the vagina acidic in the pH range of 3.5 to 4.5 (its natural range), inhibiting sperm motility.**

EFFECTIVENESS *(See Trussell's failure rates, Table 2.1, page 9)*

Typical use failure rate in first year: 21%

Perfect use failure rate in first year: 16%

Failure rates are higher for spermicides than for any contraceptive currently available.

- Cochrane review of spermicides for contraception found the probability of pregnancy varied widely in trials. A gel with 52.5 mg N-9 was significantly less effective than gels with higher N-9 doses (100 mg, 150 mg). Gel was liked more than film and suppositories in largest trial *[Grimes 2005]*

> ***Phexxi effectiveness:*** results from a 7 month clinical trial:
> **Typical use pregnancy in 7 month clinical trial:** 11%
> **Perfect Use:** 7%
> Estimated Pearl index per the package insert: 27.5%

MECHANISM OF ACTION: As barriers, the vehicles prevent sperm from entering the cervical os. As detergents, the chemicals attack the sperm flagella and body, reducing motility. Phexxi acidifies the vagina which inhibits sperm motility.

ADVANTAGES

Menstrual: None

Sexual / psychological:

- Lubrication may heighten satisfaction for either partner
- Ease in application prior to sexual intercourse
- Either partner can purchase and apply; requires minimal negotiation

Other:

- Available over the counter; requires no medical visit
- Inexpensive and easy to use
- Foam and spermicidal jelly are immediately active with placement
- May be used during lactation

DISADVANTAGES

Menstrual: None

Sexual / psychological:

- Films and suppository spermicides require 15 minutes for activation, which may interrupt or delay sex
- Must feel comfortable inserting fingers into vagina
- Some forms, e.g., gel, foam, become "messy" during intercourse
- Possible vaginal, oral, and anal irritation can disrupt or preclude sex
- Taste may be unpleasant

Cancer / tumors / masses: None

Other:

- High failure rate means spermicidal contraceptives are not effective enough to be used by women at risk for serious complications of pregnancy *(see page 75)*
- Relatively high failure rate among perfect and typical users and does not protect against transmission of HIV, GC or chlamydia. Spermicides may, in women having frequent intercourse with multiple partners, enhance transmission of HIV by irritation of vaginal mucosa and by destroying vaginal flora, e.g., lactobacilli, in nonoxynol-9 concentrations as low as 0.1% *[Van Dame 2000] [Kreiss 1992]*
- Allergic reactions and dermatitis in women and men that could decrease compliance

COMPLICATIONS

- Women and men have confused fruit jelly, e.g., grape jelly, for spermicidal "jelly"
- Women and men have attempted to use cosmetics or hair products containing non-spermicidal octoxynols and nonoxynols (nonoxynol 4, 10, 12, and 14) in lieu of nonoxynol-9

CANDIDATES FOR USE

- Willing to accept high failure rates
- Any woman and partner who presents with no prior allergy or reaction to spermicides

Adolescents:

- Readily available and not contraindicated for teens unless at high risk for HIV infection
- High failure rate should discourage long-term use as primary method

INITIATING METHOD

- Except in cases where the patient, or partner, presents with an allergy, or irritation, women can begin these methods at any time following product instructions
- Ensure ECPs are on hand at home
- Phexxi is inserted as a prefilled single-dose application up to 1 hour before each act of intercourse

INSTRUCTIONS FOR PATIENT

- Inserting person should wash and dry hands
- Spermicide has its greatest efficacy near the cervical os
- Water exposure, e.g. bathing or douching, within 6 hours after insertion or post-coitally can minimize effectiveness; reapply before next penetrative act
- Keep spermicides in cool, dry places; tablets or foam can tolerate heat, film melts at 98.6° F

Creams / foams / gels

- Apply less than 1 hour prior to sexual intercourse. With foam, shake canister vigorously. Fill plastic applicator with spermicide. Insert applicator deeply into vagina and depress plunger. Immediately active. Finish sexual intercourse within 60 minutes of application

Film, suppositories and tablets

- Insert at least 15 minutes before sexual intercourse: with film, fold the sheet in quarters and then half again (this aids insertion). Using fingers or an applicator, the inserting partner places the spermicide applicator or film deep in the vagina, near cervix. Finish sexual intercourse within 60 minutes of application

Phexxi

- Requires prescription
- Insert no more than 1 hour before sex
- Repeat with each act of intercourse
- Do not use in combination with vaginal ring
- Do not use if history of recurrent UTIs or urinary tract abnormalities

FOLLOW-UP

- Have you or your partner(s) experienced any rash or discomfort after using spermicides?
- Have you changed partners since beginning spermicides?
- Have you had sex—even once—without using spermicides?
- Would you like a more effective method?
- Did you have questions about emergency contraceptive pills?
- Do you have emergency contraceptive pills at home?
- Do you plan to have children? OR Do you plan to have more children? If yes, when?

PROBLEM MANAGEMENT

Dermatitis: Discontinue spermicides and offer another method. If spermicide was used as lubricant, recommend a water-based or silicone-based lubricant without nonoxynol-9

Changed partners: Explain STI prevention, check for STIs, and recommend condoms

Phexxi: 18% users had vaginal burning, 15% vaginal itching, 9% UTI, 9% yeast infection and 8% BV *[Thomas 2020], [package insert]*

- 10% male partners reported symptoms local discomfort

FERTILITY AFTER DISCONTINUATION OF METHOD

- No effect on baseline fertility

CHAPTER 19

COITUS INTERRUPTUS (WITHDRAWAL)

The proportion of women who have ever used withdrawal increased from 25% in 1982 to 60% in 2006-2010. *[Daniels 2013]*

EFFECTIVENESS

Typical use failure rate in first year: 20% *[Trussell 2018]*
Perfect use failure rate in first year: 4% *(See Trussell's failure rates, Table 2.1, page 9)*

MECHANISM OF ACTION: Withdrawal prior to ejaculation reduces or eliminates sperm introduced into vagina. Preejaculatory fluid is not generally a problem unless two acts of sexual intercourse are close together. It is very important that the penis is away from the introitus after withdrawal.

Are there sperm in pre-ejaculate fluid? Possibly yes.

When the penis becomes erect, pre-ejaculate, a lubricating secretion produced by the Littre or Cowper's glands, is emitted. Although two studies examining the pre-ejaculate for the presence of spermatozoa found none, two other studies found spermatozoa, though in small numbers. In one of these studies, 8 of 23 samples contained clumps of a few hundred sperm, which could theoretically have posed a risk of fertilization. In a study designed specifically to determine whether pre-ejaculate contained sperm potentially capable of fertilizing an egg, researchers examined the samples within 2 hours of production. The pre-ejaculate of 37% of men contained motile sperm, though the number of sperm in each sample was very low. Also worth noting is that this study found that subjects either consistently had sperm in their pre-ejaculate or consistently did not. The best available evidence suggests that the risk of pregnancy posed by pre-ejaculate is very low, though not zero. *[Jones 2018]*

COST: None

ADVANTAGES

Menstrual: None
Sexual / psychological:

- No barriers
- Readily available method which encourages male involvement

Cancers, tumors, and masses: None
Other: Surprisingly effective if used correctly (perfectly)

DISADVANTAGES

Menstrual: None
Sexual / psychological:

- May not be applicable for couples with sexual dysfunction such as premature ejaculation
- Requires man's cooperation and control

- May reduce sexual pleasure of woman and intensity of orgasm of man
- Encourages "spectatoring" or thinking about what is happening during sexual intercourse

Cancers / tumors / masses: None

Other: Relatively high failure rate among typical users and poor protection against STIs.

COMPLICATIONS: None

MEDICAL ELIGIBILITY CHECKLIST

- Man must be able to predict ejaculation in time to withdraw penis completely from vagina
- Premature ejaculation is a common problem that makes method less effective
- More appropriate for couples not at risk for STIs

CANDIDATES FOR USE

- Couples who are able to communicate during sexual intercourse
- Disciplined men who can ignore the instinct to continue thrusting
- Couples without personal, religious or cultural prohibitions against withdrawal
- Women willing to accept higher risk of unintended pregnancy

Adolescents: teens may have less control over ejaculation; advise use of condoms for better protection against pregnancy and STIs. While withdrawal is a relatively poor contraceptive option, especially if preventing pregnancy and infection are important, it is always available

INITIATING METHOD: Can begin at any time; provide ECPs in advance

INSTRUCTIONS FOR PATIENT

- Practice withdrawal using backup method until both partners comfortable
- Wipe penis clean of the pre-ejaculation fluid prior to vaginal penetration
- Use coital positions that ensure that the man will be capable of withdrawing easily at the appropriate time
- Use emergency contraception (preferably an IUD) if withdrawal fails

FOLLOW-UP

- Does your partner ever ejaculate/begin to ejaculate before withdrawing?
- Do you want to use a more effective method?
- Did you have any Plan B or ella at home?
- Do you plan to have children? OR Do you plan to have more children?
- Have you considered withdrawal early during intercourse, followed by putting on a condom, re-entering the vagina, then ejaculation? In one study of college males, 43% reported using withdrawal during initial phases of intercourse and then applying a condom for intra-vaginal ejaculation. *[Crosby 2002]*

PROBLEM MANAGEMENT

Failure to withdraw: Some women use emergency contraceptive pills almost everytime because the man fails to withdraw in time. Such a couple should consider another method.

FERTILITY AFTER DISCONTINUATION OF METHOD: No effect on fertility

CHAPTER 20

EMERGENCY CONTRACEPTION

THE MOST EFFECTIVE EMERGENCY CONTRACEPTION IS THE COPPER IUD

- Ten times fewer pregnancies than if emergency contraceptive pills are used
- LNG 52mg IUD recently found to have comparable efficacy
- Neither IUD type is FDA-approved for EC

FIG 20.1 ESSENTIAL FEATURES OF COMMON EC METHODS AVAILABLE IN THE UNITED STATES

Feature	Copper IUD	Ulipristal acetate 30 mg	Levonorgestrel 1.5 mg
Pregnancy risk	0.1%[1]	1.2 to 1.8%[2,3]	1.7 to 2.6%[2,3]
Timing of use relative to UPI	Typically, up to 5 days after UPI, but may be effective at any time in the menstrual cycle when urine pregnancy test is negative[1,4]	Up to 5 days after UPI[5]	Up to 3 days after UPI, although may have efficacy up to 5 days[5]
Timing of use relative to predicted ovulation	Highly effective at any time in the cycle	Effective until the LH peak[6]	Effective until the LH surge begins[6]
Availability and access	Requires office visit and clinician insertion	Requires prescription	Available OTC
Cost	Covered by insurance, though high deductible can limit access; highest cost for uninsured	Covered by insurance: • $50 self-pay at pharmacy • $67 available online	$40 to $50 OTC in pharmacies $10 to $25 online, though shipping necessitates advanced provision for some websites
Relationship to starting progestin-containing contraception	N/A, effective for contraception immediately	Wait 5 days to begin[7]	May start immediately[7]
BMI pregnancy risk	Highly effective regardless of BMI	BMI 25 to 29.9 = 1.1% BMI ≥30 = 2.6%[8]	BMI 25 to 29.9 = 2.5% BMI ≥30 = 5.8%[8]
Works to prevent pregnancy if additional UPI in same cycle	Yes	No	No

Reprinted with permission from www.uptodate.com

1. *Cleland K, Zhu H, Goldstuck N, et al. The efficacy of intrauterine devices for emergency contraception: A systematic review of 35 years of experience. Hum Reprod 2012; 27:1994.*
2. *Glasier AF, Cameron ST, Fine PM, et al. Ulipristal acetate versus levonorgestrel for emergency contraception: a randomised non-inferiority trial and meta-analysis. Lancet 2010; 375:555.*
3. *Shen J, Che Y, Showell E, et al. Interventions for emergency contraception. Cochrane Database Syst Rev 2019; :CD001324.*
4. *Turok DK, Godfrey EM, Wojdyla D, et al. Copper T380 intrauterine device for emergency contraception: highly effective at any time in the menstrual cycle. Hum Reprod 2013; 28:2672.*
5. *Emergency Contraceptive Pills: Medical and Service Delivery Guidance. International Consortium for Emergency Contraception 2018. https://www.cecinfo.org/wp-content/uploads/2018/12/ICEC-guides_FINAL.pdf (Accessed on March 09, 2019).*
6. *Noé G, Croxatto HB, Salvatierra AM, et al. Contraceptive efficacy of emergency contraception with levonorgestrel given before or after ovulation. Contraception 2011; 84:486.*
7. *Providing Ongoing Hormonal Contraception after Use of Emergency Contraceptive Pills. American Society for Emergency Contraception 2016. http://americansocietyforec.org/uploads/3/4/5/6/34568220/asec_fact_sheet-_hormonal_contraception_after_ec.pdf (Accessed on March 09, 2019).*
8. *Glasier A, Cameron ST, Blithe D, et al. Can we identify women at risk of pregnancy despite using emergency contraception? Data from randomized trials of ulipristal acetate and levonorgestrel. Contraception 2011; 84:363.*

EMERGENCY CONTRACEPTION (EC) WITH AN IUD

DESCRIPTION

- An IUD may be inserted up to 5 days after ovulation, which means insertion can occur many days after unprotected intercourse (UPI).
  - Since day of ovulation is not usually known, time of insertion is simplified to the words "up to 5 days after unprotected intercourse"
- Recent study found insertion of LNG 52-mg IUD as an EC was noninferior to Cu-IUD. *[Turok 2021]*

EFFECTIVENESS

- ***Copper T:*** less than 1 failure per 1000 Copper T insertions (0.1%)
- ***LNG 52mg IUD:*** 0.3% (or 3 failures per 1000 insertions)
- The copper T-380A IUD is the most effective EC for overweight women, efficacy not impacted by body weight

MECHANISM OF ACTION

- Prevent fertilization
- May prevent implantation

ADVANTAGES

- Insert within 5 days UPI
- Provides long-term protection against pregnancy following insertion

DISADVANTAGES

- Same disadvantages as when using an IUD as ongoing contraceptive
- Expensive if only used for EC and removal is done soon thereafter

EMERGENCY CONTRACEPTION (EC) WITH ULIPRISTAL ACETATE (UPA) (ELLA, ELLAONE, FIBRISTAL)

DESCRIPTION

- An antiprogestin taken as a 30mg single dose.
- Selective progestin receptor modulator that inhibits or delays ovulation.
- Derived from 19-norprogesterone, similar to mifepristone, but with less antiglucocorticoid activity.

EFFECTIVENESS

- Odds of pregnancy 65% lower than LNG EC if taken within 24 hours of UPI *[Glasier 2010]*
- 42% lower if taken within 72 hours of UPI *[Glasier 2010]*
- Significantly more effective than LNG EC at 72-120 hours after UPI *[Glasier 2010]*
- Rate of pregnancy in patients receiving ulipristal 1.8%
- Risk of pregnancy was more than threefold higher for obese women than non-obese
- Less risk of failure in obese women than with LNG EC. Highest risk was also related to having sex around ovulation or continued unprotected sex after taking EC.

MECHANISM: delays or inhibits ovulation

COST

- Requires a prescription so may be covered by insurance
- Approximately $50 if self-pay

ADVANTAGES

- More effective than levonorgestrel as an emergency contraceptive pill

DISADVANTAGES: requires a prescription

Menstrual: Menses delayed by an average of 2 days, which can create anxiety about pregnancy status

Sexual / Psychological:

- Women who are uncomfortable with post-fertilization methods need reassurance that use of EC with UPA is consistent with their beliefs i.e.; not abortifacient
- No STI protection

Cancer, tumors and masses: None

Other:

- Headache, nausea, abdominal pain possible.
- No protection against STIs, consider Rx for STIs if exposed.
- Use of hormonal contraception should be delayed 5 days after taking ulipristal acetate (UPA) due to concerns the contraceptive progestin may interfere with UPA action

COMPLICATIONS: None

CANDIDATES FOR USE: Same as for ECPS *see page 84*

PRECAUTIONS:

- Pregnancy and ectopic pregnancy
- Hypersensitivity to any compound of the product
- Undiagnosed abnormal uterine bleeding (be suspicious of risk of ectopic pregnancy)
- Not for repeated uses in single cycle
- Barrier contraception or abstinence is recommended immediately following use of ulipristal acetate and throughout the same menstrual cycle; efficacy of hormonal contraception may be decreased.
- Drug interactions (see package label for more details): Conivaptan, CYP3A4 inducers, Deferasirox, herbs, Tocilizumab, St. John's Wort may decrease serum levels of UPA

EMERGENCY CONTRACEPTION WITH COMBINED ORAL CONTRACEPTIVE PILLS OR PROGESTIN-ONLY PILLS

PROGESTIN-ONLY PILLS (Plan B One-Step, and many generic equivalents)*

** for simplification will use term Plan B when referring to EC with POPs*

Description

- Single oral 1.5mg dose LNG ECP available OTC without a prescription and without ID required
- Tell all patients about EC, informing them that ongoing use of an effective contraceptive is more effective than repeated use of an ECP.
- You can order a generic form of Plan B at www.afterpill.com for $20 + $5 shipping.
- FDA-approved for use within 72 hours UPI but may be used up to 5 days.

Effectiveness

- 2.6% pregnancy rate
- PLAN B or generic equivalent: take pill ASAP within 72 hours, most effective in this window, however can take up to 5 days

- Risk of pregnancy increases with increasing BMI and may not work at all in obese women
- EC guidelines in the United Kingdom state for women weighing 70kg (154.3 pounds) or more if ella (UPA) is not available or acceptable a double dose (3mg) LNG (this would be two Plan B One-Step tablets) can be used
- Pharmacokinetic study of obese women showed when dose was double, serum levels of LNG was same as normal weight women ingesting single 1.5mg dose *[Edelman 2016]*

COMBINED ORAL CONTRACEPTIVE PILLS

Description

- Two doses of COCs taken 12 hours apart with at least 100 µg of ethinyl estradiol and either 100 mcg of norgestrel or 0.50 mg of levonorgestrel in each dose.
- Norethindrone pills have slightly less effectiveness as ECPs.
- Take first dose ASAP within 120 hours after UPI; take second dose 12 hours later (second dose may be more than 120 hours after unprotected sex).

Effectiveness

- Failure rate of 2-3%

MECHANISM OF ACTION

- ECPs disrupt normal follicular development and maturation, block LH surge, and inhibit ovulation; they may also create deficient luteal phase and may have a contraceptive effect by thickening cervical mucus
- Never disrupt an implanted pregnancy, i.e. not abortifacient

COST

POPs:

- Plan B is available OTC in retail pharmacies for about $40- $50. Generics may be less costly
- Non-profit and Title X agencies may purchase POPs at $4.50 - $8.00 per treatment
- Ordering over the internet may bring cost down to $10

Yuzpe method with COCs:

- One cycle of COCs may vary from a few dollars to more than $50

Other costs:

- Cost prior to obtaining pills may vary from nothing (if dispensed in advance) to cost of full exam and pregnancy test. This may increase total cost of EC to over $100

ADVANTAGES

Menstrual: None

Sexual / Psychological:

- Offers an opportunity to prevent pregnancy after rape, mistake with method use, or barrier method failure (condom breaks or slips, diaphragm dislodges, etc.)
- Reduces anxiety about unintended pregnancy prior to next menses
- Complicated process of getting EC may lead woman to initiate ongoing contraception at EC visit

Cancers / tumors / masses: None

DISADVANTAGES

Menstrual:

- Next menses may be early (especially if taken before ovulation), on time, or late
- Notable changes in flow of next menses seen in 10-15% of women
- If no menses within 3 weeks (21 days) of taking ECPs, pregnancy test should be done

Sexual / psychological:

- Women who are uncomfortable with post-fertilization methods need reassurance that use of EC with COCs or POPs is consistent with their beliefs i.e.; not abortifacient
- No STI protection

Cancers / tumors / masses: None

Other:

- Breast tenderness, fatigue, headache, abdominal pain and dizziness
- No protection against STIs; consider treatment for possible STIs following exposure

Nausea and vomiting:

	NAUSEA	VOMITING	PRETREATMENT WITH ANTIEMETIC
POPs	23%	6%	Many clinicians use only if Hx of past problems with nausea or vomiting
COCs	50%	19%	Can reduce symptoms by 30-50%

COMPLICATIONS

- Several cases of DVT reported in women using COCs as ECPs. No increased DVT risk with levonorgestrel POPs

CANDIDATES FOR USE

- All women who have had or who may be at risk for unprotected sex.
- As a backup method for barrier methods
- Forgotten pills, late for contraceptive reinjection, fertility awareness based method miscalculation, failed withdrawal
- For the woman who has intercourse infrequently, (1-2x/yr) particularly effective if taken within one hour of otherwise unprotected sex
- NOTE: ECPs do not protect against pregnancy as well as ongoing methods

Adolescents: appropriate back-up option. Having EC available does NOT make teens less likely to use regular contraception or more likely to have unprotected sex. *[Glasier 1998] [Raine 2000] [Ellertson 2001]*

PRECAUTIONS

Plan B One Step:

- Pregnancy (no benefit; no effect)
- Hypersensitivity to any component of product
- Undiagnosed abnormal vaginal bleeding

Obesity: Increased failure rates for emergency contraceptive pills has been documented for women who are overweight and obese. For Plan B / Next Choice, the failure rates for obese women may be 4 times higher and for ulipristal, failure rates may be 2 times higher. For these women, copper IUDs should be discussed due to superior efficacy.

INITIATING METHOD: Pregnancy testing is optional, not required:

- POPs (Plan B) OTC, ID not required.
- Offer ECPs routinely to all women who may be at risk for unprotected intercourse.
- Advance provision and prescription increases use of EC
- Provide EC for all women who present after-the-fact, acutely in need. If you dispense off-label pills remove the inactive pills to reduce risk of mistake
- Patient history for prescribing EC after-the-fact:
    - LMP, previous menstrual period, dates of any prior unprotected intercourse this cycle, and date and time of last unprotected intercourse
    - Any problems with previous use of ECPs, COCs or POPs?
    - Breastfeeding or severe headaches now? History of DVT or PE? (Use POPs not COCs)
    - Any foreseeable problems if antiemetic causes drowsiness?
    - No physical exam/labs needed on a routine basis:
        - No pelvic exam is necessary. No BP measurements needed
        - Pregnancy testing useful only if concerned that prior intercourse may have caused pregnancy. ***ACOG, IPPF and CDC do not include routine pregnancy testing in their protocol***
- Advise patient about possible side effects and consider other EC options (TCu 380A IUD)
- If prescribing COCs, offer premedication with long-acting antiemetic one hour prior to first ECP dose. Take two 25 mg tablets of meclizine hydrochloride (over-the-counter Dramamine 2 or Bonine). Avoid antiemetic if drowsiness will pose safety hazard. Antiemetics not needed prior to Plan B

STARTING REGULAR USE OF CONTRACEPTIVE AFTER USE OF PLAN B

- If missed pills, restart same pill pack after ECPs taken (no need to catch up missed pills). Use condoms until next period.
- If initiating COCs, patch or ring:
    - May wait for next menses or
    - Start OCs, patch or ring next day with 7-day backup method (this will affect timing of next menses). In office, may punch out a few pills at the beginning of a pill pack to correspond with the day of the week you are seeing her. This may reduce confusion
- If starting DMPA injections, can start immediately. If so, consider having patient return in 2-3 weeks for pregnancy test
- If starting barrier methods, start immediately.
- If starting NFP, use abstinence (or barrier/spermicide) until next menses

STARTING REGULAR CONTRACEPTION AFTER USE OF ULIPRISTAL ACETATE (UPA)

- Advise to start or resume hormonal contraception no sooner than 5 days after use of UPA, and provide or prescribe the regular contraceptive method as needed. For methods requiring a visit to a health care provider, such as DMPA, implants, and IUDs, starting the method at the time of UPA use may be considered; the risk that the regular contraceptive method might decrease the effectiveness of UPA must be weighed against the risk of not starting a regular hormonal method.
- The woman needs to abstain from sexual intercourse or use barrier contraception for the next 7 days after starting or resuming regular contraception or until her next menses, whichever comes first.
- Any nonhormonal contraceptive method can be started immediately after the use of UPA.
- Advise the woman to have a pregnancy test if she does not have a withdrawal bleed within 3 weeks.

[U.S. Selected Practice Recommendations for Contraceptive Use, 2016, MMWR July 29, 2016 p.35]

SPECIAL ISSUES/FREQUENT QUESTIONS

- Give your patient a supply of EC at her annual visit.
- When in cycle should EC be offered? Anytime
- How many times a year can a woman use ECPs? No limit, but be sure to ask her why her primary method is not working
- What if a patient has had unprotected intercourse earlier in the cycle? Do urine test to rule out pregnancy. Offer EC. If concerned that your test may miss an early pregnancy, give EC and have her return in 3 weeks (if no menses) for another pregnancy test. EC will not adversely affect a developing pregnancy
- What if she used EC earlier in the month? Offer it again; she may have just delayed ovulation. Review why her primary contraceptive is failing her and offer a new method. Consider performing pregnancy test in this setting even though it may be too early to have become positive; counsel her about this possibility
- What if the pharmacy is closed or does not carry EC? Plan ahead. Encourage her to have EC on hand at home. Check with local 24-hour pharmacies

INSTRUCTIONS FOR PATIENT

- EC works best if taken as soon as possible after sex. Women at risk of pregnancy need EC at home. For advance prescription, have her fill her prescription (or obtain OTC) in advance and keep readily available.
- An antiemetic need not be taken prior to Plan B or Next Choice
- Start using contraception right away. ECPs do not reliably protect you beyond the day they are used
- Re-evaluate primary contraceptive method to make it more reliable

FOLLOW-UP

- No routine follow-up needed
- Instruct to return for pregnancy testing if no menses in 3 weeks
- If patient has persistent irregular bleeding or abdominal pain, she should return to rule out ectopic pregnancy

PROBLEM MANAGEMENT

Nausea/vomiting:

- Antiemetic may be prescribed before or after taking combined COCs as ECPs
- Vomiting that occurs due to ECPs probably indicates that enough hormones reached the bloodstream to have the desired contraceptive effect. Many experts recommend a repeat dose of ECPs if vomiting occurs within one hour of taking ECPs.
- If repeating dose because of severe vomiting and woman used COCs, switch to POPs or consider placing pills in vagina rather than taking orally (off-label) or a copper IUD. Although uptake is slower with vaginal administration, this may also be possible for woman who has experienced extreme nausea while taking COCs in the past as her regular contraceptive. No data on effectiveness of vaginal COCs used as EC
- If severe vomiting occurs, consider IUD as emergency contraceptive

Pregnancy in spite of using ECPs: If there is a pregnancy, the woman may be reassured that ECPs do not increase the risk of fetal anomalies, ectopic pregnancy or miscarriage

FERTILITY AFTER DISCONTINUATION OF METHOD: Must provide contraception for rest of cycle and beyond.

Notes for Figure 20.2

Reprinted with permission from www.uptodate.com
UPI includes instances in which no contraception was used, a method was used imperfectly, or intercourse was forced without use of contraception.
UPI: unprotected intercourse; EC: emergency contraception; IUD: intrauterine device; BMI: body mass index; LNG: levonorgestrel; DMPA: depot medroxyprogesterone acetate; UPA: ulipristal acetate.
* Pregnancy rates are 0.1% for the copper IUD, up to 1.8% for UPA, and up to 2.6% for LNG.
¶ Information on IUD device types, candidates, and device selection can be found in related UpToDate content.
Δ Contraceptive failure can include missing more than one dose of oral contraceptive pills; failure to resume the DMPA injection, patch, or vaginal ring at the correct time; having a diaphragm, cervical cap, or contraceptive sponge slip; or having a condom break.
◊ Treatment with UPA requires a prescription.
§ After receiving EC, the patient can expect her period within three weeks. Patients who do not have a period after three weeks should perform a pregnancy test.
¥ For patients in the United States, oral LNG is available over-the-counter for individuals ages 17 and older. Individuals younger than age 17 may require a prescription, which varies by state.

Figure 20.2

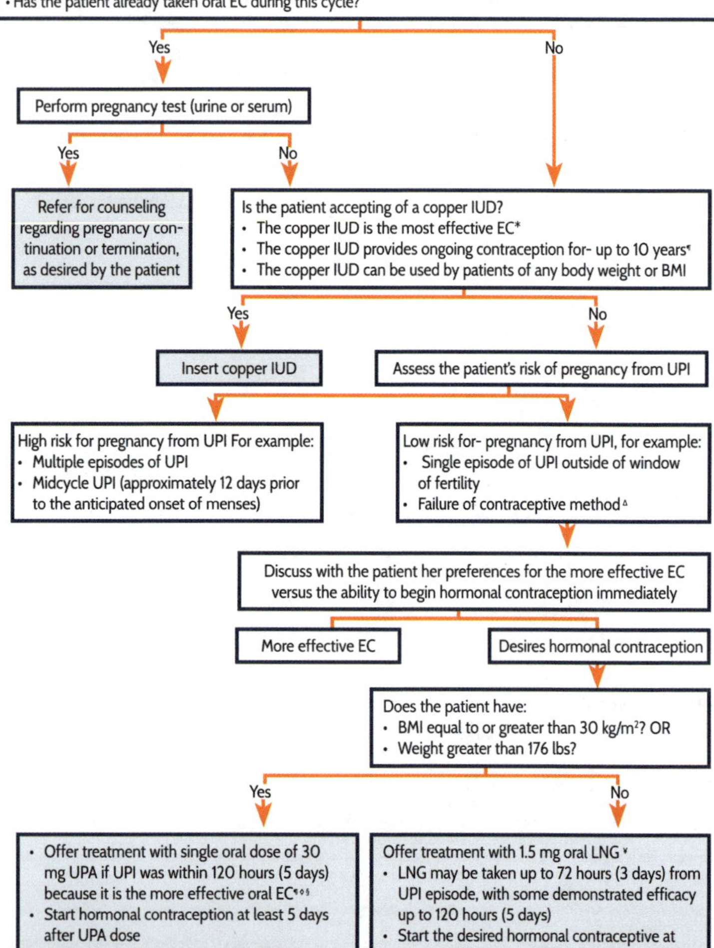

See notes on previous page

Figure 20.3

EMERGENCY CONTRACEPTION USING EMERGENCY CONTRACEPTIVE PILLS (ECPs)

POPs (Plan-B / Next Choice) ARE OTC
Educate/prescribe/provide emergency contraceptive pills (ECPs) prior to the need for them so that women and men have them available at home (or rapid access to them) in case they are needed. This is particularly important since **some pharmacies do not stock ECPs**

Start ECPs as soon as possible, after unprotected or inadequately protected sexual intercourse.
Can be used up to 5 days, but sooner is better; most effective if taken immediately or within 12 hours

No need to use anti-nausea medication if using POPs. If using a COC, first, take anti-nausea medication: 50 mg oral meclizine* has 24-hour duration of action

Brand**	Dose	
ella	1 tablet	
Plan B One-Step or equivalent	1 tablet	
One hour after antiemetic, take first dose of ECPs. Choose one of the following:		
Ogestrel, Ovral	2 white tablets per dose	**If vomiting occurs within 1 hour, repeat dose**
Levora, Low-Ogestrel, Lo/Ovral	4 white tablets per dose	
Levlen, Nordette	4 light-orange tablets per dose	
Levlen, Triphasil	4 light-yellow tablets per dose	
Trivora	4 pink tablets per dose	
Alesse, Levlite	5 pink tablets per dose	

If using one of the other COC options, repeat the same dose of ECPs 12 hours later.

Patient should (re)start ongoing method immediately and restock ECPs at home. If using ella, delay restart of hormonal methods for 5 days.

Pregnancy test if no period in 3 weeks

NOTE: if anti-nausea medication is NOT taken prior to first dose of COCs, it may be taken after the first dose, should nausea be severe or should woman vomit. Anti-nausea medication is usually not needed for women using POPs, as they do not contain estrogen.

* Meclizine hydrochloride is recommended because it has a 24-hour duration of action. It is available over the counter as Bonine and as Dramamine 2. Other medications to prevent nausea may be prescribed instead.

**Norethindrone pills recently shown to be effective but less than these levonorgestrel products.

Figure 20.4

EMERGENCY CONTRACEPTION USING COPPER IUD OR LNG 52MG IUD

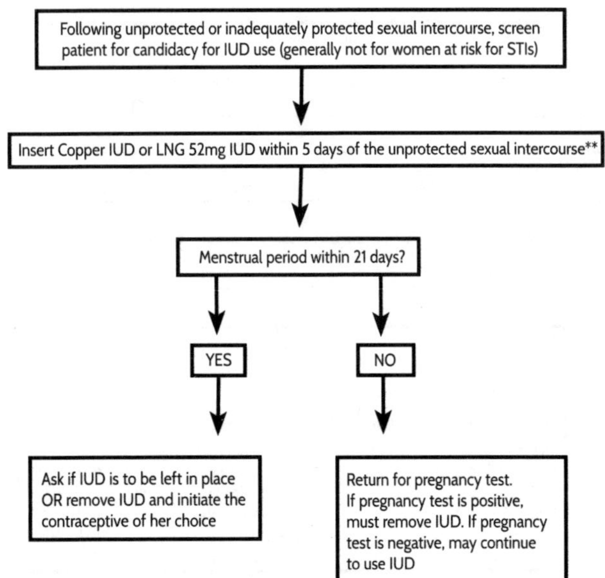

** The TCu 380A IUD may be inserted up to the time of implantation—about 5 days after ovulation—to prevent pregnancy. Thus, if a woman had unprotected sexual intercourse 3 days before ovulation occurred in that cycle, the IUD could be inserted up to 8 days after intercourse to prevent pregnancy. Instructions are simplified to say 5 days after UPI.

Postcoital Paragard insertion is the most effective emergency contraceptive. If a woman can use a TCu 380A IUD as her emergency contraceptive and leave it in as her ongoing long-term contraceptive, she may receive at least 10 or more years of excellent contraceptive protection.

CHAPTER 21

INTRAUTERINE CONTRACEPTIVES

OVERVIEW: Five intrauterine contraceptives are available in the U.S.: the copper (TCu 380A) IUD and 4 levonorgestrel IUDs.

- Continuation rates are the highest of all reversible contraceptives
- Less than 1 in 1,000 women using the TCu 380A as an emergency contraceptive becomes pregnant

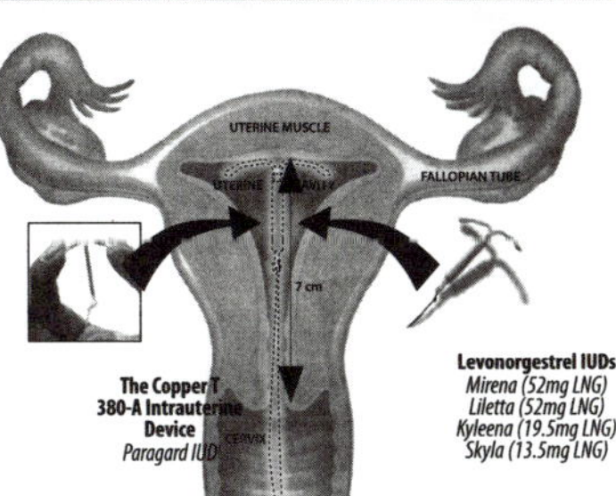

WOMEN MAY USE AN IUD IF THEY:

- are nulligravid, nulliparous or multiparous
- are young or late in reproductive years
- immediately after abortion or miscarriage
- immediately after a vaginal delivery or a C-section
- have had an STI in past
- have had an ectopic pregnancy in past
- are not in a monogamous relationship
- have fibroids that do not markedly distort the uterine cavity
- need emergency contraception
- have symptoms of endometriosis, adenomyosis, fibroids and heavy or painful periods (these conditions would suggest that an hormonal IUD be used)

Women must continue to:

- protect themselves from STI's using condoms if not in mutually monogamous relationship

CHOOSING BETWEEN COPPER AND HORMONAL IUDS:

Your patient wants an IUD. Counsel her thoroughly about the advantages and disadvantages of each IUD available. Women need to know either IUD can be removed at any time.

Copper IUD (TCu 380A):

- effective for at least 12 years
- no hormones, therefore, no hormonal side effects
- may cause heavier periods and / or more cramping
- the most effective emergency contraceptive

Hormonal IUD:

- Mirena and Liletta are effective for at least 7 years
- less pain and lighter to no periods, although irregular bleeding common
- minimal hormonal side effects
- improves symptoms from menorrhagia, endometriosis, fibroids, PCOS, and dysmennorhea
- decreased risk endometrial hyperplasia and cancer

INTRAUTERINE TCu 380A (PARAGARD)

DESCRIPTION: T-shaped intrauterine contraceptive made of radiopaque polyethylene, with two flexible arms that bend down for insertion but open in the uterus to hold solid sleeves of copper against fundus. Fine copper is wire wrapped around stem. Surface area of copper = 380 mm^2. Monofilament polyethylene tail string threaded through and knotted below blunt ball at base of stem creates double straw colored strings that protrude into vagina.

EFFECTIVENESS

- Approved for 10 years use; effective for at least 12 years

Typical use failure rate in first year: 0.8%
Perfect use failure rate in first year: 0.6% *(see Table 2.1, page 9) [Trussell 2018]*
Cumulative 12-year failure rate: 2.1 - 2.8%

MACHANISM OF ACTION:

The intrauterine copper contraceptive works primarily as a spermicide, preventing fertilization. Copper ions inhibit sperm motility and acrosomal enzyme activation so that sperm rarely reach the fallopian tube and are unable to fertilize the ovum. The sterile inflammatory reaction created in the endometrium phagocytizes the sperm. Experimental evidence suggests that the copper IUDs do not routinely work after fertilization. They are not abortifacients.

ADVANTAGES: Effective long-term contraception from a single decision
Menstrual: Menstrual cycles remain regular
Sexual / psychological

- Convenient; permits spontaneous sexual activities. Requires no action at time of use
- Intercourse may be more pleasurable with risk of pregnancy reduced

Cancers / tumors / masses

- Probable protection against endometrial cancer (6 of 7 case control studies) *[Hubacher 2002]* Possible protection against cervical cancer *[Grimes 2004]*

Other

- Highly effective
- Good option for women who cannot use hormonal methods
- Rapid return to fertility
- Private
- Convenient - single placement provides up to 12 years protection
- Cost-effective. Provides greatest net benefits of any contraceptive over a 5 year period.
- Risk for ectopic pregnancy decreased
- IUDs lead to highest levels of user satisfaction and continuation

DISADVANTAGES:

Menstrual

- Average monthly blood loss increased by up to 50%; this may be diminished by NSAIDs and may return to normal flow over time with continued use. *See Management of Bleeding, page 123*
- May increase dysmenorrhea (removal rates for bleeding and pain first year = 11.9%)
- Spotting and cramping with insertion and intermittently in weeks following insertion

Sexual / psychological

- Some women uncomfortable with concept of having "something" (foreign body) placed inside them
- Strings palpable; if strings cut too short, may cause partner discomfort

Cancers / tumors / masses: None

Other

- Increased risk of infection in first 20 days after insertion (approximately 1/1000 women will get PID)
- Offers no protection from HIV / STIs; PID
- May be expelled noticeably (with cramping and bleeding) or silently (unknowingly placing woman at risk for pregnancy). Rate of expulsion declines over time. At 5 years cumulative explusion rate (partial or complete) is 11.3%. Expulsion rate for the 5th year is 0.3%. Women who have expelled one IUD have about a one in three chance of expelling another IUD if inserted *[Grimes 2004]*
- Decreases risk of ectopic pregnancy by 70-80% vs. women not using contraception. But, if a woman gets pregnant with an IUD, rule out ectopic pregnancy. Of pregnancies in women using Paragard in FDA trials, one out of 16 pregnancies was ectopic *[WHO trial]*.

CANDIDATES FOR USE

- See CDC Medical Eligibility Criteria, *page 242*
- LARC are best for women seeking longer-term (> 1 year) method due to high initial cost
- Both parous and nulligravid women
- Good option for women who cannot or do not want to use hormones

Adolescents: appropriate candidates

- Counsel on menstrual cycle changes. Ask "Will a change in your menstrual bleeding pattern be acceptable to you?" This is particularly important for women considering LNG IUDs.

PRESCRIBING PRECAUTIONS: *See US MEC, page 242*

- Pregnancy
- Uterus < 5.5 cm or > 9 cm (package insert - some clinicians extend upper limit to 10-12 cm or greater especially if post abortion or delivery. Can insert less than 6 cm however may have higher risk of expulsion.)
- Undiagnosed abnormal vaginal bleeding
- Severe anemia (relative contraindication-levonorgestrel IUD would be a good choice)
- Active cervicitis or active pelvic infection or known symptomatic actinomycosis
- Women with current STI or PID
  - If current PID or purulent cervicitis or positive chlamydia or GC provide alternative contraception and delay IUD placement (U.S. MEC: 4). Assess if she is high risk for STIs, then risks may outweigh benefits (U.S. MEC: 3).
- Chorioamnionitis or endometritis
- Allergy to copper; Wilson's disease
- Known or suspected uterine or cervical CA - Insertion (U.S. MEC: 4), continuation (US MEC: 2)

INITIATING METHOD

- Requires placement by trained professional
- Any time in cycle when pregnancy can be ruled out; lowest overall rates of expulsion are when placement is at midcycle. No backup needed

- May be placed immediately after induced, or spontaneous abortion if no infection (increased risk of expulsion if > second trimester)
- May be placed immediately after delivery of the placenta or at any point post partum
  - Immediate (<10 minutes): U.S. MEC: 1
  - 10 min to <=4 weeks (increased risk of expulsion): U.S. MEC: 2
  - > 4 weeks post partum: U.S. MEC: 1
- May be inserted following second or third trimester loss (increased risk of expulsion)
- One IUD may be removed and a second placed at the same visit
- If indicated, test for vaginal or cervical infection, treat for symptomatic BV, yeast or trichomonas and place IUD the same day.

INSERTION TIPS: Each step should be performed slowly and gently

- Clinicians require training
- Signed consent form
- May give NSAIDs one hour prior to placement
- R/O pregnancy
- Routine antibiotic prophylaxis is not warranted; American Heart Association requires no antibiotic treatment for mitral valve prolapse, except for women at high risk for bacterial endocarditis
- Recheck position, size and mobility of uterus prior to placement
- Cleanse upper vaginal, outer cervix, and cervical os thoroughly with antiseptic
- Local anesthesia at tenaculum site: 3 approaches are 1) no anesthesia; 2) apply benzocaine 20% gel first at tenaculum site then leave a gel-soaked cotton-tipped applicator in cervical canal for 1 minute before proceeding with IUD placement; or 3) inject 1 ml of local anesthetic into the cervical lip where tenaculum will be placed
- Place tenaculum to stabilize cervix and straighten uterine axis.
- Most women will NOT need a cervical anesthetic. However, may use 10-20cc total dose of local anesthetic such as 1% lidocaine or 2% chloroprocaine inserted at the cervicovaginal junction (inject into cervix ~10mm deep) at 4 and 8 o'clock. Ensure injection is not vascular by having no return of blood prior to injection.
- Misoprostol (MIS) administered routinely prior to IUD placement does not diminish insertion pain or make placement easier. Patients may experience increased nausea and discomfort with misoprostol use.
- Sound uterus to fundus with uterine sound or pipelle.
- After placement, trim strings to about 2" (3 1/2 cm). Mark length of strings on chart for later follow-up visits to confirm that length is the same. Also chart lot number

Figure 21.1 How to insert a Copper IUD

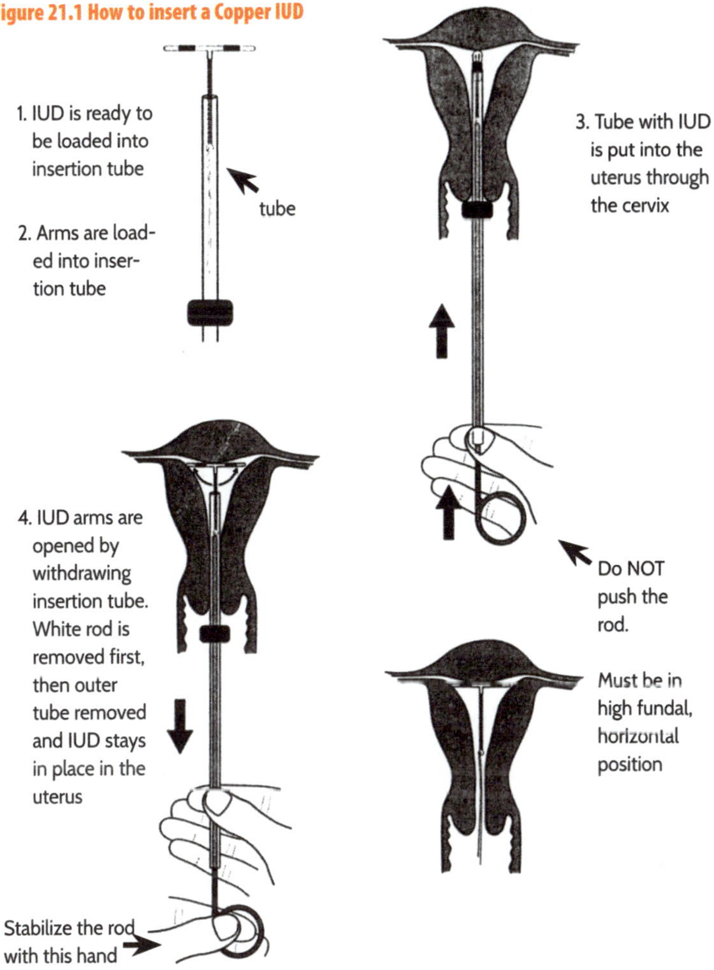

1. IUD is ready to be loaded into insertion tube

2. Arms are loaded into insertion tube

tube

3. Tube with IUD is put into the uterus through the cervix

Do NOT push the rod.

4. IUD arms are opened by withdrawing insertion tube. White rod is removed first, then outer tube removed and IUD stays in place in the uterus

Must be in high fundal, horizontal position

Stabilize the rod with this hand

POSTPLACENTAL & IMMEDIATE POSTPARTUM INSERTION

- Postplacental (within 10 minutes after expulsion of the placenta) is a convenient, effective and safe time to place TCu 380A IUDs, at either vaginal delivery and cesarean section.
- Easiest to do in women with an epidural in place
- Expulsion rates for post-placental placement are higher (7- 15% at 6 months). Advise how to detect expulsions and instruct to return for same or other method
- Postplacental IUD insertion results in a lower probability of pregnancy than delayed postpartum IUD insertion, *[Sonalker 2018]*

- The risk of infection is low with rates of 0.1% to 1.1% *[Lean 1967][Dharmeapanij 1970] [Snidvongs 1970][Cole 1984]*.
- Rates of perforation are very low during post-placental IUD placement, approximately 1 perforation in each study with patient populations ranging from 1150 to 3800 women *[Cole 1984][Edelman 1979][Phatak 1970]*
- Trim strings at level of cervix

Figure 21.2 Two techniques of postplacental IUD placement and proper location of IUD after placement

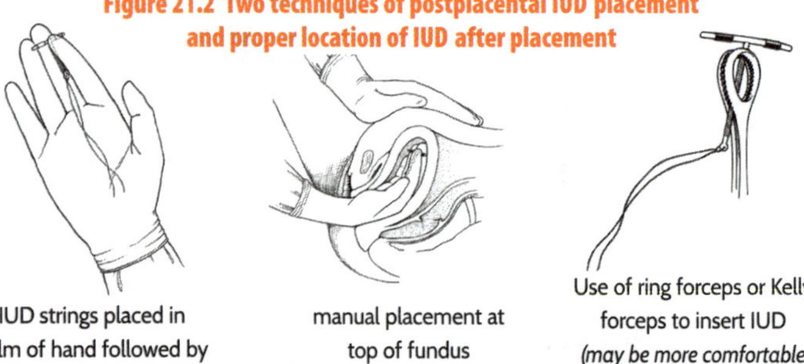

IUD strings placed in palm of hand followed by

manual placement at top of fundus

Use of ring forceps or Kelly forceps to insert IUD *(may be more comfortable for patients)*

INSTRUCTIONS FOR PATIENT

- Give patient trimmed IUD strings to learn what to check after menses each month (strings may not be apparent until a few months after post-placental placement)
- Advise patients to return if any symptoms of pregnancy, infection or expulsion

FOLLOW-UP:

- Offer condoms
- Offer to have patient return for post-insertion check about 2 months after insertion to rule out partial expulsion or other problems requiring removal. Return earlier if any problems. For those with increased risk factors for expulsion, encourage follow-up to ensure IUD is still in place.
- May be left in place during evaluation and treatment for cervical dysplasia
- Questions to assess for malposition of IUD: Can you feel your IUD strings? Have they changed in length?

PROBLEM MANAGEMENT FOR ALL IUDS

Complication	*Frequency*	*Risk factors*
PID within 20 days	1/1000	BV, cervicitis, contamination with insertion
Uterine perforation	1/1000	Immobile, markedly anteverted or retroverted uterus, breastfeeding, inexperienced, unskilled inserter
Vasovagal reaction or Fainting with insertion	Uncommon	Stenotic os, pain Prior vasovagal reaction
Expulsion	3-10%	Insertion on menses, immediately postpartum, not high enough in fundus or nulliparous, have menorrhagia
Pregnancy	LNG-52mg: 0.5% cumulative 7 yr rate TCu 380A: 2.5% cumulative 12 yr rate	Poor placement, expulsion

Uterine perforation: Perforations usually occur at insertion but may go unrecognized

- Clinical signs: pain, loss of resistance to advancement of instrument or instrument introduced deeper than uterus thought to be on bimanual exam
- Perforation by uterine sound usually occurs in midline posterior uterine wall when there is marked flexion (risk may be reduced with use of flexible plastic sound or endometrial biopsy pipelle):
  - Remove uterine sound
  - Observe for several hours. Administer antibiotics. If no bleeding seen, stable BP and pulse, patient pain-free and hematocrit stable, she may be sent home. Provide alternate contraception
  - If any persistent pain or signs of other organ damage, take or refer immediately for laparoscopic evaluation (rare)
- If IUD perforates acutely, attempt removal by gently pulling on strings
- If resistance encountered, stop and do pelvic ultrasound and/or send to surgery for laparoscopic IUD removal
- If IUD perforation noted and confirmed by ultrasound at later date, if asymptomatic, arrange for elective laparoscopic removal. Provide interval contraceptive. Can have IUD placed later (i.e. not a contraindication to future IUDs)

Spotting, frequent or heavy bleeding, hemorrhage, anemia:

- Rule out pregnancy. If pregnant, rule out ectopic pregnancy
- Rule out infection, especially if post-coital bleeding
- Rule out expulsion or partial expulsion of IUD (see below)
- May be managed with COCs for several cycles or by nonsteroidal anti- inflammatory agents (NSAIDS)
- If anemic, provide iron supplement and deal with cause
- Consider copper IUD removal and use of LNG IUD or use another method.

Cramping and/or pain:

- Rule out pregnancy, infection, IUD expulsion or partial expulsion

- Offer NSAIDs with menses or just before menses to reduce cramping
- Consider copper IUD removal and use of LNG IUD or use another method if problem.

Expulsion/partial expulsion:

- If expulsion confirmed (IUD seen by patient or clinician), rule out pregnancy. May place a new IUD
- If expulsion suspected, assess with ultrasound.
- If not seen on ultrasound, do abdominal x-ray to rule out extrauterine location
- If partial expulsion, remove IUD. If no infections and not pregnant, may replace with new IUD

Finding missing strings in non-pregnant patients:

- Check vagina for strings. Assess string length. If normal, reassure and re-instruct patient how to feel for strings
- Twist cytobrush inside cervix to snag strings which may be in canal
- Ultrasound to determine IUD presence and exact location
- If IUD in endocervix, remove and offer to replace
- If IUD correctly in uterus, IUD may be left in place or removed.
- If decision is made to remove IUD, attempt removal with IUD hook, Novak curette or alligator forceps. Use of concurrent ultrasound may be helpful . Paracervical block prior to removal attempt recommended as procedure may be painful. In non-pregnant patients who fail office removal, may also be done hysteroscopically.
- 200 mcg vaginal misoprostol the night before attempted removal may cause strings to exit cervix and facilitate removal *[Cowman 2012]*

Pregnancy with visible strings:

- Visible strings in first trimester: advise removal of IUD to reduce risk of spontaneous abortion and premature labor although counsel that removal may also precipitate these events
- Patient having miscarriage: Remove IUD. Consider antibiotics for 7 days

Missing strings in pregnant patients:

- Rule out ectopic pregnancy
- If intrauterine pregnancy, obtain ultrasound to verify IUD in situ
- If IUD is in uterus, advise patient she is at increased risk for preterm labor and spontaneous abortion but reassure her that fetus is not at increased risk for birth defects. If patient desires elective abortion, may remove IUD at procedure. Otherwise, plan for removal at delivery

Infection with IUD use:

- *BV or candidiasis:* treat routinely
- *Trichomoniasis:* treat and stress importance of condoms to prevent STIs
- *Cervicitis or PID:* IUD removal not necessary unless no improvement after antibiotic. If removal desired, give first dose of antibiotics to achieve adequate serum levels before removing IUD. *see page 108*
- *Actinomycosis:* Cultures among asymptomatic women without an IUD and among women with an IUD find that 3-4% of both are positive for Actinomyces *[Lippes 1999]*. Often suggested by Pap smear report of "Actinomycosis-like organisms". True upper tract infection with this organism is very serious and requires prolonged IV antibiotic

therapy with penicillin. However, less than half of women with such findings on Pap smears have actinomyces and those that do usually have asymptomatic colonization only. Examine patient for any signs of PID (it can be unilateral). If signs of upper tract involvement, such as pain or adrenal mass, remove IUD and treat with antibiotics (doxycycline) x 1 month.

REMOVAL

Indications: Patient request, expelling IUD, infection, pregnant, expired IUD, complications with IUD, anemia, no longer candidate for IUD.

Procedure: Grasp the strings close to external os and pull steadily

Complications

- ***Embedded IUD:*** Gentle rotation of strings may free IUD. If still stuck, may use alligator forceps with or without sonographic guidance *(see Missing Strings, page 98)*. Hysteroscopic removal may be indicated. A paracervical block reduces pain.
- ***Broken strings:*** Remove IUD with long Kelly forcep, alligator forceps, IUD hook or Novak curette

FERTILITY AFTER DISCONTINUATION OF METHOD

Immediate return to baseline fertility

IN CLINICAL TRAILS: VERACEPT

A new more flexible copper IUD with a copper surface area of 175 mm^2 is less rigid then the copper T 380-A.

This IUD is undergoing clinical trials in the United States. Its duration of effectiveness, or use for emergency contraception is not known.

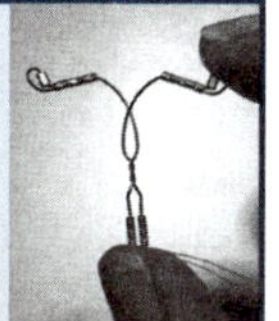

LEVONORGESTREL INTRAUTERINE SYSTEMS (MIRENA®, LILETTA®, SKYLA® AND KYLEENA)

Name	Mirena	Liletta	Kyleena	Skyla
Labeled approval	6 years	6 years	5 years	3 years
Hormone reservoir	52mg LNG	52mg LNG	19.5mg LNG	13.5mg LNG
Initial release rate	20mcg/day	18.6mcg/day	17.5mcg/day	14mcg/day
Release in later year	10mcg (5 years)		7.4mcg (5 years)	5mcg (5 yrs)
Inserter diameter	4.4mm	4.8mm		3.8mm
Length	32mm	32mm	32mm	30mm
Width of T arms	32mm	32mm	32mm	28mm
Other	Barium	Barium	Barium + silver ring on top of stem, visible by USG	Barium + silver ring on top of stem, visible by USG
First year efficacy, perfect (typical)	0.1% (0.2%)	0.1% (0.2%)	0.2%	0.4%
Cumulative efficacy	0.7% (5 yrs)	0.9% (4yrs)	0.9% (3 yrs)	1.0 (3 yrs)

DESCRIPTION: T-shaped intrauterine contraceptive with a reservoir of levonorgestel, slowly released over time.
IUDs as effective or more effective than female sterilization

MECHANISM OF ACTION:

- Levonorgestrel thickens cervical mucous preventing sperm from entry and fertilization.
- Changes in uterotubal fluid also impair sperm and ovum migration.
- Alteration (thinning) of the endometrium prevents implantation of fertilized ovum.
- The 52 mg levonorgestrel IUD has some anovulatory effect (5-15% of treatment cycles; higher in first years)

COST:

Mirena, Skyla and Kyleena:

- See *page 163* (Ordering and Stocking Device chapter). $0 if covered by Affordable Care Act.
- The Bayer Patient Assistance Foundation supplies Mirena, Skyla and Kyleena intrauterine contraceptives to providers caring for economically disadvantaged women whose insurance does not cover the device. They also provide funds for removal to qualifying individuals. Go to patientassistance.bayer.us/en/
- Units that are contaminated or must be removed in first 3 months or are expelled may be replaced free of cost. Contact Bayer: 1-866-647-3646 or 1-888-842-2937

Liletta:

- Liletta was developed as a lower-cost IUD option similar to the Mirena IUD.
- Commercial pricing approximately $650
- The company ensured that patients will pay no more than $75 of out-of-pocket costs for an IUD device and offers assistance through https://www.lilettacard.com/
- Clinics that qualify for 340b pricing can procure Liletta for approximately $50.

ADVANTAGES

Menstrual: Heavy menstrual bleeding, dysmenorrhea and endometriosis generally improves

- Menorrhagia improves: Mirena FDA-approved for treatment of heavy menstrual bleeding in women choosing IUD for contraception. At 12 months, 90% less blood loss

Sexual / psychological:

- Requires no action at time of intercourse
- Reduced fear of pregnancy can make sex more pleasurable

Cancers / tumors / masses:

- Protective against endometrial hyperplasia, endometrial cancer, fibroids
- 30% reduced risk cervical cancer in women using any type IUD
- Reduced rate of ovarian cancer with ever-use of an IUD (any type)

Other: Extremely effective

- May be used as the progestin for endometrial protection with menopausal estrogen treatment
- ***Decreased*** risk for ectopic pregnancy by 80% *[Anderson 1994]*
- Several studies show decreased PID, endometritis and cervicitis

- Reduces symptoms e.g. pain of endometriosis *[Petta 2005]*
- May be used by women at increased risk for DVT or PE and by women with Factor V Leiden and other thrombogenic mutations (U.S. MEC: 2)

DISADVANTAGES

- Menstrual changes expected (removal of Mirena for any bleeding problem in first year: 7.6%)
- Number of spotting and bleeding days is significantly higher for first few months and lower than normal after 3 to 6 months
- Amenorrhea in about 20% of Mirena / Liletta users at one year of use
- May cause cramping following insertion
- Expulsion: 2.9% in women using Mirena exclusively for contraception; 8.9% to 13.6% in women using Mirena to control heavy bleeding *[Diaz 2000] [Monteiro 2002]*

Sexual / psychological:

- Same as TCu 380A IUD except when spotting and bleeding may interfere with sexual activity
- Loss of menses means hard to keep track of menstrual cyclicity symptoms (e.g. PMS)

Other:

- Offers no protection against viral STIs like HPV or HIV
- Persistent unruptured follicles may cause ovarian cysts; most regress spontaneously
- Hormonal side effects: headaches, acne, mastalgia, moodiness including depression/ anxiety
- Brief discomfort after insertion or removal

COMPLICATIONS: *(See Problem Management page 97)*

- PID risk transiently increased after insertion (highest in first 20 days ~ 1 per 1000)
- Perforation of uterus at time of insertion approximately 1 in 1000

CANDIDATES FOR LNG IUD USE:

- Parous or nulligravid women
- Adolescents: Adolescents usually meet all the criteria for IUD use
- Indication by product label: While Mirena label says recommended for women who have had at least one child, Skyla doesn't mention this and the clinical trial enrolled 39% nulliparous women. In practice, Mirena is used by both nulligravid and nulliparous women.

Additionally:

- May be placed immediately postpartum
- Can be used in women with heavy menses, endometriosis, fibroids, cramps or anemia
- Menopausal women using estrogen, with intact uteri, who are unable to tolerate oral progestins are protected against endometrial carcinoma by using a levonorgestrel intrauterine contraceptive *[Raudaskoski 1995] [Luukkainen 2000]*
- For women wanting to avoid estrogen-containing methods

> ***CDC updated recommendations*** in the U.S. MEC in April 2020 to state that progestin-only injectable contraception, including DMPA, and intrauterine devices (including LNG-releasing and copper) are safe for use without restriction among woman at high risk for HIV infection. U.S. MEC:1

PRESCRIBING PRECAUTIONS: *(See CDC MEC, page 242)*

- May be used by woman with past history of ectopic pregnancy (U.S. MEC: 1)

INITIATING METHOD

- Counsel on menstrual changes including amenorrhea. Ask "Will a change in your menstrual bleeding pattern be acceptable to you?"
- Women using levonorgestrel IUC who received information in advance about possible bleeding changes were significantly more likely to be highly satisfied with the contraceptive. *[Backman 2002]*
- If inserted within 7 days from LMP, no backup needed. She can have it inserted any other time of cycle if reasonably certain not pregnant, but add backup or abstinence x 7 days
- Paracervical block may be helpful, especially for nulliparous women
- Advise NSAIDs for post-insertion discomfort.

INSTRUCTIONS FOR PATIENT: Similar to copper intrauterine contraceptive, *page 96*. Monthly string checks are particularly important for women using a levonorgestrol IUD for menorrhagia because of higher expulsion rates. *(see page 96)*

FOLLOW-UP: Same as TCu 380A IUD

PROBLEM MANAGEMENT: Similar to TCu 380A IUD; *see page 97*

- ***Perforation:*** A case report looked at serum LNG levels from Mirena in the omentum following uterine perforation. They were higher than POP serum levels. So, theoretically, an abdominal Mirena IUD still provides adequate contraceptive effect until it is removed. Removal of IUD still recommended.

PELVIC INFECTIONS: Same as Coppper T IUD. *see page 98*

FERTILITY AFTER discontinuation of method: Immediate return to baseline fertility

Figure 21.2

LILETTA® INSERTION TIPS:
Each step should be performed slowly and gently

This is a quick reference guide for the 1-hand inserter. For complete instructions, visit: https://www.allergan.com/assets/pdf/lilettashi_pi

Step 1 - Loading the Inserter

- Remove the inserter from the tray by gently twisting and pulling up the handle
- Ensure both sliders are pushed fully forward and aligned with their respective markings

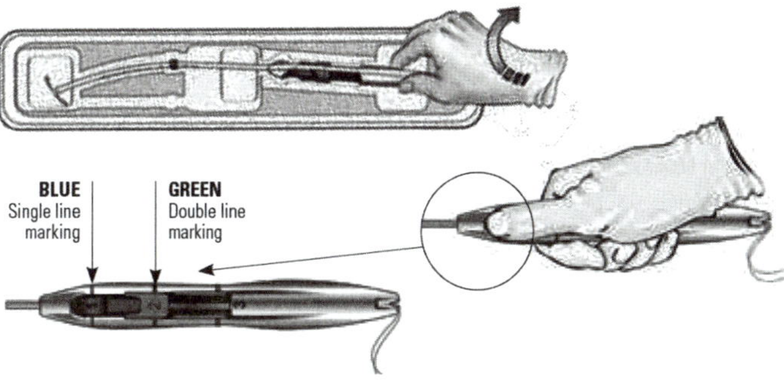

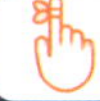 Use aseptic technique during the entire marking loading and insertion procedure.

- To load the IUS into the inserter, maintain forward pressure on the BLUE slider and gently pull the threads straight back
  - **Pull and lock** the threads into the cleft at the bottom of the handle and then stop holding the threads

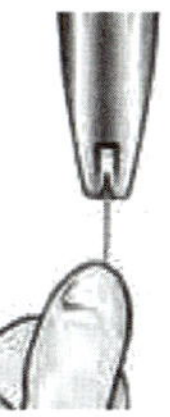
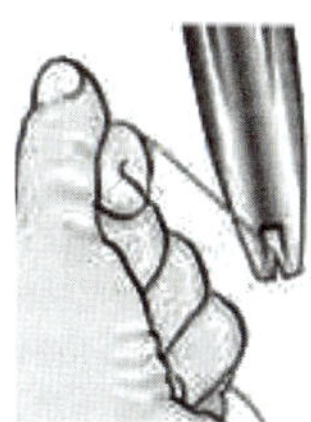

- When correctly loaded, the IUS is completely within the insertion tube, with the tips of the arms forming a hemispherical dome at the top of the tube

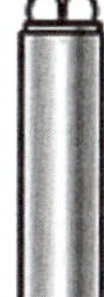

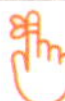 If the IUS is not correctly loaded or is discharged from the insertion tube unintentionally before insertion, DO NOT ATTEMPT INSERTION. You can repeat the loading process by pulling the threads out of the cleft and repeating the IUS loading process.

Figure 21.2 LILETTA INSTRUCTIONS -continued

Step 2 - Adjusting the Flange

- Adjust the flange to the measured uterine depth based on sounding. To adjust, place the flat side of the flange in the tray notch or against a sterile edge inside of the tray
- If required, bend or straighten the insertion tube to accommodate the anatomical orientation of the uterus
- Be careful to avoid sharp bends to prevent kinking

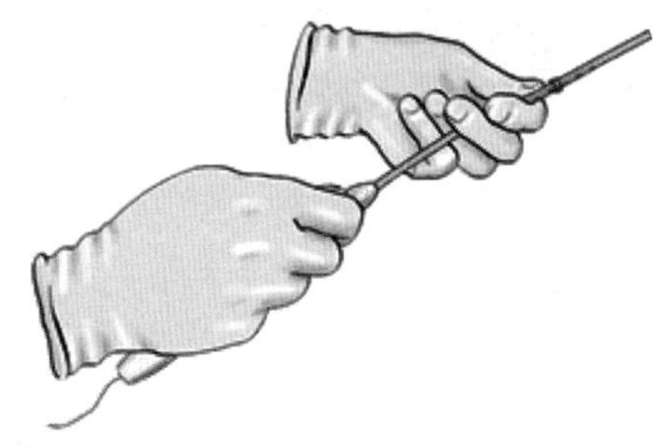

Step 3 - Inserting LILETTA into the Uterus

- Apply gentle traction on the tenaculum, as needed
- Insert the loaded tube through the cervical os
- Maintain forward pressure on the BLUE slider throughout the insertion process
- Advance until the upper edge of the flange is 1.5 to 2.0 cm from the external cervical os

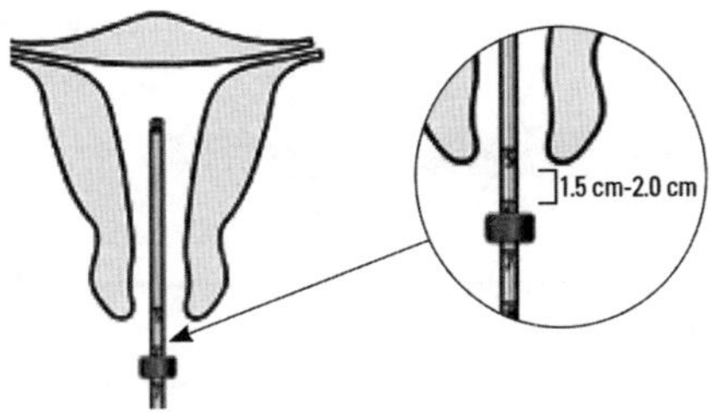

Step 4 - Releasing LILETTA in the Uterus

- Gently slide only the BLUE slider back until the BLUE and GREEN sliders form a common slider recess
- This will allow the IUS arms to open
- Wait 10 to 15 seconds to allow for the arms of the IUS to fully open

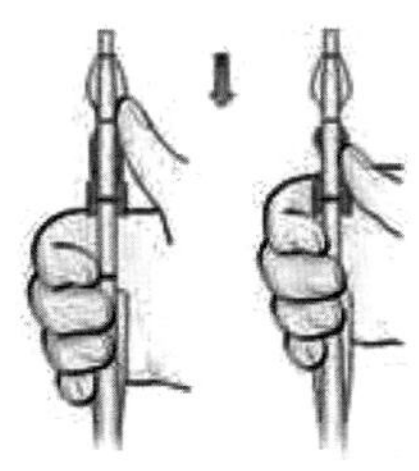

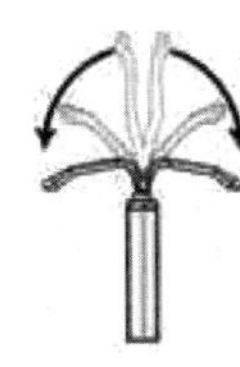

Figure 21.2 LILETTA INSTRUCTIONS -continued

Step 4 - Releasing LILETTA in the Uterus -continued

- Without moving the sliders, advance the inserter to the fundal position
  - The flange should now be at the level of the cervix

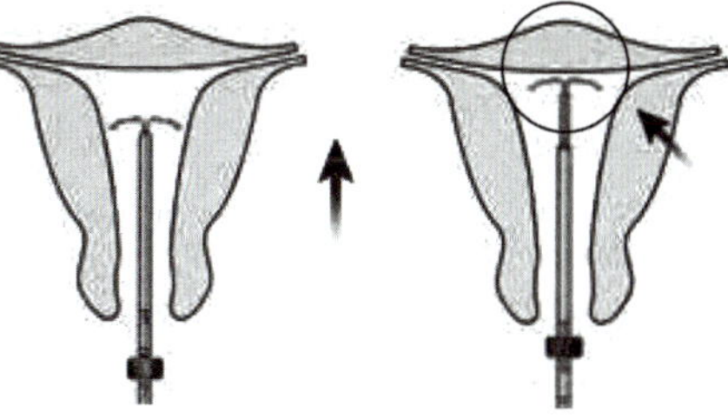

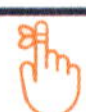

Fundal position is important to prevent expulsions.

Step 5 - Completing the Insertion

- Move both sliders down the handle until an **audible click is heard**

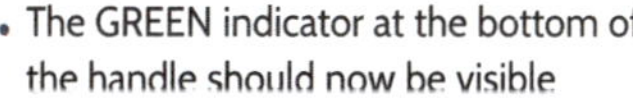

- The GREEN indicator at the bottom of the handle should now be visible
- Look at the cleft to ensure the threads were properly released; if not released, grab the threads and gently pull the threads out of the cleft
- Withdraw the inserter from the uterus

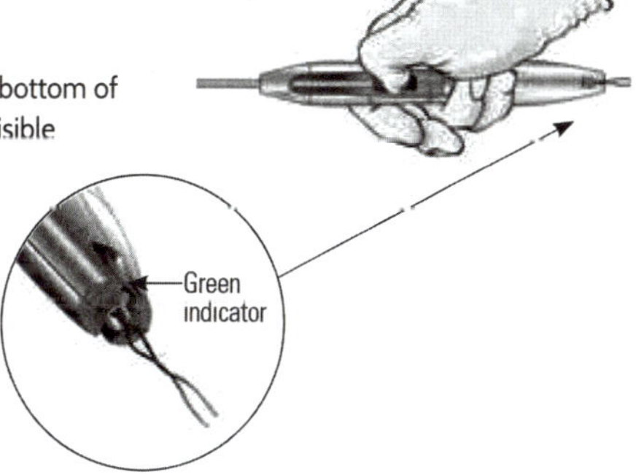

- Use blunt-tipped sharp scissors to cut the threads perpendicularly, leaving about 3.0 cm outside the cervix
- Insertion is now complete

Figure 21.3 - Insertion of Mirena, Skyla, Kyleena the same

MIRENA®, SKYLA, KYLEENA INSERTION TIPS:
Each step should be performed slowly and gently

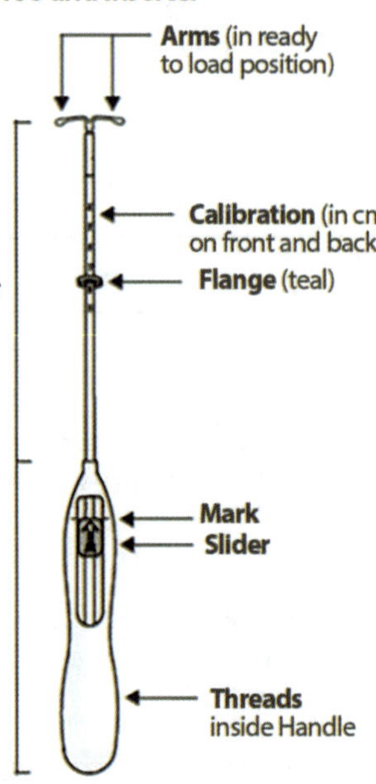

- Reconfirm signed consent
- May give NSAIDs one hour prior to insertion
- Be sure patient is not pregnant
- Routine antibiotic prophylaxis is not warranted; American Heart Association requires no antibiotic treatment for mitral valve prolapse, except for women at high risk for bacterial endocarditis
- Recheck position, size and mobility of uterus prior to insertion
- Cleanse upper vaginal, outer cervix, and cervical os and canal thoroughly with antiseptic
- Local anesthesia at tenaculum site: 3 approaches are 1) no anesthesia; 2) apply benzocaine 20% gel first at tenaculum site then leave a gel-soaked cotton-tipped applicator in cervical canal for 1 minute before proceeding with IUD insertion *[Speroff/Darney]*; 3) inject 1 ml of local anesthetic (1% chloroprocaine) into the cervical lip into which the tenaculum will be placed
- Most women will NOT need a paracervical block. However, can give 5 cc of local anesthetic at 3 and 9 o'clock
- Place tenaculum to stabilize cervix and straighten uterine axis.
- Sound uterus to fundus with uterine sound or pipelle; uterus should be at least 6 cm, but no strict limits.
- Push slider forward as far as possible retracting arms into tube
- Set flange to depth measured by sound
- Keep thumb on slider as you insert IUS into uterus
- Advance IUS until the flange is 1.5 - 2 cm from external os
- Pull back slider until it reaches mark while holding inserter steady. Wait 10 seconds to allow arms to open within uterus

Figure 21.3 IUS INSTRUCTIONS -continued

- Advance IUS until flange touches cervix allowing IUS to reach fundus
- Hold inserter in position while pulling slider down all the way.
- Withdraw IUS inserter from uterus
- Cut threads in a perpendicular position to 3 cm; requires care and sharp scissors to avoid dislodging IUS
- Hand patient cut strings so she knows what to feel for during string check

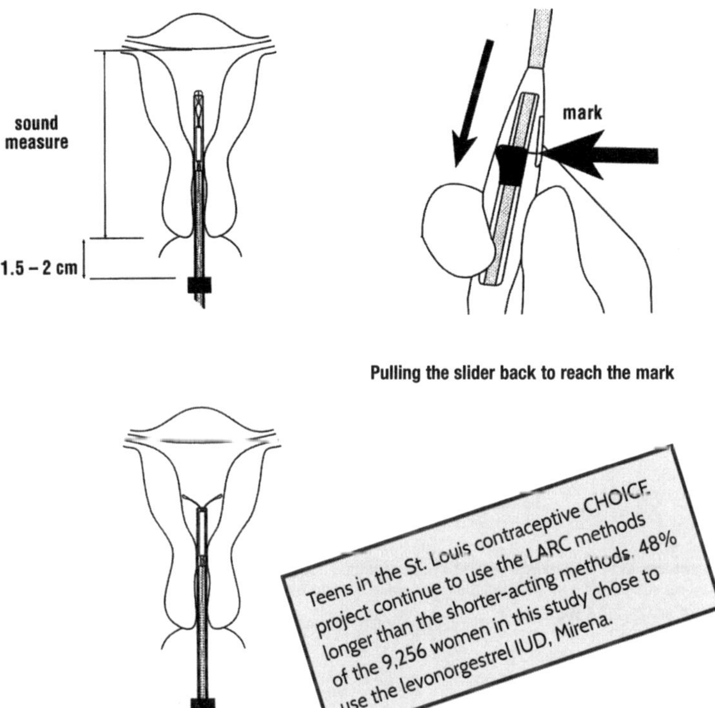

Pulling the slider back to reach the mark

The arms of the IUS being released

Figure 21.4

MANAGEMENT OF THE IUD WHEN USERS ARE FOUND TO HAVE PELVIC INFLAMATORY DISEASE
U.S. Selected Practice Recommendations (SPR 2016)

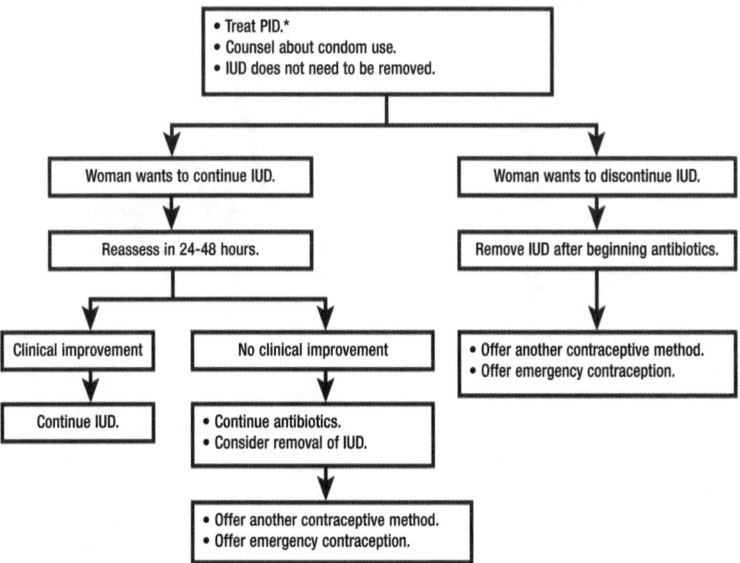

Abbreviations: IUD = intrauterine device; PID = pelvic inflamatory disease.

* Treat according to CDC's STI Treatment Guidelines (available at http://www.cdc.gov/std/treatment).

MMWR July 29, 2016, Vol. 65:No. 4

CHAPTER 22

COMBINED (ESTROGEN & PROGESTIN) CONTRACEPTIVES

DESCRIPTION

Combination hormonal contraceptives provide both an estrogen and a progestin:

- Combined birth control pills, patches *(page 128* and vaginal rings *(page 132)*

PILLS - DAILY COMBINED PILLS (COCs)

82% of women who have had sexual intercourse report using combined pills at some time in their lives. *[Daniels 2013]*

DESCRIPTION: Each hormonally active pill in combined pills contains an estrogen and a progestin.

- Ethinyl estradiol (EE) is the most commonly used estrogen
  - Other estrogens: estradiol valerate, and the newest estrogen formulation is estetrol (E4) introduced in 2021 found in the new COC called Nextstellis in combination with 3mg drospirenone (DRSP)
- Progestins include formulations of levonorgestrel (LNG), drospirenone, norethindrone, desogestrel, norgestrel, and ethinynodiol acetate.
- Traditional packs have 21 active combined pills, with or without 7 additional pills (usually placebo pills or pills with iron).
- Newer formulations have varying numbers of active pills and hormone-free pills.
- Monophasic formulations contain active pills with the same amount of hormones in each tablet.
- Multiphasic formulations contain active pills with varying amounts of progestin and / or estrogen in the hormonal pills.

EFFECTIVENESS

Perfect use failure rate in first year: 0.3% *(see Table 2.1, page 9)*

Typical use failure rate in first year: 7% *[Trussell 2018]*

Annual pregnancy rates with typical use of oral contraceptives pills are estimated to be 7% for the general population, 13% for teenagers and 30% or higher for some high-risk subgroups. *[Kost 2008] [Fu 1999]*

> ***Four ways to respond to the 5-10% typical use pill failure rate***
>
> ❶ take pills continuously (no hormone-free days), ❷ use a condom every time ❸ sign up for daily reminders at bedsider.org or use apps or alarms ❹ Give patients a full year supply of pills so refills less a problem

- Effectiveness depends on individual's success with adhering to schedule

Women were more than 20 times more likely to become pregnant in one year in the St. Louis CHOICE project if they use contraceptive pills rather than an IUD or implant. *[Winner 2007]* Teenagers in the CHOICE project were 40 times more likely to become pregnant if using pills, patches or rings than if using an IUD or implant.

MECHANISM OF ACTION

- Ovulation suppression (90% to 95% of time).
- Thickening of cervical mucus, which blocks sperm penetration and entry into the upper reproductive tract. Thin, asynchronous endometrium inhibits implantation. Tubal motility slowed.

ADVANTAGES

Menstrual:

- Menstrual regularity and predictability
- Decreased blood loss and decreased anemia
- Treatment for heavy menstrual bleeding (use of a 30mcg pill decreased HMB by 43%) *[Farquhar 2009]*.
- Decrease menstrual cramps / pain
- Eliminates ovulation pain (mittelschmerz)
- Can be used to manipulate timing and frequency of menses *(see Choice of COC, page 118 & page 122)*
- Provides progestin for women with anovulation / PCOS (reducing risk of endometrial cancer)
- Prevents and treats the pain of endometriosis *[Vercellini 2003]*.

Sexual / psychological:

- Decreased risk ovarian cancer (low and higher-dose formulations) *[Ness 2000]*.
  - Users for 5 years have 50% reduction in risk; users for 10 years have 80% reduction. Protection extends for 30 years beyond last pill use; significant reduction in risk also seen in some high risk women carrying BRCA mutations
- Decreased risk for endometrial cancer *[Grimes 2001]*
  - COC users for 1 year have 20% reduction in risk; users for 4 years have 60% reduction
  - Protection extends for 30 years beyond last pill use *[Ness 2000]*
  - Particularly important for PCOS women, obese women, and perimenopausal women
- Decreased risk of developing or dying from colorectal cancer *[Beral 1999]* The Nurses' Health Study reported a 40% reduced risk of a colorectal cancer if pills had been taken for the 8 previous years.
- Decreased risk of corpus luteum cysts and hemorrhagic corpus luteum cysts
- Breast masses: reduced risk of benign breast disease (including fibroadenomas)

ADVANTAGES OF COMBINED PILLS OVER PROGESTIN-ONLY PILLS:

- Regular withdrawal bleeding
- More dependable ovulation suppression
- Improvement in acne
- Documented reduced risk of both endometrial and ovarian cancer
- More forgiving regarding timing of ingestion of pill or missed pills

Other:

- Treatment for acne, hirsutism and other androgen excess / sensitivity states
- Reduces risk of ectopic pregnancy and risk of hospitalization with diagnosis of PID
- Reduced vasomotor symptoms and effective contraception in perimenopausal women
- Possible increased bone mineral density in perimenopausal women (not in adolescents

with hypothalamic amenorrhea). Pills with 35 mcg of estrogen used by women in their 40s have been associated with fewer postmenopausal hip fractures *[Michaelsson 1998] [Lancet 1996]*. However, low dose pills appear to not affect fracture risk. *[Vestergaard 2006]*

- Decreased pain and frequency of sickle cell disease crises

DO BIRTH CONTROL PILLS CAUSE BREAST CANCER?

- After scores of studies and 67 years, ***most experts believe that pills have minimal effect on women's risk of developing breast cancer.***
- The Women's Care Study of 4575 women with breast cancer and 4682 controls found no increased risk for breast cancer (RR: 1.0) among women currently using pills and a decreased risk of breast cancer (RR: 0.9) for those women who had previously used pills. Use of pills by women with a family history of breast cancer was not associated with an increased risk of breast cancer, nor was the initiation of pill use at a young age *[Marchbanks 2002]*
- Several studies have shown that current users of pills are slightly more likely to ***be diagnosed*** with breast cancer (Relative Risk: 1.2). *[Lancet 1996]*
- Two factors may explain the increased risk of breast cancer being diagnosed in women currently taking pills: 1) a ***detection bia***s (more breast exams and more mammography) or 2) ***promotion*** of an already present nidus of cancer cells
- Ten years after discontinuing pills, women who have taken pills are at no increased risk for having breast cancer diagnosed. *[Lancet 1996]*
- Breast cancers diagnosed in women currently on pills or women who have taken pills in the past are more likely to be localized (***less likely to be metastatic***). *[Lancet 1996]*
- By the age of 55, the risk of having had breast cancer diagnosed is the same for women who have used pills and those who have not
- The conclusion of the largest collaborative study of the risk for breast cancer is that women with a strong family Hx of breast cancer do not further increase their risk for breast cancer by taking pills. *[Lancet 1996]* This was also the conclusion of the Nurses Health Study *[Lipnick 1986] [Colditz 1996]* and the Cancer and Steroid Hormone (CASH) study. *[Murray 1989] [The Centers for Disease Control Cancer and Steroid Hormone Study 1983]*
- While there are still unanswered questions about pills and breast cancer. The very positive overall conclusion is that pills do not cause breast cancer. "***Many years after stopping oral contraceptive use, the main effect may be protection against metastatic disease.***" *[Speroff 2001] [Lancet 1996]*

DISADVANTAGES OF COMBINED PILLS

Menstrual:

- Spotting, particularly during first few cycles and with inconsistent use
- Scant or missed menses not clinically significant but can cause worry
- Post-pill amenorrhea (lasts up to 6 months). Uncommon and usually in women with history of irregular periods prior to taking pills

Sexual / psychological:

- Decreased libido and anorgasmia possible.
- Mood changes, depression, anxiety, irritability, fatigue may develop while on COCs, but no more frequent than with placebos. Rule out other causes before implicating COCs

- In a longitudinal survey of over 9000 women in Australia, OCP use was not associated with depressive symptoms *[Duke 2007]*
- Daily pill taking may be stressful (especially if privacy is an issue)

Cancers / tumors / masses:

- ***Breast cancer*** - *see boxed paragraphs on page 111*
- ***Cervical cancer:***
  - No increased risk of squamous cell carcinoma (85% of all cervical cancers) after controlling for confounding variables, such as number of sex partners, smoking and parity
  - Risk of adenocarcinoma, a relatively uncommon type of cervical cancer, is increased 60%, but no extra screening is required other than recommended Pap screening
- ***Hepatocellular adenoma:*** risk increased with > 50 µg formulations. Risk of hepatic carcinoma not increased, even in populations with high prevalence of hepatitis B

Other:

- No protection against STIs, including HIV
- Nausea or vomiting, especially in first few cycles
- Breast tenderness or pain
- Headaches
- Increased varicosities, chloasma, spider veins
- Average weight gain no different among COC users than in placebo users *(see note below)*
- See COMPLICATIONS section *page 112*
- The average woman misses 4.2 pills per cycle

Most women on antiretrovirals should use condoms since:

1. The meds may decrease the pill effectiveness if the antiretroviral induces cytochrome p450 metabolism *(U.S. MEC, page 242)*
2. GI side-effects from drugs may decrease OC effectiveness
3. It is important to avoid other infections that may facilitate HIV transmission
4. Condoms prevent the spread of HIV

COMPLICATIONS / PRECAUTIONS

- *Venous thromboembolism (VTE)*
  - The risk of VTE with COC use is less than with pregnancy:

No COC use	50/100,000 women per year
COC use	100/100,000 women per year
Pregnancy / Postpartum	200/100,000 women per year

- VTE risk is associated with the dose of estrogen; 50 µg estrogen pills is greater than 20-35 µg pills.
- The type of progestin may slightly influence VTE risk. The current labeling for desogestrel pills states that "several epidemiologic studies indicate that third-generation OCs, including those containing desogestrel, are associated with a higher risk of venous thromboembolism than certain second generations OCs. In general, these studies indicate an approximate 2-fold increased risk. However, data from additional studies have not shown this 2-fold increase in risk."

- It is not recommended to switch current users of desogestrel containing pills to other products
- A very large well-designed prospective study of the risk of VTE with drospirenone found no relative increase in risk with the use of DRSP compared with LNG pills *[Dinger 2007]*. But other large studies did find small increases in risk with DRSP vs. LNG pills *[Lidegaard 2009]*

- Blood dyscrasias such as Factor V Leiden mutation and Protein S or C abnormalities increase risk of VTE significantly. However, in the absence of strong family history screening is not necessary.
- There is no increased risk of MI or stroke for young women who are using low-dose COCs who do not smoke, do not have hypertension and do not have migraine headaches with neurological findings
- Women at risk of cardiovascular disease or stroke:
  - Smokers over 35 (MI rate of 396 per million COC users per year vs. 88 per million non-COC users per year)
  - Women with hypertension, diabetes, hyperlipidemia or obesity
  - Women with migraine with aura (only stroke risk increases)

ELEVATED BLOOD PRESSURE: A TEACHABLE MOMENT*

1. If you smoke, stop
2. Moderate exercise for 20-30 minutes each day
3. If overweight, lose weight. Reduce fat in your diet
4. Use salt in moderation
5. If you are on antihypertensive medications, take them regularly
6. Work on reducing stress in your life

* In addition to deciding if pills can be used *[see latest U.S. MEC; page 242]*

- ***Hypertension:*** 1% of users develop hypertension which usually normalizes within 1-3 months of discontinuing COCs.
- ***Neoplasia:*** COC users using early high dose pills are at higher risk of developing adenocarcinoma (rare) of the cervix and hepatic adenomas (rare).
- ***Cholelithiasis / cholecystitis:*** higher dose formulations were associated with increased risk of symptomatic gallbladder disease
  - Sub-50 mcg formulations may be neutral or have a slightly increased risk
  - Use COCs with caution in women with known gallstones. Asymptomatic (US MEC: 2), treated by cholecystectomy (US MEC: 2), symptomatic and being treated medically (US MEC: 3)
- ***Visual changes:*** Rare cases of retinal thrombosis (must stop pills). Contact lens users may have dry eyes, and may need eye drops or to switch methods

CANDIDATES FOR USE

- Most healthy reproductive aged women are candidates for COCs
- In addition to medical precautions, real world considerations such as the need for privacy, affordable access to COCs, and the requirement for daily administration should be considered

Adolescents

- Excellent candidates for contraceptive benefits if patient is able to take a pill each day.
- Many non-contraceptive effects are particularly important for adolescents.
- Failure rates are higher in teens using COCs (13% in one study).
- Encourage teens to use condoms consistently and correctly
- Be sure she has a package of Plan B One-Step or ella at home

SPECIAL CONSIDERATIONS FOR USE

- Women with medical conditions that improve with COCs: dysmenorrhea, endometriosis, menstrual migraine without aura, iron deficiency anemia, acne, hirsutism, polycystic ovarian syndrome (PCOS), ovarian or endometrial cancer risk factors, eating disorders or activity patterns that decrease menses. Consider continuous or extended COC use with a monophasic pill. *See page 116*
- Women whose reproductive health would be improved by ovulation suppression or decreased menstrual blood. Women with chronic amenorrhea (unopposed estrogen), menorrhagia or dysmenorrhea and some anticoagulated women (COCs decrease risk of internal hemorrhage with ovulation and menorrhagia)
- Women whose quality of life would be improved by reducing frequency of or eliminating menses with extended cycles or continuous COC use. *See page 116*
- Women who have difficulty swallowing pills may benefit from the **chewable** formulation *(see page 196 for chewables)*. OCs may potentially be placed in the vagina for systemic absorption, but large studies are lacking.
- Rifampin, certain anticonvulsants, certain antivirals used for HIV therapy and lamotrigine lowers the effectiveness of combined pills (U.S. MEC: 3). St. John's Wort is an over-the-counter herbal product that may decrease pill effectiveness *[Berry 2016]*

PRESCRIBING PRECAUTIONS

See latest U.S. MEC pages page 242 to Page 245

Absolute contraindications, U.S. MEC: 4

- Postpartum <21 days
- Migraine with aura any age
- Cigarette smoking ≥ 15 per day in women ≥ 35 y/o
- Multiple risk factors for CVD (older age, smoking, hyperlipidemia, DM, HTN)
- Uncontrolled HTN with either systolic BP > 160 or diastolic BP > 100
- Personal h/o DVT or PE with high risk of recurrence
  - Estrogen associated, pregnancy associated, or idiopathic DVT
  - Major surgery with prolonged hospitalization
  - H/o recurrent DVT / PE
  - Known thrombophlia including antiphospholipid syndrome or mutations (Factor V Leiden, protein S, protein C, prothrombin and antithrombin deficiency)

> **NOTE: Family history of DVT in first-degree relative, U.S. MEC: 2**

- Complicated valvular heart disease
- Ischemic heart disease

- Peripartum cardiomyopathy < 6 months
  - < 6 months everyone
  - > 6 months if residual impairment moderate or severe
- Systemic lupus erythematosis with positive or unknown antiphospholipid antibodies
- Viral hepatitis, acute or flare
- Hepatocellular adenoma or malignant hepatoma or severe cirrhosis
- Complicated solid organ transplantation
- Known or suspected vascular disease
  - H/o CVA
  - DM with vascular dz (including retinopathy or nephropathy)
  - DM > 20 year duration

Risks generally outweigh benefits, MEC: 3

- Breastfeeding 21 to <30 days postpartum (with or without other risk factors for VTE)
- Breastfeeding 30 to 42 days postpartum if have other risk factors for VTE
- Postpartum (and not breastfeeding) 21 to 42 days postpartum if have other risk factors for VTE
- Cigarette smoking < 15 cigarettes/day in women ≥ 35 y/o
- Bariatric malabsorptive procedure
- HTN, adequately controlled or mildly elevated
- Either of: systolic BP 140-150 or diastolic BP 90-99
- Personal h/o DVT / PE with low risk of recurrence (no risk factors)
- Peripartum cardiomyopathy ≥ 6 months with normal or mildly impaired cardiac function
- Breast cancer Hx with no disease for 5 yrs
- Inflammatory bowel disease with increased risk of VTE
- COC-related cholestasis or current symptomatic gall bladder
- Certain antiretrovirals, anticonvulsants

EXTENDED USE OF PILLS MAY MEAN:

A. Manipulation of a cycle to delay one period for a trip, honeymoon, or athletic event
B. Use of active hormonal pills (for more than 21 consecutive days) followed by 2-7 hormone-free days.
C. Continuous daily COCs for at least 21 pills, but after that, may break for 2-7 days when spotting or breakthrough occurs
D. Use of a monophasic pill indefinitely. Break-through bleeding (BTB) can occur at any time with this regimen. Eventually a woman develops an atrophic endometrium and BTB decreases.

CYCLIC SYMPTOMS THAT MAY IMPROVE FROM THE EXTENDED USE OF PILLS:

- Dysmenorrhea
- Symptoms of endometriosis *[Havada 2007]* even when unresponsive to cyclic regimen *[Vercellini 2003]*
- Irritability or depression. Decreased libido
- Headaches including menstrual migraine *[Sulak 2000] [Kwiecien 2003]*
- Nausea, dizziness, vomiting or diarrhea
- Cyclic yeast or other infections or cyclic nosebleeds
- Seizures, arthritis, or recurrences of asthma at the time of menses
- Cyclic symptoms associated with polycycstic ovarian syndrome

Symptoms usually occurring at midcycle:

- Spotting due to sudden fall in estradiol
- Sharp or dull pain associated with ovulation

Symptoms usually occurring just prior to menses (PMS):

- Slight to more dramatic weight gain, bloating, swollen eyes or ankles
- Breast fullness or tenderness
- Anxiety, irritability or depression, nausea or headaches
- Acne, spotting, discharge, breast fullness or tenderness
- Pain, cramping or constipation

ADVANTAGES & DISADVANTAGES OF TAKING COCS CONTINUOUSLY:

Advantages:

- May be more effective as a contraceptive
- May be easier to remember to do the same thing every day
- Less frequent menstruation *[Sulak 2000] [Glasier 2003]* and less blood loss
- Decreased expenses from tampons, pads, pain meds, and days of work missed

Disadvantages:

- More expensive and the extra packs of pills required may not be covered by insurance
- Unscheduled spotting or bleeding and the absence of regular menses
- Clinician must explain the difference: amenorrhea, while taking a progestin every day, is not harmful *[Miller 2003]* versus amenorrhea when on no hormonal contraceptive, which is a risk for endometrial hyperplasia or cancer.

INITIATING METHOD

- In asymptomatic women, **a pelvic examination is NOT necessary to start pills**
- ***Counseling is critical in helping women successfully use the pill***
- ***Timing of initiation*** *(see Table 22.1, page 120)*
  - First day of next menstrual period start **OR**
  - "**QuickStart**" (starting the day of the counseling clinic visit) when reasonably certain not pregnant, *(see page 12)*. Provide 7-day backup. Bleeding is not increased in "QuickStarters" **OR**
  - Sunday start, recommend back-up method x 7 days. Sunday start can result in no periods on weekends
- ***Choice of pill***
  - The pill that will work best for the woman is the one that she will take regularly
  - For special situations, some formulations offer advantages over others *(see Choosing cocs for women in special situations, page 118)*
  - In general, use the lowest dose of hormones that will provide pregnancy protection, deliver the non-contraceptive benefits that are important to the woman, and minimize her side effects
  - Monophasic formulations are preferable if women interested in extended cycles
  - Triphasic formulations are preferred by some clinicians to reduce some side effects (such as premenstrual breakthrough bleeding) when it is not desirable to increase hormone levels throughout the entire cycle or when it is desirable to reduce total cycle progestin levels (e.g. acne treatment).
- ***Choice of pattern of COC use***
  - 28-day cycling: Most common use pattern. Women have monthly withdrawal bleeding during placebo pills
  - *"First-day start" each cycle:* Women can start each new pack of pills on first day of menses each cycle
  - *"Bicycling" or "tricycling":* Women skip placebo pills for either 1 or 2 packs and then use the placebo pills and have withdrawal bleeding after 6 weeks (end of 2nd pack) or after 9 weeks (end of 3rd pack). Use monophasic pills
  - You may prescribe 4 packs of low dose monophasic pills omitting the placebo pills or use Seasonale, Seasonique, LoSeasonique, Jolessa, Lybrel or other pre-packaged extended cycle pills
  - *"Continuous use":* Women take only active pills and have no withdrawal bleeding. Often women must transition through bicycling or tricycling to achieve amenorrhea. Need to counsel regarding BTB and spotting
  - Studies of extended cycles have found no increased risk of endometrial hyperplasia *[Johnson 2007]*

Note: the last three options may be particularly good for:

- Women with menstrually-related problems (menorrhagia, anemia, dysmenorrhea, menstrual mood changes, menstrual irregularity, endometriosis, menstrual migraine, PMS, PMDD)
- Women on medications that reduce COC effectiveness (e.g. anticonvulsants, St. John's Wort). *See page 118*
- Women who have conceived while on COCs or who forget to take them regularly

- Women who are ambulatory but disabled and for whom menstrual bleeding may be particularly problematic
- Women who want to control their cycles for convenience
- Provide or recommend EC for when / if needed

CHOOSING COCS FOR WOMEN IN SPECIAL SITUATIONS

- *Endometriosis:* Pills taken continuously to reduce symptoms.
- *Functional ovarian cysts:* higher dose monophasic COCs may be slightly more effective. Extended or continuous use of pills may also be more effective
- *Androgen excess states:* all COCs are helpful but pills with higher estrogen / progestin ratios are preferable to reduce free testosterone and inhibit 5 alpha-reductase activity.
- *Breastfeeding women:* progestin-only methods preferable to COCs. U.S. MEC gives COC in breastfeeding a category 2 after 42 days postpartum.
- *Hypercholesterolemia:*
  - Possible negative impact on lipids but not clinically significant
  - Screening for lipids not necessary prior to prescribing COCs
  - Elevated triglycerides: Some clinicians recommend not prescribing COCs if triglycerides > 350 mg/dL because COCs increase triglycerides by approximately 30% and the risk of pancreatitis is increased (norgestimate may increase triglycerides less)
  - DSG slightly more favorable to lipids than LNG
- *Hepatic enzyme-inducing agents (e.g. anticonvulsants except valproic acid) and St. John's Wort.* Although not harmful *may reduce effectiveness of CHC, U.S. MEC: 3:* Options:
  - Encourage use of another method
  - When a COC is chosen, a formulation with a minimum of 30mcg EE should be used. Consider extended cycles.
- *Antibiotic use:*
  - U.S MEC: 1 for women on broad spectrum antibiotics
  - Rifampin U.S. MEC: 3
- *Obese patients:* Current data do not suggest different prescribing for markedly overweight women if weight is the only risk factor for heart disease. But obesity may contribute to the U.S. MEC condition "Multiple risk factors for atherosclerotic cardiovascular disease (ASCVD)". Which can mean a 3 or a 4 for the use of combined hormonal contraceptives. *(see page 242)*

BEWARE if a woman is a heavy smoker, is morbidly obese, a prediabetic and has very high blood pressure. Even if she is young, she has multiple risk factors for CVD and most clinicians would say she has a "4", meaning that combined pills would be an unacceptable health risk and should not to be used.

INSTRUCTIONS FOR PATIENT: Periodic "breaks" from pills are NOT recommended.

- Clear instructions on pill initiation, preferably written and in her primary language. If reasonably certain that she is not pregnant, use QuickStart. Have her take the first hormonally active pill immediately and use all pills. This may delay onset of next period. This will not increase the number of days of menstrual bleeding nor the number of days of spotting.

- Help her plan where to store pills, how to remember to take them and where to refill
- Explanation about possible side effects (spotting, breast tenderness, headaches, etc.) and encouragement to call or return should any become troublesome. Also highlight noncontraceptive benefits
- Warning about serious complications
- There is no clinical data that suggests generic OCs are less effective than branded OCs. Use the pill that is easiest to obtain
- Backup method: ensure patient has and knows how to use method if she needs to use one for interim protection, back-up, or as an alternate method.
- No routine follow up visit is necessary, unless a woman has multiple medical issues OR for enhanced attention OR for an adolescent
- Encourage to return with any concerns
- Each woman on birth control pills needs a package of Plan B at home
- Periodic breaks from birth control pills for several weeks to several months do NOT make pills safer. Breaks have the opposite effect because the highest risk for serious pill complications, blood clots and pulmonary emboli are in the first few weeks after starting or restarting pills.

PROBLEM MANAGEMENT

***Nausea / vomiting:* Rule out pregnancy, reassure that nausea usually improves** *(see Fig 22.6 on page 127)*

- Prescribe lower estrogen formulation
- Suggest taking pills at night (evening meal or bedtime) to sleep through higher serum levels of hormones. Suggest taking pills with morning meal if experiencing bothersome nausea during the night
- If patient vomits within one hour of taking pill, suggest antiemetic prior to taking replacement pill. Use backup method for 7 days
- Consider change to a non-estrogen containing method
- Rare abdominal pain problems possibly related to COCs: thrombosis of major intra-abdominal vessels, gallstones, pancreatitis, liver adenoma, Crohn's disease or porphyria

Spotting and / or breakthrough bleeding:

- *Women taking pills in the traditional 21/7 manner* *(See Fig. 22.2, page 123)*
  - Do not double-up on pills
- *Women taking pills for an extended period of time:*
  - Take first 21 pills every single day whether or not spotting occurs
  - Thereafter, one approach to spotting is to stop active hormonal pills on first day of spotting (after having taken pills for at least 21 days) for 2 or 3 days. Then restart pills. With any pill taken continuously, the number of days with BTB will decrease over time

Missed one pill: Instruct patient to take missed pill ASAP and take next pill as usual

Missed two or more pills:

- The most recent missed pill should be taken ASAP
- The remaining pills should be continued at usual time
- Backup for 7 days

- Consider emergency contraception (pills or IUD), may resume pills after she finishes ECPs

Missed withdrawal bleed on COCs (not on extended or continuous cycles):

- Offer pregnancy test, especially if she missed any pills in last cycle or if she has any symptoms of pregnancy
- Offer emergency contraception if any intercourse in last 5 days
- Advise patient that there are no adverse impacts of amenorrhea from COCs
- If patient prefers monthly withdrawal bleeding, consider switching to formulation with higher estrogen or lower progestin
- Otherwise, have her continue her COCs on usual schedule

New onset or significant worsening of headaches on COCs: *(see Figure 22.3, page 124)*

Hot flashes on placebo-pill week:

- Suggest starting new pill pack on first day of withdrawal bleeding or eliminate pill-free interval OR
- Offer low-dose of transdermal or oral estrogen during placebo-pill week (Mircette provides 5 days of estrogen during 4th week)
- Offer Seasonique, a formulation with 84 days of active pills, followed by 7 days of pills with 10 mcg EE or Lybrel, a formulation where all pills have hormone

If patient > 50 years old, consider checking FSH level at least 2+ weeks off the pill

MAKING THE TRANSITION FROM COCS TO HRT: *(see figure 22.4, page 125)*

FERTILITY AFTER DISCONTINUATION OF METHOD

- Immediate return of fertility: Average delay in ovulation 1-2 weeks. Post-pill amenorrhea more common in women with a past history of oligomenorrhea
  - Initiate another method immediately after discontinuing COCs unless desire pregnancy
  - Pattern of menses prior to starting pills (frequency, duration, flow, dysmenorrhea) tends to return

Pills May Help A Women become Pregnant

Taking pills for many years may actually protect a woman from some of the causes of infertility such as endometriosis, uterine fibroids, PCOS and ovarian cancer

Table 22.1 Starting Combined Oral Contraceptives*

CONDITION BEFORE STARTING	WHEN TO START COCS?
Starting (restarting) COCs in menstruating women	• Immediately, if pregnancy excluded start with first pill in package; backup needed x 7 days *(See page 118)* • First day of next menses • If within 5 days after start of her menstrual bleeding, no backup required.** • First Sunday after next menses begins ** Backup needed x 7 days
Starting (restarting) in amenorrheic women	Anytime if it is reasonably certain that she is not pregnant; abstain from sex or use backup method for the next 7 days
Postpartum and breastfeeding	• CDC Medical Eligibility Criteria *(see page 242)* ◆ <21 days: U.S. MEC:4 ◆ 21-<30 days: U.S. MEC: 3 ◆ 30-42 days: U.S. MEC: 3 (if has other risk factors for VTE) ◆ 30-42 days: U.S. MEC: 2 (no other risk factors for VTE) ◆ >42 days: U.S. MEC: 2
Postpartum and not breastfeeding	• CDC Medical Eligibility Criteria *(see page 242)* ◆ <21 days: U.S. MEC:4 ◆ 21-42 days: U.S. MEC: 3 (if other risk factors for VTE); U.S. MEC: 2 (no other risk factors for VTE) ◆ >42 days: U.S. MEC:1
After 1st or 2nd trimester (< 24 weeks) pregnancy loss or termination	• Start the same day (U.S. MEC: 1 *see page 242*)*** No backup contraception needed
Switching from another hormonal method	• Start COCs immediately if she has been using hormonal method correctly and consistently, or if it is reasonably certain she is not pregnant. No need to wait until next period. No additional contraceptive needed. If > 5 days from LMP, back-up for 7 days. • If previous method was an injectable, start COCs at the time repeat injection would have been given
Switching from a non-hormonal method (other than IUD)	• Can start immediately or at any other time if it is reasonably certain that she is not pregnant. Use backup method for the next 7 days unless it is the first day of menses*
Switching from an IUD (including hormonal)	• Start pills within 5 days of start of mentrual bleeding, no additional contraceptive needed & IUD can be removed at that time • Start pills at any other time if it is reasonably certain she is not pregnant. If sexually active in this menstrual cycle and more than 5 days since menstrual bleeding started, start coc and remove IUD at time of next menstrual period OR give EC, then start COCs immediately; backup x 7 days

* Selected Practice Recommendations for Contraceptive Use. 2016

** Back-up method needed for 7 days after starting COCs if it has been more than 5 days since menstrual bleeding started

*** See summary of U.S. Medical Eligibility Criteria on page 242 to page 246)

Figure 22.1

CHOOSING A PILL

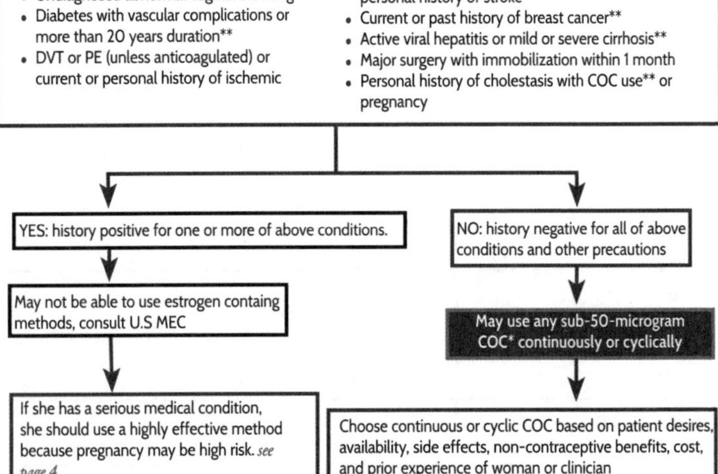

- The World Health Organization and the Food and Drug Administration both recommend using the lowest dose pill that is effective. All combined pills with less than 50 µg of estrogen are considered "low-dose" and are effective and safe.
- There are no studies demonstrating a decreased risk for deep vein thrombosis (DVT) in women on 20-µg pills. Data on higher dose pills have demonstrated that the lower the estrogen dose, the lower the risk for DVT
- All COCs lower free testosterone. Class labeling in Canada for all combined pills states that use of pills may improve acne
- To minimize discontinuation due to spotting and breakthrough bleeding, counsel women in advance, reassure that spotting and breakthrough bleeding become better over time. *(See Figure 22.2, page 123)*

*The package insert for women on Yasmin and Yaz states *[Berlex 2001]*: "Yasmin is different from other birth control pills because it contains the progestin drospirenone. Drospirenone may increase potassium. Therefore, you should not take Yasmin if you have kidney, liver or adrenal disease, because this could cause serious heart and health problems. Other drugs may also increase potassium. If you are currently on daily, long-term treatment for a chronic condition with any of the medications below, you should consult your healthcare provider about whether Yasmin is right for you, and during the first month that you take Yasmin, you should have a blood test to check your potassium level: NSAIDs (ibuprofen [Motrin®, Advil®], naproxen [Naprosyn®, Aleve®, and others] when taken long-term and daily for treatment of arthritis or other problems]; potassium-sparing diuretics (spironolactone and others); potassium supplementation; ACE inhibitors (Capoten®, Vasotec®, Zestril® and others); Angiotensin-II receptor antagonists (Cozaar®, Diovan®, Avapro® and others); heparin"

**These are conditions that receive a US MEC:3 or a US MEC: 4 *(See page 242)*

Figure 22.2

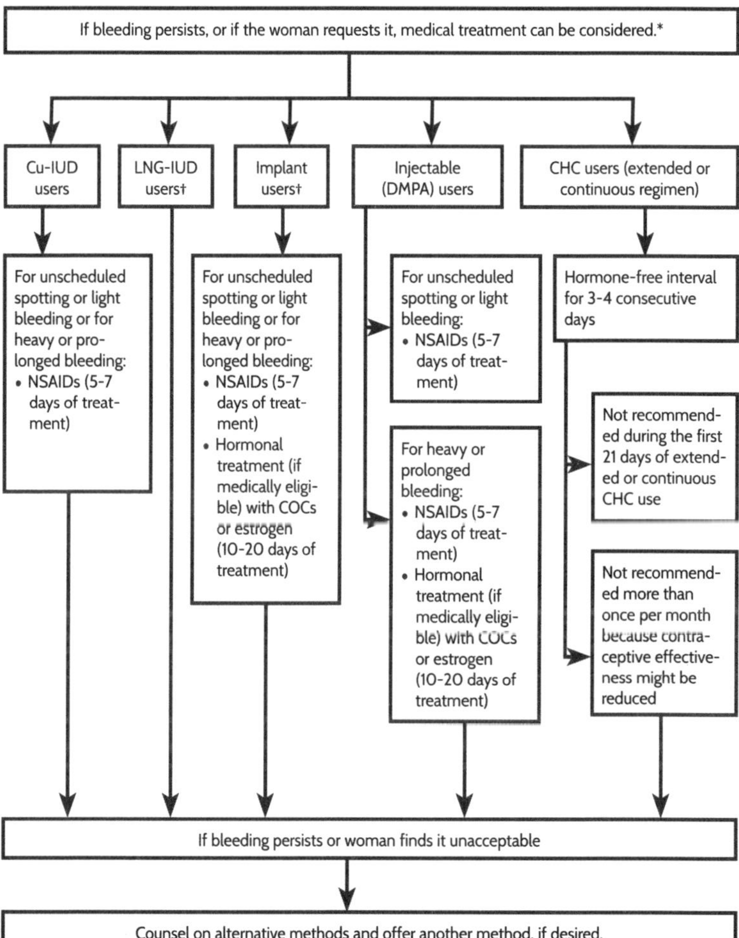

Abbreviations: CHC = combined hormonal contraceptive; COC = combined oral contraceptive; Cu-IUD = copper-containing intrauterine device; DMPA = depot medroxyprogesterone acetate; LNG-IUD= levonorgestrel-releasing intrauterine device; NSAIDs =nonsteroidal antiinflammatory drugs.

* If clinically warranted, evaluate for underlying condition. Treat the condition or refer for care.

† Heavy or prolonged bleeding, either unscheduled or menstrual, is uncommon.

CDC MMWR June 29, 2016, Vol. 65:No. 4

Figure 22.3

NEW ONSET OR WORSENING HEADACHES IN COC USERS

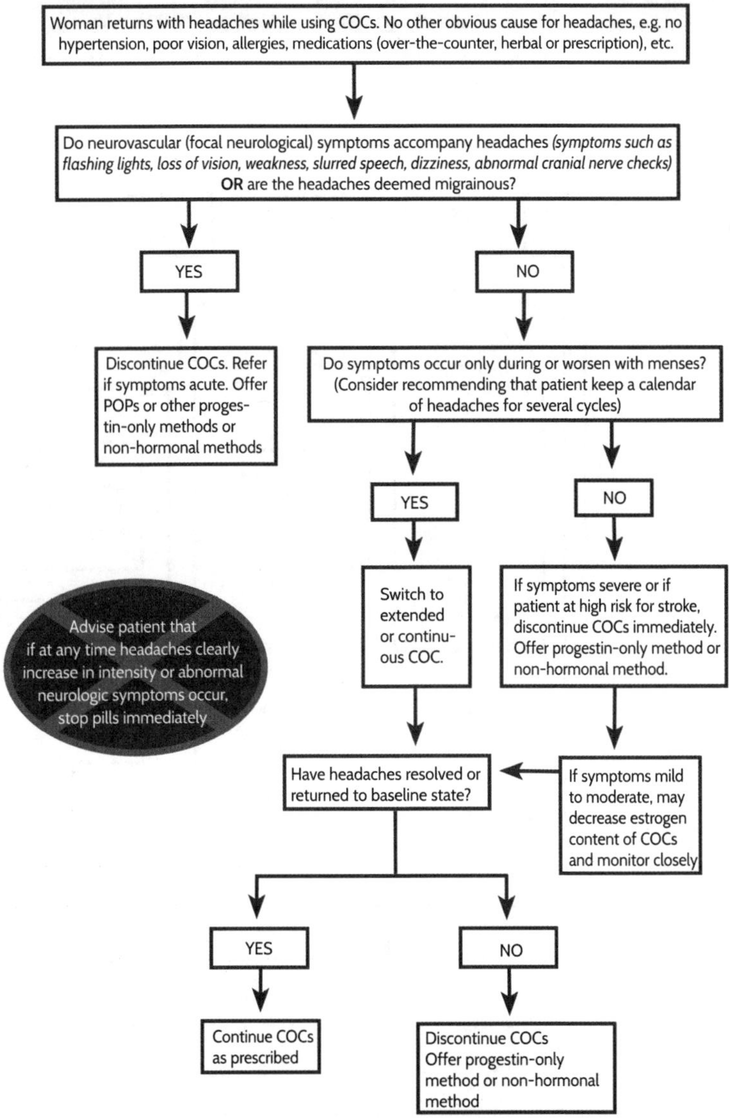

Woman returns with headaches while using COCs. No other obvious cause for headaches, e.g. no hypertension, poor vision, allergies, medications (over-the-counter, herbal or prescription), etc.

↓

Do neurovascular (focal neurological) symptoms accompany headaches *(symptoms such as flashing lights, loss of vision, weakness, slurred speech, dizziness, abnormal cranial nerve checks)* **OR** are the headaches deemed migrainous?

- **YES** → Discontinue COCs. Refer if symptoms acute. Offer POPs or other progestin-only methods or non-hormonal methods
- **NO** → Do symptoms occur only during or worsen with menses? (Consider recommending that patient keep a calendar of headaches for several cycles)
  - **YES** → Switch to extended or continuous COC. → Have headaches resolved or returned to baseline state?
  - **NO** → If symptoms severe or if patient at high risk for stroke, discontinue COCs immediately. Offer progestin-only method or non-hormonal method. → If symptoms mild to moderate, may decrease estrogen content of COCs and monitor closely → Have headaches resolved or returned to baseline state?

Have headaches resolved or returned to baseline state?

- **YES** → Continue COCs as prescribed
- **NO** → Discontinue COCs Offer progestin-only method or non-hormonal method

Advise patient that if at any time headaches clearly increase in intensity or abnormal neurologic symptoms occur, stop pills immediately

Figure 22.4

MAKING THE TRANSITION FROM COCs TO MENOPAUSE, WITH OR WITHOUT HORMONE THERAPY (HT)

The transition from COCs to menopause, with or without HT may be accomplished in a number of ways. Some reviewers of this algorithm switch to a 20 or 25-mcg pill if the patient is going to use COCs into their early 50s.

This algorithm does NOT include testing for a woman's menopausal status using lab tests.

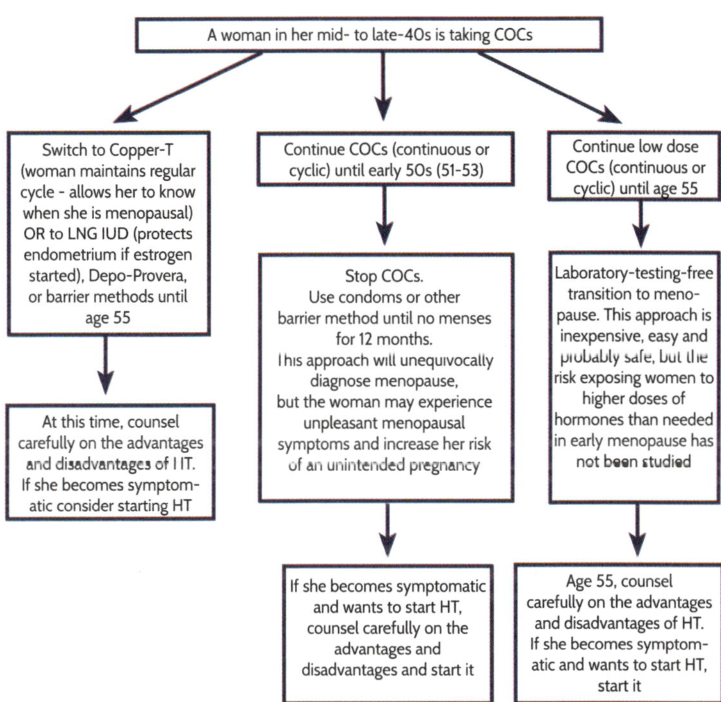

Figure 22.5

RECOMMENDED ACTIONS AFTER LATE OR MISSED COMBINED ORAL CONTRACEPTIVE
U.S. Selected Practice Recommendations (SPR 2016)

If one hormonal pill is late: (<24 hours since a pill should have been taken)

If one hormonal pill has been missed: (24 to <48 hours since a pill should have been taken)

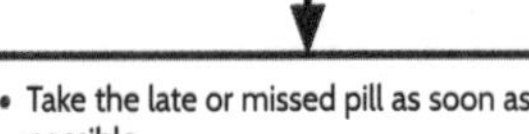

- Take the late or missed pill as soon as possible.
- Continue taking the remaining pills at the usual time (even if it means taking two pills on the same day).
- No additional contraceptive protection is needed.
- Emergency contraception is not usually needed but can be considered (with the exception of UPA*) if hormonal pills were missed earlier in the cycle or in the last week of the previous cycle.

If two or more consecutive hormonal pills have been missed: (≥48 hours since a pill should have been taken)

- Take the most recent missed pill as soon as possible. (Any other missed pills should be discarded.)
- Continue taking the remaining pills at the usual time (even if it means taking two pills on the same day).
- Use back-up contraception (e.g., condoms) or avoid sexual intercourse until hormonal pills have been taken for 7 consecutive days.
- If pills were missed in the last week of hormonal pills (e.g., days 15-21 for 28-day pill packs):
  - Omit the hormone-free interval by finishing the hormonal pills in the current pack and starting a new pack the next day.
  - If unable to start a new pack immediately, use back-up contraception (e.g., condoms) or avoid sexual intercourse until hormonal pills from a new pack have been taken for 7 consecutive days.
- Emergency contraception should be considered (with the exception of UPA*) if hormonal pills were missed during the first week and unprotected sexual intercourse occurred in the previous 5 days.
- Emergency contraception may also be considered (with the exception of UPA) at other times as appropriate.

**UPA = ulipristal acetate*

CDC MMWR July 29, 2016, Vol. 65:No. 4

Figure 22.6

RECOMMENDED STEPS AFTER VOMITING OR DIARRHEA WHILE USING COMBINED ORAL CONTRACEPTIVES
U.S. Selected Practice Recommendations (SPR 2016)

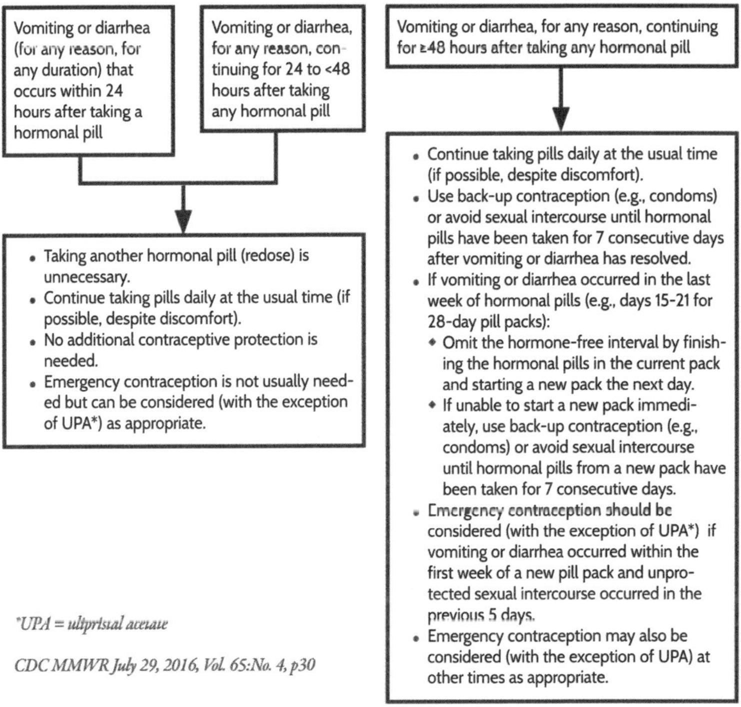

Vomiting or diarrhea (for any reason, for any duration) that occurs within 24 hours after taking a hormonal pill

Vomiting or diarrhea, for any reason, continuing for 24 to <48 hours after taking any hormonal pill

→

- Taking another hormonal pill (redose) is unnecessary.
- Continue taking pills daily at the usual time (if possible, despite discomfort).
- No additional contraceptive protection is needed.
- Emergency contraception is not usually needed but can be considered (with the exception of UPA*) as appropriate.

Vomiting or diarrhea, for any reason, continuing for ≥48 hours after taking any hormonal pill

→

- Continue taking pills daily at the usual time (if possible, despite discomfort).
- Use back-up contraception (e.g., condoms) or avoid sexual intercourse until hormonal pills have been taken for 7 consecutive days after vomiting or diarrhea has resolved.
- If vomiting or diarrhea occurred in the last week of hormonal pills (e.g., days 15-21 for 28-day pill packs):
    - Omit the hormone-free interval by finishing the hormonal pills in the current pack and starting a new pack the next day.
    - If unable to start a new pack immediately, use back-up contraception (e.g., condoms) or avoid sexual intercourse until hormonal pills from a new pack have been taken for 7 consecutive days.
- Emergency contraception should be considered (with the exception of UPA*) if vomiting or diarrhea occurred within the first week of a new pill pack and unprotected sexual intercourse occurred in the previous 5 days.
- Emergency contraception may also be considered (with the exception of UPA) at other times as appropriate.

**UPA = ulipristal acetate*

CDC MMWR July 29, 2016, Vol. 65:No. 4, p30

PATCHES - WEEKLY - XULANE, ZAFEMY (previously marketed as Ortho Evra) AND TWIRLA

DESCRIPTION

- One combined hormonal patch is worn for one week for 3 consecutive weeks, on the lower abdomen, buttocks, upper outer arm or to the upper torso (except for the breasts). The fourth week is patch-free to permit withdrawal bleeding.
- ***Xulane*** 4.5 cm square patch delivers 20 mcg of ethinyl estradiol and 150 mcg of the progestin, norelgestromin (EE/N patch) daily. *[Grimes 2001]*
    - It takes 3 days to achieve steady states or plateau levels of hormones after application of the patch with sufficeint hormone for 9 days
    - Delivers about 60% more estrogen over a 21-day period than a 35 mcg EE. but ~25% lower peak levels of EE. AUC may be more comparable to a 50 mcg EE pill.
- ***Twirla*** is a 28cm^2 weekly patch approved in 2020.
    - Releases 30 mcg EE and 120 mcg LNG per day (EE/LNG patch)
    - Releases hormonal doses to COCs with same formula.

MECHANISM: Prevents pregnancy in the same manner as combined pills

EFFECTIVENESS

EE/N Patch (Xulane):

Perfect use failure rate in the first year of use: 3-6 in 1,000 women (0.3-0.6%) (users who apply transdermal contraceptive patches on schedule and each patch remains in place for the full week), *Table 2.1 on page 9.*

Typical use failure rate in the first year of use: 7%, with data suggesting increased failures in overweight women

EE/LNG Patch (Twirla):

Clinical trial pregnancy rate: 3.5% in normal weight, 5.7% in overweight and 8.6% in obese women. Therefore this patch is contraindicted in obese women. *[USFDA Product Information]*

ADVANTAGES

Menstrual: Like combined pills

Sexual / psychological:

- May enhance sexual enjoyment due to diminished fear of pregnancy
- Convenient for women who forget to take pills
- Does not interrupt intercourse

Cancers / tumors / masses: No data yet; benefits probably comparable to combined pills

Other:

- Option throughout the reproductive years:
  Each patch contains enough hormone to suppress ovulation for up to 9 days.
- May bathe, swim and do normal activities

DISADVANTAGES

Menstrual: In the first cycle, about one-fifth of patch users experienced breakthrough bleeding or spotting. This improved with time

Sexual / psychological: Similar to pills. *See page 111*

Cancers / tumors / masses: Same as COCs *See page 112*

Other:

- Lack of protection against sexually transmitted infections
- Among 812 women on the EE/N patch, 3 serious adverse events were considered possible or likely related to use of the patch, including 1 case of pain and paraesthesia in the left arm, 1 case of migraine and 1 case of cholecystitis *[Audet 2001]*
- Must remove and replace patch weekly.
- Application site problems in EE/N trial include partial detachment (2.8%) or complete detachment (1.8%) and skin irritation (1.1%) *[Audet 2001]*.
- The St. Louis CHOICE study found 1, 2 and 3 year continuation rates for the EE/N patch of 49%, 40% and 28% *[Diedrich 2015]*.

In one multicenter three-cycle study, almost half the women reported that their patch fell off at least once. *[Crenin 2018]*.

- Pigment changes (hyper and hypo) have been noted (under 1%) under the site of patch application.
- Border of patch may become dirty, picking up lint, hairs or fabric. Remove with baby oil after patch is changed
- Nausea occurred in 20.4% of EE/N patch users vs 18.3% of COC users
- Breast discomfort was greater in EE/N patch vs OC users in cycles 1 and 2 (15.4% vs 3.5% in cycle 1 and 6.6% vs 1.5% in cycle 2) and was similar thereafter *[Audet 2001]*
- Headaches were as likely in women on EE/N patch (21.9%) as in women on pills (22.1%)
- Irritation or allergic skin reaction while using the EE/N patch (19%)

COMPLICATIONS *(See page 112)*

- Due to higher EE levels with the EE/N patch, users should be informed of the possiblity of an increase in risk of adverse events, particularly VTE although studies show either no increased risk or an approximate doubling of risk of VTE *[Jick 2006, 2007 Package Insert] [Cole-2007]*. Currently available data do not show an increased risk of MI or stroke
- Other complications similar to COCs

PRESCRIBING PRECAUTIONS

- Precautions same as for COC *(see page page 114)*
- Women weighing more than 90 kg (198 lbs) should be told that the EE/N patch is less effective as compared to its use in women < 198 lbs and that they should consider using a backup or another method.
- EE/LNG: inform about increasing failures with increasing body weight and contraindiction with obesity. Not for use if BMI > 30

CANDIDATES FOR USE

- Women wanting to avoid daily pill-taking or a sex-related method like condoms
- Women wanting regular menstrual periods. May be used by individuals allergic to latex

Adolescents: **Excellent option, particularly for women unable to remember to take pills daily** *[Archer 2002]*

INITIATING METHOD

- With the 1st pack of patches, the patient is eligible for up to three free replacement patches. Write prescription for "replacement patch" with the first box of patches
- **A pelvic examination is not necessary prior to starting this method**
- Ask patient, "What day of the week is the easiest for you to remember?" and start then
- ***QuickStart:*** Start anytime with backup for 7 days, if reasonably sure the woman is not pregnant. If started on day one of cycle, backup not needed.
- Women switching from DMPA should start when the next injection is due
- But as with pills, provide or recommend EC for when / if needed

INSTRUCTIONS FOR PATIENT

- If the patch-free interval is more than 9 days (late restart), apply a new patch and use backup contraception for 7 days *(see page 131)*
- No band-aids, tattoos, or decals on top of patch as this might alter absorption of hormones
- Smooth the edges down when you first put it on
- Avoid placing patch on exactly the same site 2 consecutive weeks
- Location of patch should not be altered in mid-week
- Women should check the patch daily to make sure all edges remain closely adherent to skin
- Single replacement patches are available through pharmacies.
- Disposal: fold over self. Place in solid waste, preferably in a sealed plastic bag to minimize hormone leakage into waste site. Do not flush down toilet

FOLLOW UP

- How are your menstrual periods?
- Have you experienced skin irritation?
- Has your patch ever come off partially or completely?
- Have you had problems remembering to replace your patch on schedule?
- Offer condoms

PROBLEM MANAGEMENT *(See page 119)*

FERTILITY AFTER DISCONTINUATION OF METHOD: Same rapid return of fertility as COCs

Figure 22.7

RECOMMENDED ACTIONS AFTER DELAYED APPLICATION OR DETACHMENT* WITH COMBINED HORMONAL PATCH
U.S. Selected Practice Recommendations (SPR 2016)

Delayed application or detachment* for <48 hours since a patch should have been applied or reattached

↓

- Apply a new patch as soon as possible. (If detachment occured <24 hours since the patch was applied, try to reapply the patch or replace with a new patch.)
- Keep the same patch change day.
- No additional contraceptive protection is needed.
- Emergency contraception is not usually needed but can be considered (with the exception of UPA**) if delayed application or detachment occurred earlier in the cycle or in the last week of the previous cycle.

Delayed application or detachment* for ≥48 hours since a patch should have been applied or reattached

↓

- Apply a new patch as soon as possible.
- Keep the same patch change day.
- Use back-up contraception (e.g., condoms) or avoid sexual intercourse until a patch has been worn for 7 consecutive days.
- If the delayed application or detachment occurred in the third patch week:
  - Omit the hormone-free week by finishing the third week of patch use (keeping the same patch change day) and starting a new patch immediately.
  - If unable to start a new patch immediately, use back-up contraception (e.g., condoms) or avoid sexual intercourse until a new patch has been worn for 7 consecutive days.
- Emergency contraception should be considered (with the exception of UPA**) if the delayed application or detachment occurred within the first week of patch use and unprotected sexual intercourse occurred in the previous 5 days.
- Emergency contraception may also be considered (with the exception of UPA) at other times as appropriate.

**If detachment takes place but the woman is unsure when the detachment occurred, consider the patch to have been detached for : ≥48 hours since a patch should have been applied or reattached.*

***UPA = ulipristal acetate*

CDC MMWR July 29, 2016, Vol. 65:No. 4

VAGINAL CONTRACEPTIVE RINGS - MONTHLY - NUVARING AND ANNOVERA

DESCRIPTION:

- **NuvaRing** (EE / ENG) combined hormonal contraceptive, 5.4 cm (2 inches) diameter flexible (not hard) ring, 4 mm (1/8 inch) in thickness.
  - Made of ethylene vinylacetate polymer.
  - Left in place in the vagina for 3 weeks (or 1 month) and then removed for a week to allow withdrawal bleeding. May be used continuously with no hormone-free days (off-label).
  - Releases low doses of ethinyl estradiol (EE 15 mcg daily) and etonogestrel (ENG 120 mcg daily) the active form of desogestrel (120 mcg daily).
  - Maintains a steady, low release rate for 42 days while in place, even in obese women *[Dragoman 2013]*
  - Releases less estrogen daily at a steadier rate than pills or patches
- **Annovera** is a new combined hormonal contraceptive containing segesterone acetate / ethinylestradiol (SA/EE) measuring 5.6 cm (2.2 inches) in diameter and 8.4 mm (1/4 inch) in thickness. It is a flexible ring that is slightly thicker than the NuvaRing. One Annovera ring lasts for a year. It is placed into the vagina for 21 days, removed and washed, and then the same ring is replaced into the vaginal after 7 hormonal-free days. It does not require refrigeration.
  - In a recent clinical trial of 2,308 women, a perfect-use failure rate was 3 per 100 woman per year. As of this time, there is not a typical-use failure rate for Annovera.

MECHANISM OF ACTION: Similar to combined pills. *see COCs, page 110*

EFFECTIVENESS

NuvaRing: Overall perfect use pregnancy rate of 0.3 *[Trussell 2004]* to 1.2 per 100 woman-years (all first-year users) in clinical trials. *[Oddson 2005]* Typical use pregnancy rate estimated as 7% *(see page 9)*

Annovera: Overall pooled pregnancy rate 3% in recent clinical trials

ADVANTAGES: No daily fluctuation in hormone levels

Menstrual:

- Better withdrawal / spotting pattern than COCs probably due to not forgetting pills and the steady blood levels
- Irregular bleeding is low in the first cycle of use (6%) and continues to be low throughout subsequent cycles *[Dieben 2002]*

Sexual / psychological: Decreased fear of pregnancy may increase pleasure from intercourse

Cancers / tumors / masses: Probably similar to COCs

Other: May be easier to adhere to schedule than daily pill *[Bjarnadottir 2002]*

- 85% of women and 71% of partners say they cannot feel it *[Dieben 2002]*
- The lowest serum levels of estrogen and progestin in any combined hormonal method
- Ok to use water-based lubricants and spermicides but not oil-based (including silicone-based) lubricants
- Privacy - no visible patch or pill packages. Particularly helpful for some teens
- Little weight gain associated with ring use *[O'Connel 2005]*

DISADVANTAGES

Menstrual: Withdrawal bleeding continued beyond the ring-free interval in about one quarter of ENG/EE cycles, usually spotting (20% to 27%) *[Roumen 2001]*.

- Although not necessary, some women may rinse the ring. Also, ring can be accidentally pulled out by a tampon

Sexual / psychological: Some women dislike placing / removing objects into / out of vagina

- May feel discomfort from the ring during intercourse. If bothersome, ring may be removed and reinserted within 3 hours

Cancers / tumors / masses: None

Other: Adverse events reported by ENG/EE vaginal contraceptive ring users that were judged by the investigators to be possibly device-related are headache (6.6%), nausea (2.8%), weight increase (2.2%), dysmenorrhea (1.8%), depression (1.7%), leukorrhea (5.3%), vaginitis (5.0%), and vaginal discomfort (2.2%) *[Roumen 2001]*

- Expulsion in 20% women in first three months of use

COMPLICATIONS: Similar to combined pills

PRESCRIBING PRECAUTIONS

- The CDC Medical Eligibility Criteria for the combined rings are the same as for COCs
- Women who are hesitant about touching their genitalia or who have difficulty inserting or removing ring may not be good candidates
- Pronounced pelvic relaxation
- Data on efficacy in obese women are limited but do not suggest increased failures. The initial NuvaRing's trials excluded such women and the Annovera trials excluded them after two women with BMI > 29 developed VTE.

CANDIDATES

- Women wanting to avoid having to do something daily, or at the time of intercourse
- Women wanting regular menstrual periods
- Women satisfied with OCs but willing to try the patch or ring were happier with the ring than their OC *[Creinin 2007]*

Adolescents: Requires less discipline than taking pills daily

INITIATING METHOD: ***Teach women to insert and remove ring in office. Ask women if they would like you to insert a ring after you do an exam to demonstrate***

- New ring can be inserted at any time in cycle if reasonably certain woman is not pregnant; use backup x 7 days (CDC)
  - Manufacturer of NuvaRing recommends back up for 7 days if not intiated on first day of menses while CDC SPR states no back up if within 5 days LMP.
- Provide or recommend EC for when / if needed
- QuickStart of Nuvaring has been studied with high levels of satisfaction by users *[Schafer 2006]*.

INSTRUCTIONS FOR PATIENT

- The ring is removed at the end of 3 (or 4) weeks of wear; then, after one ring-free week, the woman inserts a new ring of ENG/EE or same SA/EE ring
- The woman's menstrual period (withdrawal bleed) occurs during the ring-free week

- Ring removal during intercourse is not recommended; however, may be removed without using a backup if < 3 hours a day
- Should not be used in combination with diaphragm, cervical cap or female condom.
- Check for presence frequently, especially after intercourse due to risk of expulsion
- No special accuracy is required for ring placement; absorption is fine from anywhere in the vagina
- Because the ring is small and flexible, most women do not notice any pressure or discomfort, and it is not likely to be uncomfortable for their partners during intercourse
- Advantageous to have 2 rings on hand in case one is lost
- Avoid douching with ring in place. Douching is not recommended for any woman
- Data from NuvaRing suggest increased hormonal levels with oil based vaginal creams. Therefore use water-based products.
- Tampons, water-based lubricants and water based vaginal yeast creams can be used with the ring in place
- Rings may be stored at room temperature avoiding extreme heat for up to 4 months. If a woman has more than a 4-month supply of rings, they may be stored in a refrigerator. Avoid freezing
- A ring that falls into the toilet can be washed with soap and water and reinserted
- If the ring is left in place longer than three weeks, the user is still protected from pregnancy for up to 35 days by the same ENG/EE ring, allowing flexibility. For example, the ring could be reinserted on the first of the month each month with no hormone-free interval (similar to taking combined pills with no hormone-free days)
- Extended use of the ENG/EE ring has been studied. The number of bleeding and spotting days combined was similar in shorter and extended cycles *[Miller 2005]*. Extended use decreased menstural flow and cramping *[Sulak 2008]*. If breakthrough bleeding occurs after 21 days use, instruct the patient to remove the ring, store it for 4 days, then reinsert *[Sulak 2008]*
- Dispose of ring with solid waste, preferably in a sealed plastic bag to minimize leakage into waste site

FOLLOW UP: Ask about difficulty during removal or insertion or frequent expulsion. Women may need closer follow-up if they have: genital prolapse, severe constipation, or frequent vaginal infection (i.e. recurrent yeast infection). Otherwise, follow-up is similar to women on pills. Offer condoms.

FERTILITY AFTER DISCONTINUATION: Excellent and immediate. Average return to ovulation: 11 days (range 8-21 d) *[Mulders 2002]*

FROM ANNOVERA PRESCRIBING INFORMATION:

"The use of water-based vaginal miconazale cream resulted in no change in exposure to EE or SA from the vaginal system. However, the use of either the 1-day or 3-day oil-based miconazole suppository was associated with an overall increase in exposure up to 67% for EE and 32% for SA. Concurrent use of oil based vaginal suppositories should not occur with Annovera use.

CHAPTER 23

PROGESTIN-ONLY CONTRACEPTIVES

Progestin-only pills, Depo-Provera injections, implants and the LNG IUD *(see chapter 21)*

LOW DOSE PROGESTIN PILLS, MINI-PILLS OR POPS

DESCRIPTION: Progestin-only pills (POPs) contain only a progestin. Each progestin-only pill contains 0.35 mg norethindrone (NET) or 4 mg drospirenone. Usage in U.S. is low, estimated at 0.4% of contraceptors from NSFG data *[Hawks 2012]* and 4% from claims data *[Liang- 012]*.

- NET POPs taken daily with no hormone free days
- Drospirenone packaged as 24 active pills with 4 inert pills (Slynd)

EFFECTIVENESS *[Trussell- 018]*

Typical use failure rate in first year: 7.0%
Perfect use failure rate in first year: 0.3% *(See Table 2.1, page 9)*
Slynd: clinical trials pearl index from 0.7-4.0

MECHANISM OF ACTION

- Primarily thickens cervical mucus to prevent sperm entry
- Inhibition of ovulation, approximately 40% of women ovulate normally
- ***Timing is critical:*** thickening of cervical mucus happens about 2 to 4 hours AFTER a NET POP is taken and lasts for about 22 hours.
  - NET pills - if more than 3 hours late, take pill and add backup for 2 days.
- ***Slynd:*** missed pill window extended from 3 hours to 24 hours.

ADVANTAGES

Menstrual:

- Decreased menstrual blood loss, cramps and pain. Amenorrhea occurs in 10% of women and is more likely with punctual dosing
- Decrease in ovulatory pain (Mittelschmerz) in cycles when ovulation suppressed

Sexual / physiological:

- May enhance sexual enjoyment due to diminished fear of pregnancy
- No disruption at time of intercourse; facilitates spontaneity

Cancers / tumors / masses:

- Protection against endometrial hyperplasia and endometrial cancer

Other:

- Rapid return to baseline fertility
- Possible reduction in PID risk due to cervical mucus thickening
- Good option for women who cannot use estrogen but want to take pills
- May be used by smokers over age 35
- May be used by breastfeeding women
- Likely to be the first over-the-counter pill in the United States

Advantages of progestin-only pills over combined pills:

- Only one absolute contraindication "4" in the U.S. MEC: Breast cancer within 5 years *(see box below)*
- Safer for those with thromboembolic conditions
- May be used by breastfeeding women immediately postpartum

DISADVANTAGES

Menstrual: Irregular menses ranging from amenorrhea to increased days of spotting and bleeding but with reduced blood loss overall

Sexual / psychological:

- Spotting and bleeding may interfere with sexual activity
- Intermittent amenorrhea or concerns about pregnancy
- Possible increase in depression, anxiety, irritability

Cancers / tumors / masses: None

Other:

- Must take pill at same time each day (3-hour delay of NET is a "missed pill," and 24 hour window for Slynd)
- Effect on cervical mucus decreases after 22 hours and is gone after 27 hours

U.S. MEC - 2016: What the numbers mean

1. No restrictions (method can be used)
2. Advantages generally outweigh theoritical or proven risk
3. Theoretical or proven risks usually outweigh the advantages
4. Unacceptable health risk (method not to be used)

COMPLICATIONS

- Allergy to progestin pill is rare
- Amenorrhea
- Latina, breast-feeding women who had gestational diabetes may be at higher risk of developing overt diabetes in first year postpartum *[Kjos 1998]*

CANDIDATES FOR USE *(See U.S. MEC Medical Eligibility Criteria, page 242)*

- Almost every woman who can take pills on a daily basis can be a candidate for POPs
  - POPs are particularly good for women with contraindications to or side effects from estrogen:
    - Women with personal history of thrombosis (DVT or PE) (U.S. MEC: 2 - *see box above*)
    - Recently postpartum women (U.S. MEC: 1)
    - Women who are exclusively breastfeeding (<1 month U.S. MEC: 2, ≥ 1 month U.S. MEC: 1)
    - Smokers over age 35 (U.S. MEC: 1)
    - Women who have had or are afraid of having chloasma, hypertriglyceridemia (U.S. MEC: 2) or other estrogen-related side effects
    - Women with hypertension (U.S. MEC: 1,2)

PRESCRIBING PRECAUTIONS

Progestin-only pills can be used by all women willing and able to take daily pills except:

- Slynd should be used with caution in those at risk for hyperkalemia.
- Suspected or demonstrated pregnancy (although there are no proven harmful effects for the fetus)

- Current breast cancer or breast cancer less than 5 years ago (U.S. MEC: 4)
- Inability to absorb sex steroids from gastrointestinal tract (active colitis, etc.)
- Taking medications that increase hepatic clearance (U.S. MEC: 3 for rifampin, anticonvulsants carbamazepine, oxcarbazepine, phenytoin, phenobarbital, primidone, and topiramate.)

SPECIAL SITUATIONS

History of pregnancy while using POPs correctly:

- Switch to more effective method e.g. IUD, implant or DMPA injections
- Continue POPs but add condoms or other backup with every act of coitus

Use with a broad-spectrum antibiotic such as tetracycline or erythromycin:

- Few studies support antibiotics' role in contraceptive failure. *(See U.S. Medical Eligibility Criteria page 242 for "other antibiotics")*

INITIATING METHOD

- **A pelvic examination is not necessary prior to initiation of this method**
- ***New starts:*** Offer condoms either for back-up or for use should patient stop POPs. Also encourage advance obtaining of Plan B
- ***Post-partum:*** May initiate immediately regardless of breast-feeding status (U.S. MEC: 2)
- ***After miscarriage or abortion:*** Start immediately (U.S. MEC: 1)
- ***Menstruating women:*** No backup if started within 5 days of LMP. If > 5 days, recommend at least 2 day back-up barrier method
- ***Switching from IUD, COCs, DMPA, to POPs:*** Start immediately if reasonable certain not pregnant *(seepage 12)*. If more than 5 days from LMP, abstain or use backup for 2 days.
- ***Switching from IUD:*** If the woman has had sexual intercourse since the start of her current menstual cycle and it has been > 5 days since menstrual bleeding started, theoretically, residual sperm might be in the genital tract, which could lead to fertilization if ovulation occurs. Here are options on day of visit:
  - Retain IUD for at least 2 days after POPs initiated, then remove.
  - Advise woman to abstain or use backup for 7 days, remove IUD and if she has had intercourse in past 7 days provide Plan B (not ella), start POP immediately after EC.

INSTRUCTIONS FOR PATIENT

- Take one pill daily at same time until end of pack. Start next pack the next day
- If at risk for infection, use condoms with every act of intercourse
- If you miss a pill by more than 3 hours from regular time, take the missed pill(s) and use backup for 48 hours. Consider using emergency contraception if sex in past 5 days. Obtain a package of Plan B to have at home.

FOLLOW-UP COUNSELING QUESTIONS

- How many pills do you typically miss or are late taking per pack? (average in U.S.: 4.2)
- Have you missed any pills in last 5 days? (candidate for EC)
- Have you missed any periods or experienced any symptoms of pregnancy?
- What has your menstrual bleeding been like?
- Have you had any increase in headaches, or change in mood or libido?
- What are you doing to protect yourself from STIs?
- Offer condoms

PROBLEM MANAGEMENT

- Amenorrhea: Rule out pregnancy after any missed period or if symptoms of pregnancy have been noted. If not, reassure.
- Irregular bleeding: After finding out if missing pills, rule out STIs, pregnancy, cancer. If no evidence of underlying pathology, reassure.
- Heavy bleeding: Rule out STIs, pregnancy, cancer, anemia.
- Abdominal pain: Consider pelvic pathology (ectopic pregnancy, torsion, appendicitis, PID) and refer for treatment. Progestin slows follicular atresia so there is increased risk of ovarian cysts. May usually be managed conservatively unless pain is severe. Recheck in 6 weeks and anytime her symptoms worsen

FERTILITY AFTER DISCONTINUATION OF METHOD: Fertility returns to baseline promptly

DMPA INJECTIONS (DEPO-PROVERA) - EVERY 3 MONTHS

DESCRIPTION

- IM DMPA: 0.1 cc of a crystalline suspension of 150 mg DMPA injected deep intramuscularly into the deltoid or gluteus maximus muscle every 13 to 15 weeks.
- SQ DMPA: – 104 mg subcutaneous injections every 13-15 weeks. Women may self-administer at home
  - Available in prefilled syringe of 0.6ml with 26-gauge x 3/8 inch needle
  - Self administration is safe, feasible, and off-label *[NFPRHA 2020]*
  - In May 2021, CDC stated self-administration DMPA-SC should be offered

EFFECTIVENESS *[Trussell-2018]*

Typical use failure rate in first year: 6%

Perfect use failure rate in first year: 0.2% *(See Table 2.1, page 9)*

Continuation at 1 year: 23% *[Westfall 1996]* 42% *[Polaneczky 1996]* 56% Continuation rates for Depo are the lowest of any current contraceptive.

Subcutaneous Depo-Provera

Despite the lower dose of Sub Q DMPA (104 vs 150 mg), no pregnancies occurred among the 44% of study subjects who were overweight (26%) or obese (18%). In fact, there were no pregnancies at all in 720 women over one year. 55% were amenorrheic at the end of one year. *[Jain 2004]* Research indicates that use of subcutaneous depot medroxyprogesterone acetate (DMPA-SC, marketed as Sayana Press) may help women to continue using injectable contraception longer than women who receive traditional intramuscular injections. *[Burke 2018]* CDC state "existing recommendations in the U.S. MEC and U.S. SPR for provider-administered DMPA also apply to self-administered DMPA-SC" *[Curtis 2021]*

MECHANISM OF ACTION: Suppresses ovulation by inhibiting LH and FSH surge, thickens cervical mucus blocking sperm entry, slows tubal and endometrial mobility, and causes thinning of the endometrium.

ADVANTAGES

Menstrual:

- Less menstrual blood loss, anemia, or hemorrhagic corpus luteum cysts
- After 1 year of use, 50% of women develop amenorrhea; 80% develop amenorrhea in 5 years. For this to be an advantage, it must be clearly explained at first and at each subsequent visit.
- Decreased menstrual cramps, pain and ovulation pain. May also decrease PMS
- Improvement in endometriosis. Depo-subQ provera 104 is also FDA approved for management of endometriosis pain

Sexual / psychological:

- Intercourse may be more pleasurable without worry of pregnancy
- Convenient: permits spontaneous sexual activity; requires no action at time of intercourse

Cancers / tumors / masses:

- Decreased blood loss in women with fibroids
- Significant reduction in risk of endometrial hyperplasia and of endometrial cancer
- Reduction in risk of ovarian cancer (increased protection with increased time use)

Benefits for women with medical problems:

- Suppresses ovulation, bleeding and menstrual blood loss in anticoagulated women and women with bleeding diathesis; decreases anemia
- Reduces acute sickle cell crises by 70% *[de Abood 1997]*
- Excellent method for women on anticonvulsant drugs; may actually decrease seizures, and effectiveness of DMPA is not compromised by anticonvulsants *(see U.S. MEC on inside of back cover of this book, page 242)*.
- Amenorrhea and prolonged effective contraception may be helpful for developmentally or physically challenged women.

Other:

- Significantly reduces risk for ectopic pregnancies and slightly decreases risk of PID
- Convenient: single injection provides 15 weeks protection
- Most protocols call for administration anytime between 11 and 15 weeks.
- Less user-dependent than POPs, COCs
- Good option for women who cannot use estrogen
- Private: no visible clue that patient is using contraception. This may prevent physical abuse of a woman by a partner who does not want her using a contraceptive.
- May be used by nursing mothers
- Return to baseline fertility may be delayed, but is ultimately unaffected
- Recent data found no increased risk of HIV transmission

DISADVANTAGES

Menstrual:

- Irregular menses during first several months: many women experience unpredictable spotting and bleeding, occasionally blood loss reported to be heavy but unlikely to cause anemia. After 6-12 months, amenorrhea more likely (50% after 1 year)
- Very rare: high dose progestins can cause accumulation of a thick endometrium which, when expelled, can be quite painful, called membranous dysmenorrhea.

Sexual / psychological: *(Also see weight gain, below)*

- Spotting and bleeding may interfere with sexual activity
- Amenorrhea may raise uncertainty about whether a woman is pregnant
- Hypoestrogenism can (infrequently) cause dyspareunia, hot flashes or decreased libido
- Possible increase in depression, anxiety, irritation, PMS, fatigue or other mood changes, but DMPA may also reduce risk of these disorders
- Fear of needles may make this an unacceptable choice

Cancers, tumors, and masses: none

Other:

- See boxed message: Depo Provera & Bone Mineral Density *page 141*
- No protection against STIs: must use condoms if at risk
- Must return every 11-15 weeks for injection
  - Women have been taught to give themselves deep intramuscular injections
  - No contraceptive requires more return visits than Depo-Provera injections
- Long-acting and not immediately reversible
  - Slow to return to baseline fertility: average 10 months from last injection with variability in time to return to ovulation (15-49 weeks)
- Occasionally, hypoestrogenism (E2 < 25) may develop as a result of FSH suppression. Potential for decreased bone mineral density if used for prolonged period without opportunity for recovery prior to menopause. May have more effect on teen bones. *See Box on page 141*
- Headaches may occur
- Acne, hirsutism may develop
- Possible increase in diabetes risk in amenorrheic breastfeeding Latina women with diagnosis of gestational diabetes during first year postpartum *[Kjos 1999]*
- Metabolic impacts: glucose (slight rise), LDL (slight rise or neutral), HDL (may decrease)
- Other hormone-related Sx: breast tenderness, bloating, hair loss, vasomotor symptoms
- Associated with modest weight gain in most women

COMPLICATIONS

- Specific individuals and certain ethnic groups may have significant weight gain e.g. Navajo women, obese individuals when initiating.
- Adolescent girls who were obese when starting DMPA gained significantly more weight (mean 9.4 kg) than obese girls starting OCs (mean 0.2 kg) and controls (mean 3.5 kg) *[Ziegler 2006]*
  - A woman who is thin when she starts receiving the DMPA and then does not gain weight during her first year on DMPA is far less likely to gain weight on DMPA in subsequent years
  - Weigh users at initiation and first few reinjections to identify weight gain
- Worsening depression (rare)
- Severe allergic reaction, including anaphylaxis (very rare). May consider having women wait in or near office for 20 minutes after injection.

CANDIDATES FOR USE

Woman who:

- Want privacy, convenience, and high efficacy.
- Want intermediate-to-long-term contraception and can return every 11-15 weeks
- Do not plan a pregnancy soon after DMPA discontinuation
- Want or need to avoid estrogen:
  - Personal history of thrombosis (U.S. MEC: 2) or strong family history of venous thromboembolism (U.S. MEC: 1)
  - Recently postpartum women (U.S. MEC: 1)
  - Breastfeeding: <1 month U.S. MEC:2, ≥1 month U.S. MEC: 1
  - Smokers over age 35 (U.S. MEC: 1)
  - Fear of chloasma or had vomiting, hypertriglyceridemia, or other estrogen-related side effects on estrogenic contraceptives
- Use drugs which affect liver clearance (except aminoglutethimide)
- With anemia, fibroids, seizure disorder (U.S. MEC: 1), sickle cell disease (U.S. MEC: 1), endometriosis, hypertriglyceridemia (U.S. MEC: 2)
- Physically compromised women for whom irregular bleeding is a burden

Adolescent women: (U.S. MEC: 2)

- Only 4 appointments each year
- Extremely effective even if patient returns up to 15 weeks after last injection
- Decreases menstrual cramps and pain
- May be associated with significant weight gain, acne, complexion changes

CDC updated recommendations in the U.S. MEC in April 2020 to state that progestin-only injectable contraception, including DMPA, and intrauterine devices (including LNG-releasing and copper) are safe for use without restriction among woman at high risk for HIV infection. U.S. MEC:1

Bone Mineral Density (BMD) and Depo-Provera

Depo-Provera received a black box warning from the FDA in 11/04 due to this issue.

"Women who use DMPA may lose significant BMD. Bone loss is greater with increasing duration of use and may not be completely reversible. It is unknown if use of DMPA during adolescence or early adulthood, a critical period of BMD accretion, will reduce poor bone mass and increase risk of osteoporotic fracture in later life. DMPA should not be used as a long-term birth control method (e.g. longer than two years) unless other methods are considered inadequate."

Organizations that do not advocate limiting use as above:

- ACOG, CDC, Society for Adolescent Health and Medicine (SAHM), WHO
- Best available data suggests DMPA use does not reduce peak bone mass or increase risk of fractures later in life
- Effect is largely reversible, even after > 4 years of DMPA use, comparable to the effect and reversal seen after lactation *[Petitti 2000]*.
- Longitudinal studies of DMPA use in teens found a significant difference in BMD between DMPA users and non-users due to a decrease in users and an increase in nonusers. By 12 months after discontinuation, BMD of former users was the same as for non-users. *[Scholes 2005]*

PRESCRIBING PRECAUTIONS:

- Women unwilling to accept a change in their menstrual periods should not use this method.
- Pregnancy
- Undiagnosed abnormal vaginal bleeding
- Unable to tolerate injections; afraid of shots
- History of breast cancer, MI or stroke
- Current venous thromboembolism (unless anticoagulated)
- Active viral hepatitis
- Known hypersensitivity to DMPA
- Wanting to become pregnant soon after stopping DMPA
- Women in their mid to late thirties would be wise to discontinue DMPA and switch to another contraceptive 12 to 24 months prior to trying to become pregnant

DRUG INTERACTIONS: Aminoglutethimide (Cytodren), used to treat Cushings disease, reduces DMPA efficacy

INITIATING METHOD *(see Figure 23.1, page 146)*

A pelvic exam is NOT necessary prior to the initiation of this method

Cycling women:

- Preferred start time is during first 7 days from the start of menses, no backup needed
- Alternative: inject anytime in the cycle if not pregnant, back-up x 7 days

Postpartum women: May give injection prior to hospital discharge. Special considerations:

- After severe obstetrical blood loss, may want to delay injection until lochia stops
- If patient has history or high risk for severe postpartum depression, may want to delay injection at least 4-6 weeks
- May start DMPA immediately whether breastfeeding (U.S. MEC: 2) or not (U.S. MEC: 1). *see page 242*

Women who have spontaneous or therapeutic abortion: May initiate immediately.

Women switching methods:

- If > 7 days from LMP, abstain or use backup for 7 days
- ***Switching from IUD:*** If the woman has had sexual intercourse since the start of her current menstrual cycle and it has been >5 days since menstrual bleeding started, theoretically, residual sperm might be in the genital tract, which could lead to fertilization if ovulation occurs. Options are:
  - Advise the women to retain the IUD for at least 7 days after the injection and return for IUD removal.
  - Advise the woman to abstain or use back-up for 7 days before removing the IUD and switching to DMPA.
  - If the woman cannot return for IUD removal and has not abstained or used back-up for 7 days, advise to use ECPs (with the exception of UPA) at the time of IUD removal

INSTRUCTIONS FOR PATIENT: ***Some women may be able to self-administer DMPA-SC***

- Do NOT massage area where shot was given for a few hours (massaging may hasten absorption and reduce duration of action and thereby effectiveness)

- Expect irregular bleeding / spotting in beginning. Usually decreases over time. Return at any time spotting or bleeding is bothersome.
- It is not harmful or dangerous if you do not have periods while you use DMPA
- Be sure to take in 1000 mg (women over age 25) to 1200 mg (adolescent women) of calcium every day to strengthen bones. Take calcium tablets like calcium carbonate or TUMS daily if your diet does not include enough calcium. Calcium is best absorbed when 500 mg is taken late in the day with a glass of orange juice. Get weight bearing and muscle-strengthening exercise at least 3 times a week (preferably 20 minutes daily)
- Return within 15 weeks for your next injection. Use abstinence, condoms, and EC, if necessary, if you are late coming for your re-injection
- Pregnancy is rare; return if you develop pregnancy symptoms other than amenorrhea
- Serious complications with DMPA are rare, but return if you develop severe headaches, heavy bleeding, depression or problems at the shot site (pus, pain, allergic reaction)
- If a woman becomes pregnant when she starts or while using Depo as her contraceptive, there is no increase in birth defects
- Monitor weight at home and contact provider if significant change is noted

WEIGHT GAIN IN A WOMAN ON DEPO: A TEACHABLE MOMENT

Nutritional Counseling:

1. Eat balanced diet with lots of fruits and vegetables and minimal saturated fats, chips, cookies, pasta, rice, and other carbohydrates
2. Exercise more and every day
3. Find patterns of eating and exercising that you enjoy. You won't do them for long unless you enjoy the process
4. Drinking calories leads as quickly to obesity as eating them. Avoid juice and sweetened drinks
5. Drink 8-10 glasses of water daily.

FOLLOW-UP VISIT QUESTIONS

- Are you experiencing spotting or irregular bleeding? Have you missed periods or had very light periods? Are you concerned about your pattern of bleeding?
- Did you have pain at the injection site after previous injection?
- Have you felt depressed or had major mood changes?
- Have you gained 5 pounds or more? Weigh patients at each visit.
- Consider measuring height and calculating a BMI
- Do you have any increase in your headaches?
- Have you had the feeling that you may be pregnant?
- Did you have any problems returning on time for this injection?
- Do you plan to have children? OR Do you plan to have more children?
- Offer condoms to all women on DMPA

PROBLEM MANAGEMENT

Allergic reaction or vasovagal reaction: Support as needed. Benadryl may reduce pruritus and swelling. Most allergic manifestations subside in 1 week or so. Avoid future injections and help her choose a different method. Anaphylaxis extremely rare.

Vaginal dryness, dyspareunia, or atrophic vaginitis: May be due to low estrogen levels. Consider giving vaginal estrogen. Dyspareunia may be relieved with water soluble or silicone lubricants.

Pain or infection at injection site: Offer anti-inflammatory medications. Rule out infection or needle damage to nerve, etc. Provide appropriate antibiotics if cellulitis present

Patient returns early (<11 weeks) wanting reinjection (eg b/c of travel): Administer DMPA

Patient returns late (>15 weeks) for reinjection: *See Figure 23.1 on page 146*

Switching to another method (eg OCs, IUD, etc) from DMPA: Initiate new method at any time convenient for patient. Preferred time would be near end of effectiveness of last DMPA injection unless switching to OCs, patch or vaginal rings to control menstrual disorders on DMPA. **Do NOT wait until next menses to start pills.** She may have amenorrhea for a number of months after DMPA

Transitioning perimenopausal women: *See Figure 23.2 on page 147*

Weight gain: Advise to watch caloric intake and to increase exercise. Be ready to discontinue method if weight gain is excessive or unacceptable *(See Nutritional Counseling onpage 143)*

Heavy bleeding:

- Rule out pregnancy, cervical infection or neoplasia and other causes
- Rule out anemia - recommend iron-rich foods and / or supplements
- May treat with NSAIDs or low-dose estrogen supplements:
  - Ibuprofen 800 mg orally every 8 hours for 3 days
  - Mefenamic acid: 500 mg once, then 250 mg every 6 hours for 2-3 days
  - Conjugated equine estrogen (2.5, 1.25 or 0.625 mg) orally once a day up to four times per day for 4-6 days OR ethinyl estradiol x 21 days (expensive)
  - COCs for 1-2 months (in addition to DMPA use)

Irregular bleeding and spotting *(see algorithm on page 123)*:

- Reassure that cumulative blood loss is usually less not more than no method use
- Rule out infection or cervical lesions as source
- Reassure that irregular spotting and bleeding is to be expected in first several months
- May use same therapies as outlined in heavy bleeding section above

Amenorrhea:

- Reassure her it does not require medical treatment. Do pregnancy test if she has other symptoms of pregnancy, if a women's bleeding pattern changes abruptly to amenorrhea or in some instances, to ensure she is not pregnant. *[U.S. Selective Practice Recommendations 2016]*
- Switch method if patient desires regular menses (consider patch, ring, COCs). Even if she stops DMPA, menses may not return for months

Depression:

- Evaluate suicidal ideation and refer immediately, if indicated
- Explain that DMPA usually does not worsen depression. Start antidepressant therapy, if needed. Discontinue DMPA if any concern

FERTILITY AFTER DISCONTINUATION OF METHOD

- Because anovulation may last for more than 1 year, women who know they will want to become pregnant within one year of cessation of use should consider another option, especially women over 35 years of age

- Fertility may return after 3 months; however, conception rates overall are lower than women discontinuing other contraceptive methods. After last shot, 50% of women are pregnant after 6-7 months (compared to 4 months with other methods). Delay not increased with increased duration of use. More than 90% of women become pregnant within 2 years.
- Women who do not want to await spontaneous return of ovulation will require gonadotrophin therapy to induce ovulation. Gonadotropins will not overcome effect of DMPA on cervical mucus.

FIGURE 23.1 Initial Injection or Late Reinjection (more than 2 weeks since scheduled return visit at 13 weeks) of DMPA or Switching From DMPA to COCs or Another Hormonal Method*

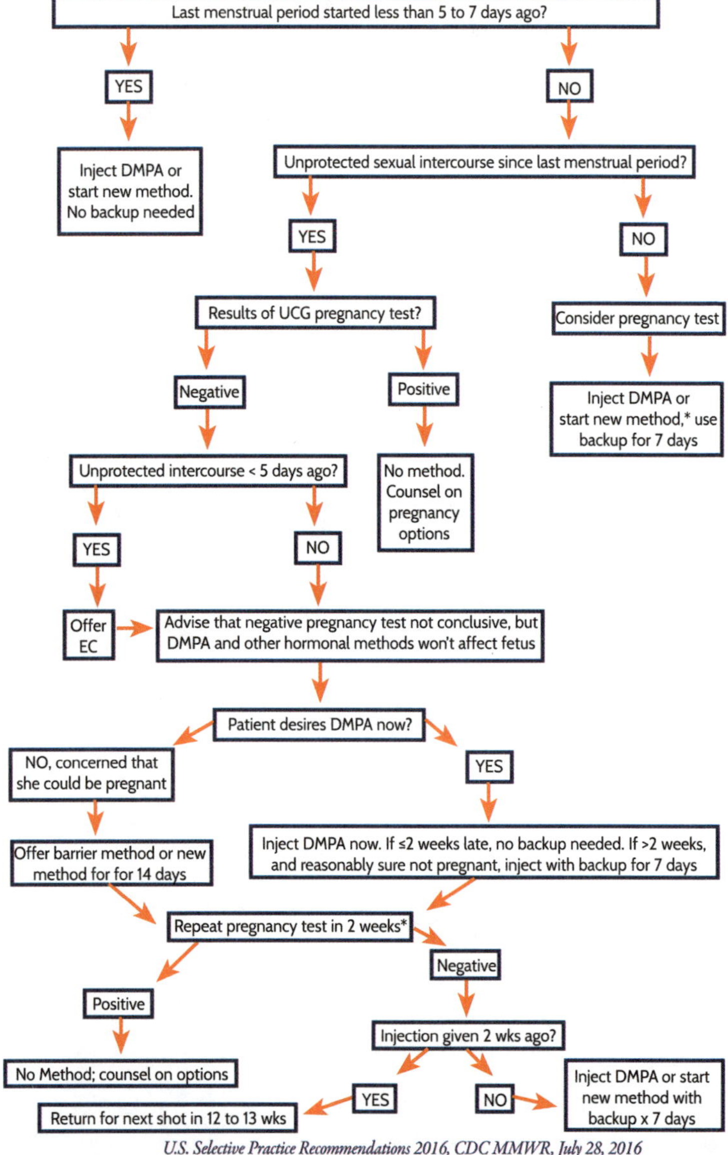

U.S. Selective Practice Recommendations 2016, CDC MMWR, July 28, 2016

Figure 23.2 Making Transition from DMPA to Menopause, With or Without Hormone Therapy (HT) with Estrogen or Estrogen-progestin

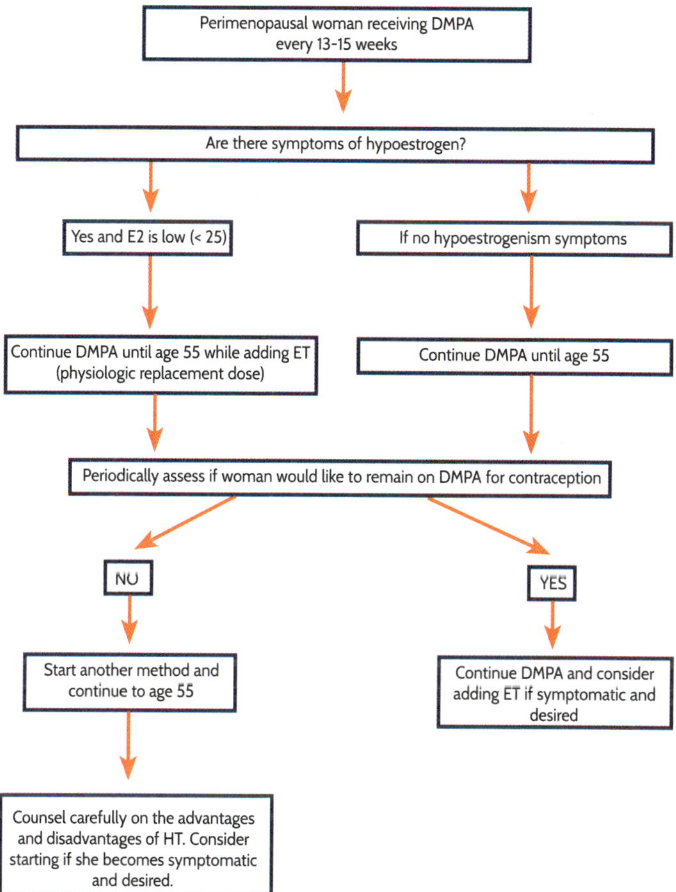

* DMPA suppresses gonadotropins, so measuring FSH may not be informative of menopausal state. DMPA use decreases endogenous estrogen levels. Some researchers recommend that, at age 50, 2 FSH measurements be done at the time of the injection visit to assess menopausal status. If 2 consecutive levels are > 35-40 m IU/ml, this is suggestive of menopause *[Juliato 2007]*

The two-rod LNG implants, Jadelle and Sinoplant. were modeled after Norplant. Used globally, clients in U.S. may request removal which may be approached in same way as Nexplanon removal. Jadelle effective for 5 years.

IMPLANTS: NEXPLANON - THE SINGLE ETONOGESTREL IMPLANT

DESCRIPTION

- 4 cm long and 2 mm in diameter with a membrane of ethylene vinyl acetate (EVA) and with a core of 68 mg of etonogestrel (3-ketodesogestrel)
- Initial release 60 mcg per day decreasing to 25-30 mcg/day by end of year 3. Implant is effective for at least 3 years
- Placed under the skin of upper arm with a 16-gauge disposable, preloaded inserter
- Radiopaque: barium sulfate replacing some of the EVA core

EFFECTIVENESS

Perfect use: .038 pregnancies per 100 years of use

Many of the pregnancies are due to insertions not complying with menstrual timing recommendations or even non-insertions.

Drugs that may lower Nexplanon effectiveness include the anticonvulsants phenytoin, carbamazepine, barbiturates, primidone, topiramate, and oxcarbazepine. *[2016 U.S. MEC: 2]*

Studies have supported efficacy through 5 years including one study of 200 women. *[Alimetal 2016]*

MECHANISM OF ACTION

- Within 24 hours of insertion thick cervical mucus prevents normal sperm transport
- Inhibition of ovulation. Effect decreases with prolonged use; however does not result in pregnancy.
- Cause atrophic endometrium

ADVANTAGES

Menstrual: Decreased menstrual and ovulatory cramping or pain; overall, less bleeding than with Norplant and more amenorrhea (15% at one year).

Sexual / psychological:

- Sexual intercourse may be more pleasurable because fear of pregnancy is reduced
- Usage not linked to sexual intercourse—allowing spontaneity

Cancers / tumors / masses: None

Other:

- High continuation rate in clinical trials. Cyclic headaches may improve
- Single implant is easier and faster to insert and remove than multiple implants. Removal is usually accomplished with only a #11 scalpel and gentle finger pressure with < 1.0 cc ml of local anesthetic (use tuberculin syringe)

DISADVANTAGES

Menstrual:

- Unpredictable / irregular menstrual bleeding frequent and may persist but usually is light and well-tolerated
- Amenorrhea and oligomenorrhea common

Sexual / psychological:

- Irregular bleeding may inhibit sexual intercourse

Cancers / tumors / masses: None

Other:

- No STI protection
- Hormonal side effects: headache is most common
- May develop acne (or acne may improve)
- Insertion and removal require procedures and special training

COMPLICATIONS:

- Removal difficulties (although less frequent than with Norplant)
- Rarely, sonographic or MRI localization is required
- Rare infections

CANDIDATES FOR USE:

- Nexplanon is particularly good for women with contraindications to or side effects from estrogen:
  - Women with personal history of thrombosis (U.S. MEC: 2)
  - Recently postpartum women (U.S. MEC: 1)
  - Women who are exclusively breastfeeding, no effects on breast milk or breastfeeding infants (<30 days U.S. MEC: 2, ≥30 days U.S. MEC: 1) *[Reinprayoon 2000] [Taneepanichskul 2005]*
  - Smokers over age 35 (U.S. MEC: 1)
  - Women who had or fear chloasma, hypertriglyceridemia (U.S. MEC: 2) or other estrogen-related side effects
  - Women with hypertension (U.S. MEC: 1, 2)

PRESCRIBING PRECAUTIONS, MEDICAL ELIGIBILITY CHECKLIST, INITIATING METHOD:

Same precautions as for progestin-only pills

INITIATING METHOD:

- If placed within 5 days of LMP, no backup needed. Can be placed any time of cycle if reasonably certain not pregnant. If later than 5 days from LMP, use backup x 7 days
- Switching from IUD: same as DMPA *(see page 142)*

Instructions for Patient: Irregular bleeding is to be expected and persists while rod is in place. If your pattern of bleeding is unacceptable, there are treatments that may make your bleeding pattern more acceptable (periodic COC, patch, ring use). Amenorrhea more likely than with Norplant, but less likely than with DMPA

FOLLOW-UP: Routine GYN follow-up

PROBLEM MANAGEMENT:

Amenorrhea: Pregnancy test if symptoms of pregnancy

Spotting / breakthrough bleeding: to be expected; not harmful. If bothersome may provide several cycles of low-dose pills, patch, rings or NSAIDs

Arm pain after insertion

- Rule out nerve damage or infection
- If due to bruising, advise her to make sure bandage is not too tight
- Apply ice packs for 24 hours
- Take acetaminophen or NSAID

Infection in insertion area

- *No abscess:* cellulitis only. Do not remove, clean infected area with antiseptic. Oral antibiotics for 7 days. (Recheck in 24-48 hours to make sure improving)
- *Abscess:* Preload with antibiotics; prepare infected area with antiseptic, make incision, drain pus, and remove implant. Continue antibiotic therapy and wound care

Difficult to locate rod: may be found by ultrasound or X-ray. This requires experienced sonographer using tranducer of 10 MHz or greater. Rarely, there may be a failure of provider to insert the rod (implant left in inserter)

Fertility After discontinuation of use: Return to baseline fertility is rapid and complete; 94% ovulate within 3-6 weeks of removal

NEXPLANON INSERTION
PREPARATION FROM MANUFACTURER

Prior to placing Nexplanon carefully read the instructions for insertion as well as the full prescribing information.

Before placement of Nexplanon, the healthcare provider should confirm that:

- The woman is not pregnant nor has any other contraindication for the use of Nexplanon
- The woman has had a medical history and physical examination; gynecologic examination not necessary.
- The woman understands the benefits and risks of Nexplanon
- The woman has received a copy of the patient labeling included in packaging
- The woman has reviewed and completed a consent form to be maintained with the woman's chart
- The woman does not have allergies to the antiseptic and anesthetic to be used during insertion.

The following equipment is needed for the implant insertion:

- An examination table for the woman to lie on
- Sterile surgical drapes, sterile gloves, antiseptic solution, sterile marker (optional)
- Local anesthetic, needles and syringe
- Sterile gauze, adhesive bandage, pressure bandage

Placement Procedure

Step 1: Have the woman lie on her back on the examination table with her non-dominant arm flexed at the elbow and externally rotated so that her wrist is parallel to her ear or her hand is positioned next to her head (Figure 1).

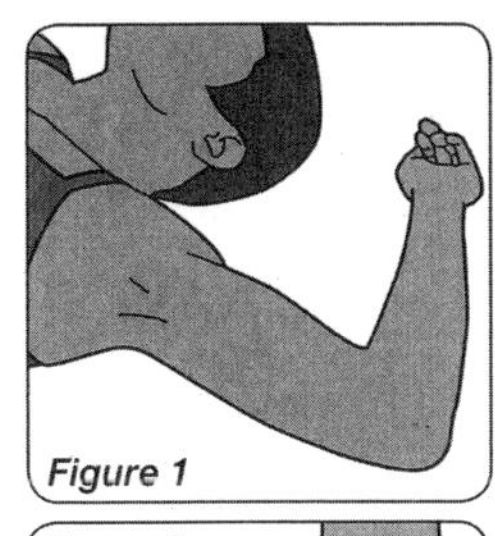
Figure 1

Step 2: Identify the insertion site, which is at the inner side of the non-dominant upper arm about 8-10 cm (3-4 inches) above the medial epicondyle of the humerus (Figure 2). **The implant should be placed subdermally just under the skin to avoid the large blood vessels and nerves that lie deeper in the subcutaneous tissue. The implant should be placed at the level of the triceps muscle, NOT in the sulcus between the biceps and triceps muscles as previously instructed.**

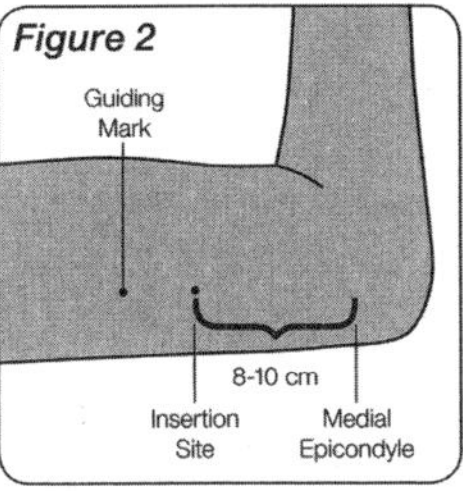

Figure 2

Step 3: Make two marks with a sterile marker: first, mark the spot where the etonogestrel implant will be inserted, and second, mark a spot a few centimeters proximal to the first mark (Figure 2). The second mark will later serve as a direction guide during placement.

Step 4: Clean the insertion site with an antiseptic solution.

Step 5: Anesthetize the insertion area (for example, with anesthetic spray or by injecting 2 mL of 1% lidocaine just under the skin along the planned insertion tunnel).

Step 6: Remove the sterile preloaded disposable Nexplanon applicator carrying the implant from its blister. The applicator should not be used if sterility is in question.

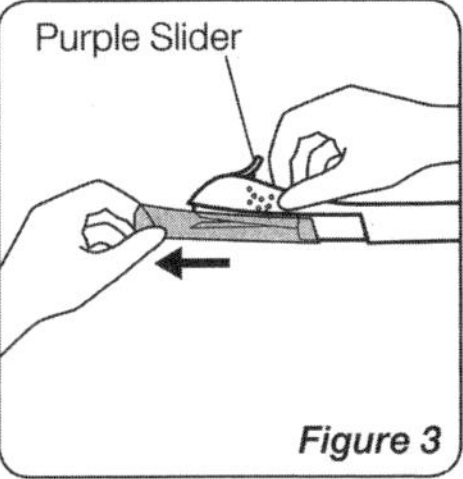

Figure 3

Step 7: Hold the applicator just above the needle at the textured surface area. Remove the transparent protection cap by sliding it horizontally in the direction of the arrow away from the needle (Figure 3). If the cap does not come off easily, the applicator should not be used. You can see the white colored implant by looking into the tip of the needle. Do not touch the purple slider until you have fully inserted the needle subdermally, as it will retract the needle and prematurely release the implant from the applicator.

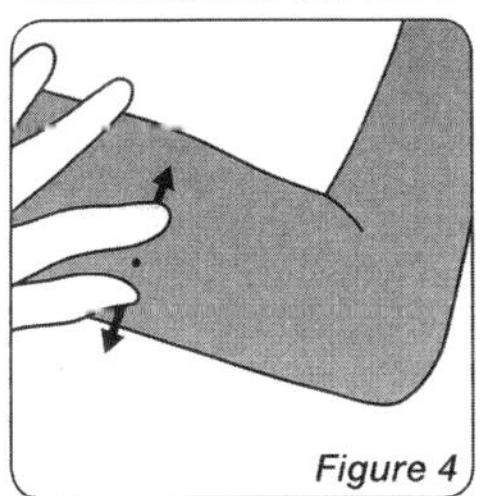
Figure 4

Step 8: With your free hand, stretch the skin around the insertion site with thumb and index finger (Figure 4).

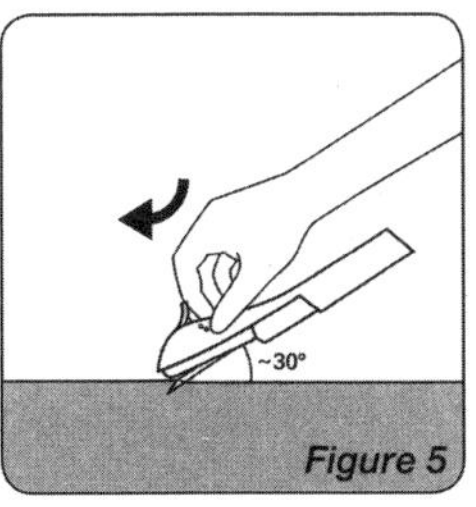

Figure 5

Step 9: Puncture the skin with the tip of the needle angled about 30° (Figure 5).

Step 10: Lower the applicator to a horizontal position. While lifting the skin with the tip of the needle (Figure 6), slide the needle to its full length. You may feel slight resistance but do not exert excessive force. If the needle is not inserted to its full length, the implant will not be placed properly.

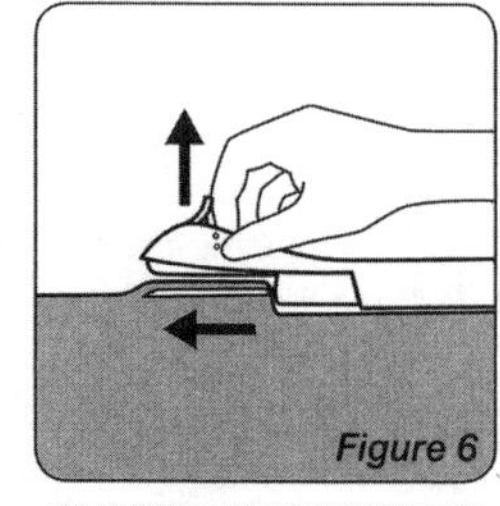
Figure 6

You can best see movement of the needle if you are seated and are looking at the applicator from the side and NOT from above. In this position, you can clearly see the insertion site and the movement of the needle just under the skin.

Step 11: Keep the applicator in the same position with the needle inserted to its full length. If needed, you may use your free hand to keep the applicator in the same position during the following procedure. Unlock the purple slider by pushing it slightly down. Move the slider fully back until it stops (Figure 7). The implant is now in its final subdermal position, and the needle is locked inside the body of the applicator. The applicator can now be removed. If the applicator is not kept in the same position during this procedure or if the purple slider is not completely moved to the back, the implant will not be inserted properly.

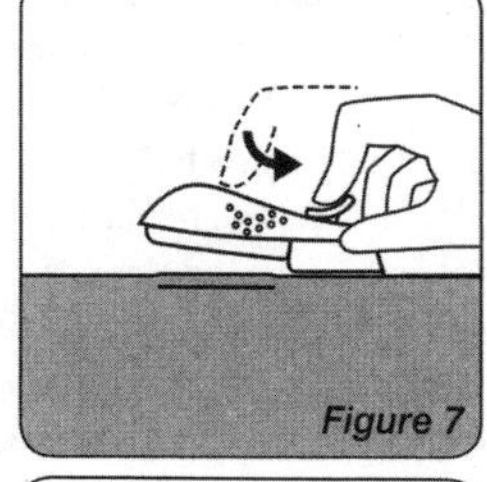
Figure 7

Step 12: Always verify the presence of the implant in the woman's arm immediately after insertion by palpation. By palpating both ends of the implant, you should be able to confirm the presence of the 4 cm rod (Figure 8).

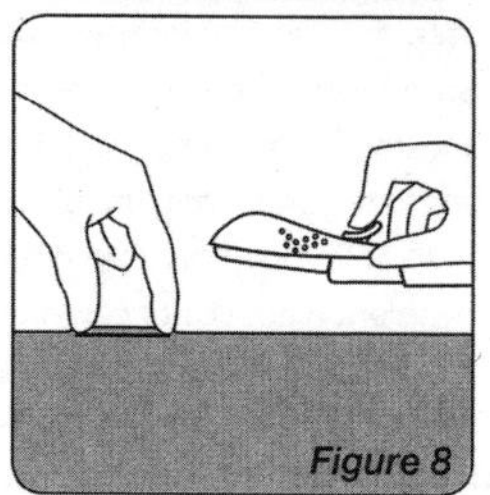
Figure 8

CHAPTER 24

FEMALE STERILIZATION: TUBAL LIGATION OR OCCLUSION

DESCRIPTION: Surgery to remove (salpingectomy) or to interrupt the patency of fallopian tubes. In 2011-2013 in the USA, 44.2% of women aged 35-44 were relying on tubal sterilization for contraception and 18% on their partner's vasectomy *[National Health Statisctics Reports 2015]*. Approximately half of sterilizations in the U.S. are done postpartum, within 48 hours of delivery *[Peterson 1998]*.

EFFECTIVENESS: Failure rates vary depending on sterilization method and patient's age.

Table 24.1 Cumulative 10-year failure rates for some methods of voluntary female sterilization methods*

Method	Failure rate (highest rate)
Postpartum partial salpingectomy	0.8%*
Silastic bands over loop of tube	1.8%*
Interval partial salpingectomy	2.0%*
Bipolar cautery	2.5%*
Spring clip application	3.7%*
Filshie clip (7 years)	0.9%+

For each sterilization method, at least 50% more failures were ascertained AFTER 2 YEARS as had been identified in the 2 years immediately following the sterilization procedure

** U.S. Collaborative Review of Sterilization. The risk of pregnancy after tubal sterilization. Am J Obstet Gynecol 1996;174:1161-70.*

+ Filshie clip (0.9% failure rate - 7 years) [Chi-Chen 1987]

- Younger women had higher failure rates
- All methods require proper application to maximize effectiveness
- Teaching institution rates (above study) may differ from private settings

Hysteroscopic tubal occlusion: No longer available in U.S.

MECHANISM OF ACTION: remove or block fallopian tubes

- Since it is theorized many ovarian cancers originate in the fimbria of the distal fallopian tubes, serious consideration should be given to removal of fallopian tubes by salpingectomy as the tubal sterilization procedure of choice.

LAPAROSCOPIC STERILIZATION: TRANSABDOMINAL

- Enables inspection of abdomen
- Typically performed under general anesthesia
- Risk of organ or vascular injury

Bipolar cautery:

- Apply to at least 3 cm of isthmic portion of the fallopian tube (at least 2 cm from uterotubal junction). Thoroughly cauterize tissue using bipolar cutting current of 25 Watts passing through jaws of instrument. Use of a current meter ensures complete coagulation. Bipolar cautery has the highest risk of subsequent fistualization and ectopic pregnancy.

Silastic band: (Fallope Ring, Yoon Band)

- ***Silicone Band (Fallope Ring):*** apply over knuckle of tube at least 2 cm from utero-tubal junction. Loop of banded tube should clearly contain two complete diameters of tube
- ***Spring-loaded clip (Hulka-Clemens):*** Apply to isthmic portion of tube. 1-2 cm distal to cornu at an angle of 90% relative to long axis of tube. Destroys <1 cm tissue. Highest failure rate

Filshie clip:

- Hinged titanium clip with cured silicone rubber lining. Apply to isthmic portion of tube, 1 to 2 cm from cornu. Destroys 5mm tube. Should see hook end of clip through filmy mesosalpinx. May apply postpartum with special applicator (0.9% failure vs. 0.4% failure for interval application) *[Penfield 2000]*

Figure 24.1 Laparoscopic Technique Diagrams

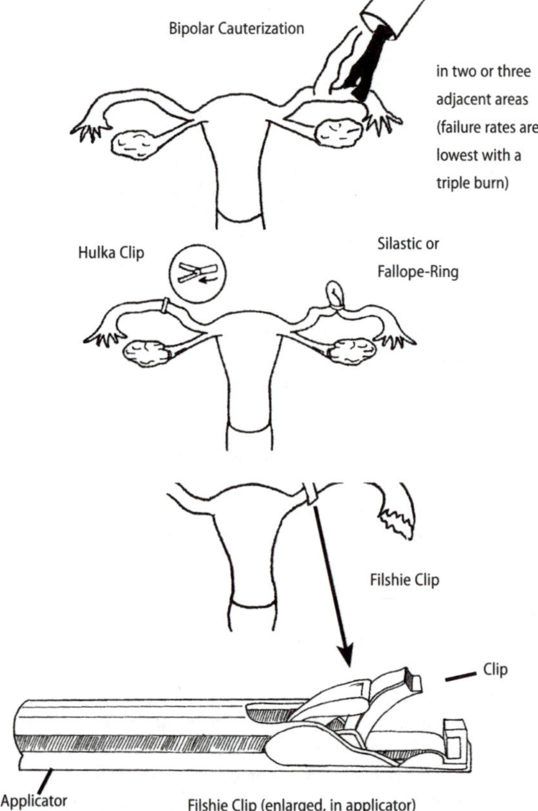

POSTPARTUM OR INTERVAL MINI-LAPAROTOMY METHODS

Modified Pomeroy:

- Ligation at the base of a loop of isthmic portion of tube with plain absorbable catgut suture (2 separate ties) followed by excision of the knuckle of tube. Segment is histologically confirmed to contain tubal ostia.

Modified Parkland:

- Excision of segment of isthmic portion of tube after separate ligation of cut ends, no "knuckle" formed

Irving, Uchida and Fimbriectomy are rarely performed

Figure 24.2

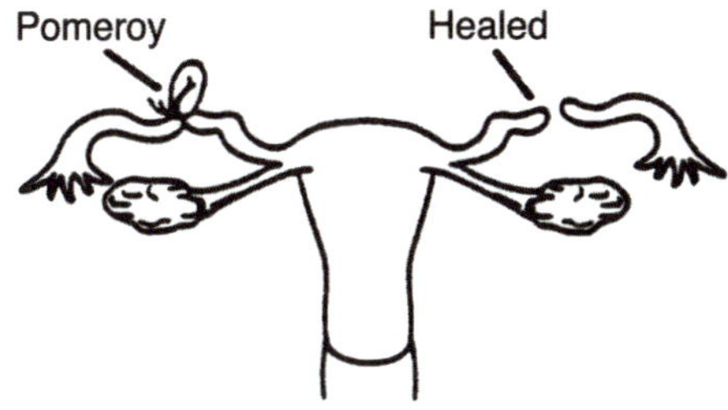

ADVANTAGES

Menstrual: None

Sexual / psychological: Enhanced enjoyment of sex by reducing worry of pregnancy

Cancers / tumors / masses:

- Decreased risk of ovarian cancer. Women with BRCA 1 mutations who have undergone a tubal ligation have a 60% lower risk of developing invasive ovarian cancer. *[Narod 2001]*. Overall 40% reduction in risk of ovarian cancer. ***Salpingectomy may be the best procedure to reduce a women's risk of ovarian cancer.***

Other:

- Permanent and highly effective

DISADVANTAGES

Menstrual:

- Reported "tubal ligation syndrome" includes changes in menstrual pattern or pain, however, data from 9,514 women who underwent tubal sterilization by 6 techniques and followed for up to 5 years suggest no increases in the amount or duration of menstrual bleeding or menstrual pain. *[Peterson 2000]*

Sexual / psychological:

- Regret may occur especially with young patients; counsel well and offer reversible methods if any hesitancy *(see Fig. 24.3, page 159)*

Cancers / tumors / masses: None

Other:

- Requires outpatient surgery (usually with general anesthesia); expensive in short term
- If failure occurs, higher risk of ectopic pregnancy (30%)
- Not readily reversible
- Does not prevent spread of HIV and STIs
- Obstacles to performing postpartum sterilization prevent 50% of women from getting procedure.
    - As many as 17% of these women will have an unintended pregnancy within a year *[ACOG 2013]*

COMPLICATIONS *[Peterson 1997]*

	Minilaparotomy	Laparoscopy
Minor	11.6%	6.0%
Major	1.5%	0.1-3.5%

- Minor complications include infection, wound separation
- Major complications include conversion to laparotomy, hemorrhage, viscus injury especially with cautery, anesthetic complications
- Major vessel injury risk with laparoscopy 3-9/10,000 procedures
- Mortality: 1-2/100,000 procedures (leading cause is general anesthesia)

LONG-TERM RISKS

- Statistically higher risk for subsequent hysterectomy, but only in women who had gynecologic complaints prior to sterilization
- Regret (0.9% - 26.0%). Risk factors include: age under 30, low parity, sterilization at time of cesarean delivery, change in marital status, poverty, minority status, misinformation about permanence or risks, hurried decision. If sterilized < 30 years old, 40% requested information on reversal, 20% expressed regret but only 1% had a reversal done *[Schmidt 2000]*. This issue requires careful counseling

CANDIDATES FOR USE

- Woman who is certain she wants no more children
- Woman over age 21 (only required for Medicaid reimbursement, not for medical requirements or for California state funding)
- Woman for whom surgery is considered safe

Adolescents: Not a preferred method, generally higher regret and higher failure rates

COMPONENTS OF PRESTERILIZATION COUNSELING

- Permanent nature of procedure, not intended to be reversible
- Alternative methods available, esp. LARC and vasectomy
  - Vasectomy is safer, more effective and less expensive
  - LARC as effective, reversible, and have less morbidity and mortality
- Procedural details including risks / benefits of anesthesia
- Possibility of failure and risk of ectopic pregnancy
- Need for condoms for protection from STIs and HIV
- Complete informed consent process
- Local regulations regarding waiting period between consent and procedure. Consider gauging patient interest earlier on during pregnancy to allow for consideration and forms.

**Adapted from ACOG Technical Bulletin, Benefits and Risks, No. 208, February 2013.*

INITIATING METHOD

- Obtain informed consent.
- Any time in cycle with certainty of no conception, otherwise follicular timing preferred.
- The routine provision of antibiotics is generally NOT recommended *[see ACOG Practice Bulletin No. 23, January, 2001]*

FOLLOW-UP

- For women having interval occlusion procedure, follow up in two weeks for post-op wound check is typical. Routine annual gynecology exams

MANAGEMENT OF PROBLEMS

- Anesthesia complications, wound infections, intraperitoneal adhesion formation, hydrosalpinx – managed with standard approaches
- Although some women report irregular menses or dysmenorrhea after tubal sterilization, several studies have demonstrated that a syndrome of irregular menses or dysmenorrhea following tubal sterilization does NOT exist *[Peterson 2000]*. These problems are not apt to develop at any higher rates in sterilized women. They are most likely age-related or related to discontinuation of prior hormonal method that controlled bleeding and pain.

Although the Essure female sterilization system is no longer marketed, individuals may present with Essure in place. Consult www.essure.com for information about management of problems or removal of Essure coils.

FERTILITY AFTER TUBAL STERILIZATION

- Women must desire to be permanently sterile because reversal is costly and results are unpredictable. In vitro fertilization may be possible, but many cannot afford this procedure and it is not always successful

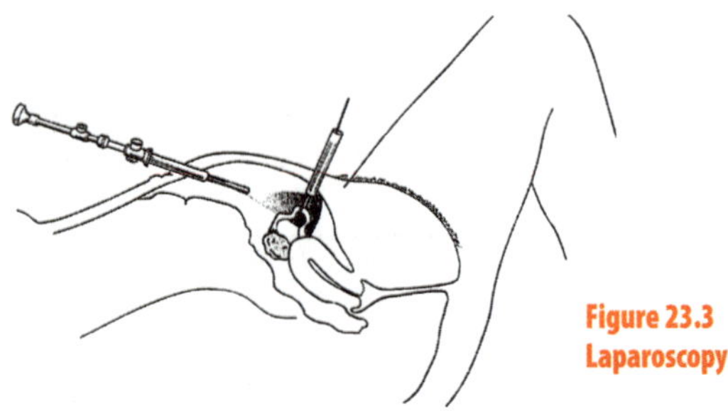

Figure 23.3 Laparoscopy

Five methods of birth control that appear to protect a woman from ovarian cancer:

1. Combined birth control pills
2. Progestin-only birth control pills
3. Depo-Provera injections
4. Tubal sterilization by ligation, clips, burning or removal of a segment of the fallopian tubes
5. Tubal sterilization by salpingectomy (complete removal of the tubes and fimbria)

Figure 24.3 Sterilization Requested by Young Woman

Inform that risk of regret following tubal sterilization is higher if individual is:

- Young
- Unmarried (single, separated or divorced)
- Unmarried now but is married later on, especially if new partner wants a child with her
- Married now but becomes divorced later
- On Medicaid or low income
- African-American or Latinx
- After the end of a pregnancy (postpartum, post-therapeutic abortion or post-miscarriage)
- Thinking that tubal sterilization is easy to reverse (it is both very expensive and only about 60% effective).

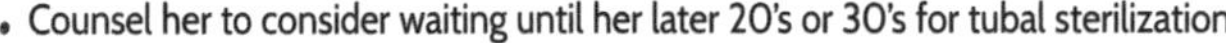

- Counsel her to consider waiting until her later 20's or 30's for tubal sterilization
- Offer use of effective long-term reversible contraceptive
- Be sure client knows that the final decision is hers to make, not yours or her partner's
- Ask if partner is interested in vasectomy

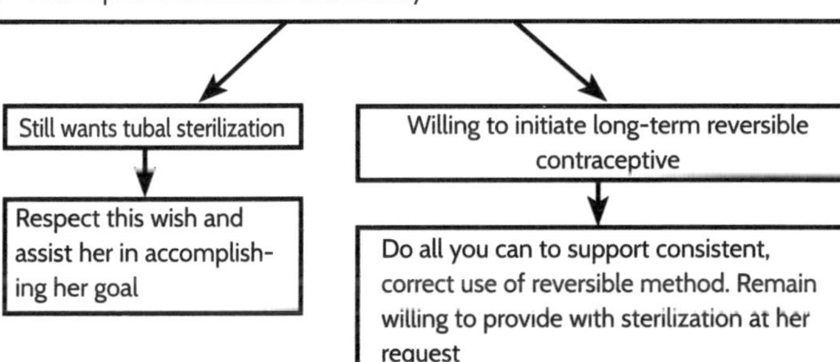

CHAPTER 25

MALE STERILIZATION: VASECTOMY

DESCRIPTION:

- Quick, outpatient surgical procedure in which the vas deferens, which carry the sperm from the testicles to the urethra, are disrupted on both sides.
- Considered a permanent method
- Among married men aged 15-44, 13.1% report having had a vasectomy
- Fourth most common birth control method
- Commonly performed by urologists.

> Although vasectomy is safer and potentially more effective than tubal sterilization, as of mid-2000, there are only 4 nations in the world where vasectomies exceeded tubal sterilizations: Great Britain, the Netherlands, New Zealand and Bhutan

EFFECTIVENESS *(See Table 2.1, page 9)*

Typical use failure rate in first year: 0.15%
Perfect use failure rate in first year: 0.10%
[Trussell 2018]

ADVANTAGES

Sexual / psychological:

- Sexual intercourse may be more enjoyable because fear of pregnancy decreased
- Frequency of intercourse is increased in half or more of patients and decreased in only 5% of men *[Smith 2010][Shain in Goldsmith 1986][Hofmeyer 2002]*
- No interference with sexual intercourse and no contraceptive burden for female partner

Cancers / tumors / masses: None

Other:

- Simpler, safer (only 0.5 deaths per 100,000 patients) and more effective than female sterilization
- Shares contraception responsibility with partner
- No supplies or further clinic visits needed after sperm count documented to be zero
- Only local anesthesia required

DISADVANTAGES: Not effective immediately. Approximately 25% to 50% of failures occur during time after surgery but before sperm are cleared.

Sexual / psychological:

- Some men resist vasectomy fearing that it will interfere with sexual function (it doesn't) or because they feel contraception is solely the woman's responsibility (it should not be)
- Will need back-up method until there are no motile sperm. Female partner may still need contraception if she has other partner(s) or needs STI protection
- Regret at a later time possible: up to 20% of men who have had a vasectomy end up desiring children in the future, and 2% of men have reversal procedure done.

Cancers / tumors / masses: None

Other:

- Does not reduce risk for STIs; condoms necessary for at-risk partners
- Short-term post-operative discomfort, bruising, and swelling
- May require legal paperwork prepared in advance depending on state sterilization laws

COMPLICATIONS

- Hematoma, bruising, wound infection, or adverse reaction to local anesthesia
- Severe chronic pain (1-2%) *[Valcencic 2003]*. Pain usually responds to prostaglandin inhibitors. Pain usually limited to less than 1 year. Pain may start months or years after operation. A vasectomy reversal likely improves pain in medication-refractory cases.

CANDIDATES FOR USE: Men / couples who desire a permanent method

INITIATING METHOD

- Take preoperative history; make general health assessment
- Ask if history of genital infections or anomalies
- Obtain informed consent. In general, try to involve partner
- Carefully counsel, especially about permanence of method
- Advise patient to bathe genital area and upper thighs prior to surgery; wear clean, loose-fitting clothes to facility; no food for 2 hours before procedure
- Patients should consult their doctors about the risks and benefits of avoiding aspirin, NSAIDs, and blood-thinners the week before the procedure.
- Scrotal support for at least 2 days. Avoid ejaculation for 1 week; avoid strenuous activity for 1 week.

PRECAUTIONS

- Current infection of penis, prostate, or scrotum
- Fear of needles or scalpels (scalpels not required if no-scalpel vasectomy)

INSTRUCTIONS FOR PATIENT

- Plan to rest for 48 hours and wear scrotal support
- Apply ice pack to incision site to decrease swelling, pain and bruising. Small packages of frozen peas conform well around the scrotum
- Keep area dry for two days – wear snug underwear and pants to provide support where needed
- If any symptoms or signs of infection develop, seek help immediately.
- Return as directed for sperm counts. Over 80% of men are azoospermic after 20 ejaculations and 3 months. If there are still sperm present at 3-month follow-up, check again within 2 months.
- The American Urological Association guidelines recommend stopping additional contraceptive back-up methods when a semen specimen shows azoospermia or only rare nonmotile sperm .
- If motile sperm are found 6 months post-operatively, the vasectomy should be considered a failure and repeat vasectomy should be considered

PROBLEM MANAGEMENT

Wound infection: Treat with antibiotics. Drain and treat any abscesses

Hematoma: Apply warm moist packs to scrotum. Provide scrotal support

Granuloma: Observe; usually it will resolve itself. Occasionally requires surgery

Pain at site: If no infection, provide scrotal support and analgesics

Chronic persistent pain considered to be severe: 1-2% First line treatment with NSAIDs. Vasovasostomy or reversal can be considered for refractory pain.

FERTILITY AFTER VASECTOMY

- Patient must accept that vasectomy is permanent at time of consent; however, reversal is often possible.
- Microsurgical techniques of reversal now result in return of sperm to ejaculate in over 90% of men, but in pregnancy rates of only 50% or above. Successful reversal rates decrease as time since procedure increases
- Factors that may have an effect on success of conception after reversal:
  - skill of microsurgeon
  - length of time since vasectomy
  - presence of antisperm antibodies (man)
  - partner's fertility
  - manner in which vasectomy was performed (amount of vas removed or cauterized)

CHAPTER 26

ORDERING AND STOCKING DEVICES: LILETTA, NEXPLANON, MIRENA / SKYLA / KYLEENA, PARAGARD

ORDERING AND STOCKING DEVICES: Telephone numbers below are for ordering devices, speaking with customer service, reporting adverse events.

LILETTA

- Call 1-855-Liletta to order, www.Liletta.com
- Most specialty pharmacies have Liletta on formulary
- No special training is required to order. You can request training at https://www.lilettahcp.com
- Covered as either a medical (both IUD and procedure are covered) or pharmacy (only IUD is covered) benefit
- Replacement policy can be found at: *https://www.lilettaaccessconnect.com/#resources/!ResourceSupport/Replacement*

NEXPLANON

- Call 877-467-5266 to order Nexplanon; www.nexplanon.com for information and ordering and https://www.organonconnect.com/nexplanon/dosing-administration/ for training.
- Nexplanon dispensed by three pharmacies: CuraScript, TheraCom and CVS Caremark
- To set up account, need state license number and DEA number
- Pharmacy verifies that health care provider (HCP) has attended a company sponsored Implanon or Nexplanon training program
- Nexplanon is usually a "medical benefit"; sometimes a pharmacy benefit
- If Nexplanon contaminated prior to insertion or touching the patient, there is no replacement by the company.
- Out-of-pocket cost for Nexplanon averages at $981.56. However, most people with private insurance, Medicare or Medicaid will receive it for free.
- You can request training on how to insert Nexplanon from this webpage *http://www.nexplanon-usa.com/en/hcp/services-and-support/request-training/index.asp*

MIRENA / SKYLA / KYLEENA

- Call 1-866-647-3646, www.mirena-us.com
- To set up an account, clinician needs license. Bayer verifies that the HCP has been trained. If not, a training kit will be included in the order
- Verify insurance coverage
- Clinicians can order through CVS Caremark at www.whcsupport.com/documents/PP-290-US-0345_SP_Prescription_Request.pdf or by calling 1-866-638-8312. Clinicians fax prescription and CVS Caremark determines insurance eligibility and calls patient to confirm out-of-pocket costs. The Mirena is shipped to HCP

- If no coverage, patients can pay by credit card with Mirena shipped to HCP.
- If Mirena is contaminated upon insertion, or removed early for a medical reason, no general replacement policy exists. However, by calling the hotline or their Bayer sales consultant, they will consider each event on a case-by-case basis.
- ***Cost of Mirena*** if no insurance: $999 (single payment). 95% of patients with commercial insurance will receive a Mirena for free
- ***Cost of Skyla*** if no insurance: $650-780

PARAGARD

- Call 1-877-727-2427, *www.Paragard.com*
- To set up an account, a clinician needs a state license number
- Verify patient insurance coverage prior to insertion
- If no coverage, patients can pay by credit card / Paragard shipped to HCP
- Replacement policy: If a clinician contaminates the IUD prior to touching the patient (e.g., drops on floor), call the hotline within 7 days AND save the product to ship back to them. They will send a replacement.
- If the woman has the Paragard removed for a medical reason within 90 days (and reported within 30 days of removal) they will replace the product if the patient desires. If patient paid for IUD – she will be reimbursed. If she paid and is not satisfied with the IUD, she can get a full refund within the first 150 days
- ***Cost*** of IUD if no insurance: $754-$900. Most patients with commercial insurance will receive a Parapard for free

CHAPTER 27

SEXUALLY TRANSMITTED INFECTIONS (STIs)

2021 CDC GUIDELINES FOR TREATMENT*

Since women and men seeking contraceptives are also at risk for sexually transmitted infections, below are recommendations excerpted from the 2021 CDC guidance. Consult the CDC website for more information.

CLINICAL PREVENTION GUIDELINES

STIs are on a rise in the United States. The 2019 STI Surveillance Report documented significant increases in reported STIs between 2015 and 2019 (increased chlamydia by 20%, gonorrhea by 50%, and syphilis by 70%). It is still unknown how the COVID-19 pandemic will affect these rates. Highly concerning are the growing reports of antibiotic resistant STIs and a resurgence of syphilis.

Also troubling are health disparities. Racial and ethnic minorities had STI rates several times higher thane whites, and youth (15-21 y/o) comprised significant proportions of cases across all groups. Gay, bisexual and other MSM have higher rates of syphilis and gonorrhea than heterosexual men.

The prevention and control of STIs are based on the following five major strategies:

- Accurate risk assessment and education and counseling of persons at risk on ways to avoid STIs through changes in sexual behaviors and use of recommended prevention services
- Pre-exposure immunization for vaccine preventable STIs
- Identification of asymptomatically infected persons and persons with symptoms associated with STIs
- Effective diagnosis, treatment, counseling, and follow up of infected persons
- Evaluation, treatment, and counseling of sex partners of persons who are infected with an STI

For complete guidelines, see the CDC STI website

Prevention Methods

A new condom should be used for each sex act (oral, vaginal or anal)

- ***Male Condoms***
  - Used consistently and correctly, latex condoms are effective in preventing the transmission of HIV infection and reduce the risk for other STIs
  - Polyurethane condoms provide comparable protection against STIs / HIV and pregnancy to latex condoms
  - Use only water-based lubricants with latex condoms
- ***Female Condoms***
  - Female condoms can provide protection from acquisition or transmission of STIs, although data are limited
  - Although more costly, this method offers the advantage of being controlled by the receptive partner
- ***Condoms and Spermicides***
  - Condoms lubricated with spermicides are no more effective than other lubricated condoms in protecting against HIV and STIs
  - Vaginal spermicides containing N-9 do not protect against HIV and STIs and have been associated with increased risk of HIV infection
- ***Nonbarrier Contraception, Surgical Sterilization, and Hysterectomy***
  - Non-barrier contraception offer no protection against HIV or other STIs. The ECHO study observed no difference in HIV incidence rates among women randomly assigned to DMPA, LNG-implant or TCu 380A
  - Women who use hormonal or intrauterine contraception, have been surgically sterilized, or have had hysterectomies should still be counseled about HIV / STI protection
- Male circumcision has been shown to reduce the risk for HIV and some STIs in heterosexual men
- Post exposure prophylaxis (PEP) may reduce HIV and STI risk after sexual exposure
- Antiretroviral therapy for persons infected with HIV can prevent HIV infection in partners. An exposed individual or clinician can call the Postexposure Prophylaxis Hotline: 1-888-448-4911
- Preexposure prophylaxis (PrEP) is effective at reducing the risk of HIV infection among uninfected individuals. U.S. Public Health Service recommends TDF/FTC for PrEP among individuals who are at high-risk for HIV through sexual activity or injection drug use. Comprehensive guidance on PrEP can be found at www.cdc.gov/hiv/risk/prep/

SPECIAL POPULATIONS

Detailed guidelines are available in the CDC STI treatment guidelines for specific screening recommendations for persons in correction facilities, men who have sex with men, women who have sex with women, transgender men and women. As many of these populations are diverse, it is imperative to focus on the specific sexual history and risk behaviors and symptoms of the individual and target counseling and treatment accordingly.

Pregnant Women

- ***Recommended Screening Tests***
- ***Syphilis:*** all pregnant women at first prenatal visit; high risk (high areas of syphilis morbidity) retested at 28 weeks and at delivery. Some states require all women to be screened at delivery
- ***Hepatitis B surface antigen (HbsAg):*** all pregnant women first visit. HbsAg-positive pregnant women should be reported to the local and / or state health department; household and sexual contacts of HbsAg-positive women should be tested and immunized it negative
- ***Neisseria gonorrhea:*** first visit for women at risk or living in an area of high prevalence
- ***Chlamydia trachomatis:*** all women at first prenatal visit and in the third trimester for women at increased risk (i.e., women aged <25 years and women who have a new or more than one sex partner or whose partner has other partners)
- HIV screening test: encouraged for all pregnant women as routine prenatal test at the first prenatal visit. If high risk retest in 3rd trimester before 36 weeks
- Bacterial vaginosis (BV) and Trichomonas vaginalis: Only symptomatic women. Current evidence does not support universal testing for BV
- ***Papanicolaou (Pap) smear:*** Test at same frequency as non-pregnant women / management differs
- Hepatitis C antibodies at the first prenatal visit for women at high risk (intravenous drug users, blood transfusions, organ transplant)
- ***HSV:*** In the absence of lesions during the third trimester, routine serial culture for herpes simplex virus (HSV) is not indicated for women who have a history of recurrent genital herpes. Prophylactic cesarean section is not indicated for women who do not have active genital lesions at the time of delivery. The presence of genital warts is not an indication for cesarean delivery unless size obstructs delivery in labor (rare)

Adolescents

- With limited exceptions, all U.S. adolescents can consent to the confidential diagnosis and treatment of STIs.
- All male and female children and adolescents along with females up to 26 years old should get the HPV vaccine
- Health-care providers who care for adolescents should integrate sexuality education into clinical practice. Providers should counsel about sexual behavior associated with STIs and educate on evidence-based strategies. USPSTF recommends high-intensity behavioral counseling for all sexually active adolescents to prevent STIs.

Transgender Women

- High incidence of HIV (27.7% among all TW and 56.3% among black TW)
- Be sure to understand whether the patient has had bottom surgery to give more effective counseling

DISEASES CHARACTERIZED BY GENITAL ULCERS

Management of Patients Who Have Genital Ulcers

- In the United States, most young, sexually active patients who have genital ulcers have genital herpes or syphilis, although an ulcer may have more than one organism. Ulcerative infections have been associated with an increased risk for HIV infection and transmission
- The evaluation of all patients who have genital ulcers should include :
  1. Syphilis serology and darkfield examination from lesion or NAAT if available
  2. NAAT or culture for herpes type 1 or 2 AND
  3. Serology testing for HSV
- In areas where chancroid is prevalent, obtain NAAT or culture for Haemophilus ducreyi.
- HIV testing should be performed in all persons with an ulcer who are not already known to have HIV.
- The clinician should administer treatment based on a presumptive diagnosis according to clinical presentation

CHANCROID (SHAN-kroyd)

Organism: H. ducreyi

Presents with: ulcers and tender, suppurative inguinal adenopathy

Diagnosis: Culture on special medium of H. ducreyi, or if all of the following criteria are met: ***a)*** patient has 1 or more painful ulcers; ***b)*** no evidence of syphilis on lab exam after at least 7 days after the appearance of ulcers; ***c)*** the clinical picture is typical of chancroid and d) test for HSV is negative.

Treatment: Recommended Regimens

Azithromycin.............................1 g orally in a single dose, OR
Ceftriaxone ....250 mg intramuscularly (IM) in a single dose, OR
Ciprofloxacin ....500 mg orally twice a day for 3 days, OR
Erythromycin base.................500 mg orally three times a day for 7 days.

Follow-up: Re-examine in 3-7 days. If no improvement consider whether a) the diagnosis is correct, b) the patient is coinfected with another STI, c)the patient is infected with HIV, d) the treatment was not taken as instructed, or e) the H. ducreyi strain causing the infection is resistant to the prescribed antimicrobial. Patients with HIV are more likely to experience treatment failure and require repeated or longer antibiotic courses.

- The time required for complete healing:
  - Depends on the size of the ulcer; large ulcers may require >2 weeks
  - Healing is slower for some uncircumcised men who have ulcers under the foreskin
  - Resolution of fluctuant lymphadenopathy is slower than that of ulcers and may require drainage, even during otherwise successful therapy
  - Although needle aspiration of buboes is a simpler procedure, incision and drainage of buboes may be preferred because of less need for subsequent drainage procedures

Management of Sex Partners: Should be examined and treated regardless of symptoms if they had sexual contact within 10 days of the onset of symptoms

Special Considerations: Pregnancy. Ciprofloxacin is low risk to the fetus during pregnancy but has potential for toxicity during breastfeeding. No adverse effects of chancroid on pregnancy outcome or on the fetus have been reported.

GENITAL HERPES SIMPLEX VIRAL (HSV) INFECTION (Her-pes)

HSV is a common, chronic, life-long infection. Most persons shed the virus intermittently and are unaware that they are infected and are asymptomatic at the time of transmission.

Organisms: HSV-1 and HSV-2

Diagnosis: Painful multiple vesicular or ulcerative lesions are common for those presenting with HSV, however these symptoms may be absent in infected individuals. Recurrences and subclinical shedding are more common for HSV-2.

- If genital lesions present, perform type specific testing from lesion using culture or NAAT
- Type specific serology can be done in absence of lesions
- All persons with HSV should be tested for HIV
- PCR is test of choice for systemic infections, not for genital herpes

Counseling: Counseling of these patients should include the following:

- Patients should be advised to abstain from sexual activity when lesions or prodromal symptoms are present and encouraged to inform their sex partners
- Latex condoms, when used consistently and correctly, can reduce but not eliminate the risk for genital herpes
- Sexual transmission of HSV can occur during asymptomatic periods
- Daily use of valacyclovir can reduce transmission among persons without HIV
- The risk for neonatal infection should be explained to all patients, including men. Childbearing-aged women who have genital herpes should be advised to inform healthcare providers who care for them during pregnancy about the HSV infection
- Risk of neonatal HSV is low except when genital herpes is acquired late in pregnancy or if prodrome or lesions are present at delivery
- Patients having a first episode of genital herpes should be advised that a) Episodic antiviral therapy during recurrent episodes might shorten the duration of lesions and b) Suppressive antiviral therapy can prevent recurrent outbreaks
- Patients may be directed to websites such as: *http://www.ashasexualhealth.org*

Treatment: Clinical recurrences and subclinical shedding are much less frequent for HSV-1 than HSV-2 genital infection

HSV, Recommended Regimens for First Clinical Infection*

Acyclovir........................ 400 mg orally three times a day for 7-10 days, OR
Famciclovir..................... 250 mg orally three times a day for 7-10 days, OR
Valacyclovir.................... 1.0 g orally twice a day for 7-10 days

**Treatment can be extended if healing incomplete after 10 days.*

**Acyclovir 200 mg orally five times a day for 7-10 days (is effective but not recommended because of the frequency of dosing)

HSV, Recommended Regimens for Episodic Therapy for Recurrent HSV-2 Genital Herpes Infection

Acyclovir........................ 800 mg orally twice a day for 5 days, OR
Acyclovir........................ 800 mg orally three times a day for 2 days, OR
Famciclovir..................... 125 mg orally twice a day for 5 days, OR
Famciclovir..................... 1000 mg orally twice a day for 1 day, OR
Famciclovir..................... 500 mg orally once followed by 250 mg twice daily for 2 days,

OR

Valacyclovir..................... 500 mg orally twice a day for 3 days
Valacyclovir..................... 1.0 g orally once a day for 5 days

HSV, Recommended Regimens for Daily Suppressive Therapy for Recurrent HSV-2 Genital Herpes

Acyclovir.......................... 400 mg orally twice a day, OR
Famciclovir..................... 250 mg orally twice a day, OR
Valacyclovir..................... 500 mg orally once a day, OR
Valacyclovir..................... 1.0 g orally once a day

- Famciclovir somewhat less effective for suppression of viral shedding

Severe Disease: IV therapy should be provided for patients who have severe disease or complications necessitating hospitalization, such as disseminated infection, pneumonitis, hepatitis, or complications of the central nervous system (e.g., meningitis or encephalitis)

- ***HSV, Recommended Regimen for Persons with Severe Disease***

Acyclovir.......................... 5-10 mg/kg body weight IV every 8 hours until clinical resolution is attained followed by high dose oral therapy to complete 10 days total therapy

Special Considerations for HSV:

- ***HIV:*** patients taking antiretroviral therapy generally have fewer outbreaks
  - Immunocompromised patients can have prolonged or severe episodes of genital, perianal or oral herpes.
  - Recommended Regimens for Episodic Infection in Persons with HIV:
    Acyclovir................... 400 mg orally three times a day for 5-10 days, OR
    Famciclovir .... 500 mg orally twice a day for 5-10, OR
    Valacyclovir .... 1 g orally twice a day for 5-10 days
  - Recommended Regimens for Daily Suppressive Therapy in Persons with HIV:
    Acyclovir................... 400-800 mg orally twice to three times a day, OR
    Famciclovir .... 500 mg orally twice a day, OR
    Valacyclovir .... 500 mg orally twice a day,
- ***Antiviral-resistant HSV***
  - Clinical management remains challenging and should be done in consultation with an infectious disease specialist
- ***Pregnancy***
- All pregnant women should be asked if they have a history of genital herpes. Available data does not indicate an increased risk for major birth defects in women treated with acyclovir
- Suppressive acyclovir treatment late in pregnancy reduces the frequency of cesarean delivery among women with recurrent infection
- Recommended Regimens for Daily Suppressive Therapy in pregnant women with recurrent genital herpes*:
  Acyclovir....................... 400 mg orally three times a day, OR
  Valacyclovir................. 500 mg orally twice a day,

** Treatment recommended starting at 36 weeks gestation*

- ***Perinatal Infection***
  - The risk for transmission to the neonate from an infected mother is high (30% - 50%) among women who acquire genital herpes near the time of delivery and is low (<1%) among women who have a history of recurrent herpes at term and women who acquire genital HSV during the first half of pregnancy
  - Therefore, prevention of neonatal herpes should emphasize prevention of acquisition of genital HSV infection during late pregnancy
  - Susceptible women whose partners have oral or genital HSV infection, should be counseled to avoid unprotected genital and oral sexual contact during late pregnancy
  - At the onset of labor, all women should be examined and carefully questioned about whether they have symptoms of HSV. Infants of women who do not have symptoms or signs of HSV infection or its prodrome may be delivered vaginally
  - Cesarean delivery does not completely eliminate the risk for HSV infection in the neonate but is recommended in presence of any lesions (even recurrent)

GRANULOMA INGUINALE (DONOVANOSIS) (gran-u-LO-ma in-gwi-NAL-e, don-o-van-O-sis)

Organism: Klebsiella granulomatis, formerly known as Calymmatobacterium granulomatis, is an intracellular, gram-negative bacterium. It is seen rarely in the USA. Presents as a painless, slowly progressive, vascular, ulcerative lesion without regional lymphadenopathy. Subcutaneous granulomas (pseudobuboes) might occur.

Diagnosis: Visualization of Donovan bodies from tissue of lesion or biopsy

Treatment: Appears to halt progressive destruction of tissue. Prolonged duration of therapy often required to enable granulation and re-epithelialization of the ulcers. Therapy should be continued at least 3 weeks and until all lesions have healed completely. Relapse can occur 6-18 months after apparently effective treatment

- ***Granuloma Inguinale, Recommended Regimens***

  Azithromycin 1 g orally per week or 500 mg daily for at least 3 weeks and until all lesions healed.
- ***Granuloma Inguinale, Alternative Regimens: all for at least 3 weeks and until all lesions healed***

  Doxycycline ....100 mg orally twice a day, OR
  Erythromycin base ....500 mg orally four times a day, OR
  Trimethoprim- sulfamethoxazole.......One double-strength tablet orally twice a day

NOTE: For any of the above regimens, the addition of another antibiotic should be considered if lesions do not respond within the first few days of therapy. Pregnant women should be treated with macrolide (erythromycin or azithromycin).

- All persons should be tested for HIV
- Sexual partners within 60 days before onset should be examined and offered therapy

LYMPHOGRANULOMA VENEREUM (LGV) (lim-fo-gran-u-LO-ma ve-nar-E-um)

This is most frequently manifested in heterosexuals as unilateral tender inguinal and / or femoral lymphadenopathy. Rectal exposure can result in proctocolitis, mimicking inflammatory bowel disease with mucoid and / or hemorrhagic discharge, pain, constipation, fever and / or tenesmus. If untreated, LGV proctocolitis can lead to colorectal fistulas or strictures

Organism: Invasive strains L1, L2, or L3 of Chlamydia trachomatis

Diagnosis: NAATs for C. trachomatis at the symptomatic site, along with exclusion of other etiologies. NAAT can detect both LGV strains and non-LGV strains of c. trachomatis.

Treatment: Presumptive treatment should be started at initial visit. Treatment cures infection and prevents ongoing tissue damage, although tissue reaction can result in scarring. Buboes may require aspiration through intact skin or incision and drainage to prevent the formation of inguinal / femoral ulcerations.

- ***LGV, Recommended Regimen***
  Doxycycline.......................... 100 mg orally twice a day for 21 days OR
- ***Alternative Regimen***
  Erythromycin base.............. 500 mg orally four times a day for 21 days OR
  Azithromycin.......................... 1 gm orally once weekly for 3 weeks*
- Persons with LGV diagnosis should be tested for HIV, gonorrhea, and syphilis and retested for chlamydia in 3 months. Sexual partners within 60 days should be evaluated and tested for chlamydia. Asymptomatic partners should be presumptively treated for chlamydia.
  **This treatment has not been validated so a test of cure 4 weeks after treatment can be considered*

SYPHILIS (SIF-i-lis)

Organism: Treponema pallidum (tre-po-NE-ma PAL-e-dum)

Diagnosis: Darkfield exams from exudate are definitive. A presumptive diagnosis of syphilis requires use of two tests: a nontreponemal test (i.e. VDRL or RPR) and a treponemal test (i.e. FTA-ABS, TP-PA, various immunoassays, chemiluminescence immunoassays, immunoblots or rapid treponemal assays). Use of only one type of test is insufficient and can result in false-negative results in persons during primary syphilis and false-positive results in persons without syphilis. Nontreponemal test antibody titers correlate with disease activity and are used to follow treatment response. For further detail, see CDC guidelines.

Treatment:

- Parenteral penicillin G is preferred drug for Rx of all stages of syphilis. The preparation(s) used (i.e., benzathine, aqueous procaine, or aqueous crystalline), the dosage, and the length of Rx depend on the stage and clinical manifestations of disease
- Parenteral penicillin G is the only therapy with documented efficacy for syphilis during pregnancy. Patients who report a penicillin allergy, including pregnant women with syphilis in any stage, should be desensitized and treated with penicillin
- The Jarisch-Herxheimer reaction is an acute febrile reaction often accompanied by headache, myalgia, and other symptoms that might occur within the first 24 hours after any therapy for syphilis; patients should be advised of this possible adverse reaction

PRIMARY AND SECONDARY SYPHILIS AMONG ADULTS

- ***Recommended Regimen for Adults***
  Benzathine penicillin G............. 2.4 million units IM in a single dose

Management Considerations: All patients who have syphilis should be tested for HIV infection. In areas in which the prevalence of HIV is high, patients who have primary syphilis should be retested for HIV after 3 months if the first HIV test result was negative, and they should be offered PreP at time of negative result.

Follow-up: Patients should be reexamined clinically and serologically at both 6 and 12 months. For expected response, see CDC Guidelines, *"NOTES: (including cases you have seen)" on page 242*

Management of Sex Partners: Sexual transmission of T. pallidum has occurred only when mucocutaneous syphilitic lesions are present; such manifestations are uncommon after the first year of infection. However, persons exposed sexually to a patient who has syphilis in any stage should be evaluated clinically and serologically and treated according to recommendations available on CDC website.

Special Considerations

- ***Penicillin Allergy:*** Nonpregnant penicillin-allergic patients who have primary or secondary syphilis can be treated with one of the following regimens. Close follow-up of such patients is essential. Limited clinical studies suggest that ceftriaxone may be effective for early syphilis. The optimal dose and duration of therapy have not been defined, however, 1 gm daily IM or IV for 10-14 days has been shown effective.
- ***Recommended Regimens***
  Doxycycline .... 100 mg orally twice a day for 2 weeks,
  Tetracycline .... 500 mg orally four times a day for 2 weeks
- Pregnant patients who are allergic to penicillin should be desensitized, if necessary, and treated with penicillin.

LATENT SYPHILIS:

See most recent CDC Guidelines

TERTIARY SYPHILIS:

See most recent CDC Guidelines

DISEASES CHARACTERIZED BY URETHRITIS AND CERVICITIS

Management of Patients Who Have Nongonococcal Urethritis

Diagnosis: NAAT Testing for chlamydia and gonorrhea is strongly recommended because a specific diagnosis might improve compliance, reduce complications and re-infection and partner notification. Men with NGU should be tested for syphilis and HIV.

Treatment:

- ***Nongonococcal Urethritis, Recommended Regimens***
  Doxycycline .... 100 mg orally twice a day for 7 days
- ***Nongonococcal Urethritis, Alternative Regimens***
  Azithromycin .... 1 g orally in a single dose, OR
  Azithromycin .... 500 mg orally in single dose; then 250 mg orally daily for 4 days

Follow-up: If symptoms persist, patients should be instructed to return for reevaluation and to abstain from sexual intercourse even if they have completed the prescribed therapy

- Cases with documented GC, CT, or T. vaginalis should be (CT, GC reported to the health department) re-tested 3 months after treatment because of high reinfection rates

- Men treated for NGV should abstain until partners have been treated

Partner Referral: Patients should refer all sex partners within the preceding 60 days for evaluation and empiric treatment with a regimen effective against CT.

- ***Recurrent / Persistent Urethritis, Recommended Treatment***
  Consider retreatment with initial regimen if noncompliant or reexposed. Otherwise, do NAAT for T. vaginalis and consider presumptive treatment. Recent studies have shown that the most common cause of persistent NGU is M. genitalium. More information on CDC website.

In areas with prevalent T. vaginalis, men should be treated with metronidazole 2 g orally in a single dose or tinidazole 2 g orally in a single dose, with partner referral.

CHLAMYDIAL INFECTION IN ADOLESCENTS AND ADULTS

Several important sequelae can result from Chlamydia trachomatis (kla-MID-e-a tra-KO-ma-tis) infection in women; the most serious of these include PID, ectopic pregnancy, and infertility. Some women who have apparently uncomplicated cervical infection already have subclinical upper reproductive tract infection. Chlamydial infection is much more common in women under age 25 than in older women. **All women ≤25 years old should be screened annually, and older women at risk.**

Diagnosis: See complete CDC Guidelines. Urogenital C. trachomatis can be diagnosed with swabs from either vaginal, cervical or first-void urine samples. NAAT tests are most sensitive.

Treatment:

- Treatment of infected patients prevents transmission to sex partners and, for infected pregnant women, usually prevents transmission to infants during birth
- Treatment of sex partners helps to prevent reinfection of the index patient and infection of other partners.
- Patients should abstain until their partner(s) have been adequately treated (i.e. 7 days after completion of antibiotics)
- Individuals should be tested for syphilis, HIV, syphilis, and gonorrhea
- MSM who are HIV negative with rectal chlamydia should be offered PreP.
- ***Chlamydia Infection, Recommended Regimens***
  Doxycycline 100 mg orally twice a day for 7 days
- ***Chlamydia Infection, Alternative Regimens***
  Azithromycin........................1 gm orally in a single dose OR
  Levofloxacin.........................500 mg orally once daily for 7 days

Follow-up: Patients do not need to be retested for chlamydia after completing treatment with doxycycline or azithromycin unless symptoms persist or reinfection is suspected because these therapies are highly efficacious. Retesting is recommended for chlamydia infection 3 months after treatment due to high prevalence of reinfection.

Management of Sex Partners: Patients should be instructed to refer their sex partners for evaluation, testing, and presumptive treatment, if they had sexual contact with the patient during the 60 days preceding onset of symptoms in the patient or diagnosis of chlamydia, and the most recent contact should be tested even if > 60 days ago

- Partner therapy should be considered as permitted by law.

Special Considerations:

- ***Pregnancy:***
  - Clinical experience and studies suggest azithromycin is safe and effective
  - Doxycycline is contraindicated in second trimester for pregnant women
  - Levofloxacin is low risk in pregnancy but contraindicated when breastfeeding
  - Repeat testing, preferably NAAT, 4 weeks after completion of therapy with the following regimens is recommended because sequelae to mom and infant
  - Women <25 years old and those at increased risk (e.g., new partner) should be screened at first prenatal visit and rescreened in third trimester
- ***Recommended Regimens for Pregnant Women***

  Azithromycin..............................1 g orally in single dose
- ***Alternative Regimens for Pregnant Women***

  Amoxicillin...................................... 500 mg orally three times a day for 7 days

GONOCOCCAL INFECTION IN ADOLESCENTS AND ADULTS

Gonorrhea was traditionally treated using ceftriaxone and azithromycin. Due to increasing azithromycin resistance in gonorrhea strains, the CDC updated it's recommendation to treatment with monotherapy of ceftriaxone at a higher dose for uncomplicated gonorrheal infections. All women <25 should be screened annually and older women at risk.

Uncomplicated Gonococcal Infections of the Cervix, Urethra, and Rectum

- ***Recommended Regimens***

  Ceftriaxone............................500 mg IM in a single dose for persons weighing <150 kg

  Ceftriaxone............................1 g IM in a single dose for persons weighing >150 kg

  Doxycycline..........................100 mg orally 2 times per day for 7 days if chlamydia has not been excluded
- ***Alternative Regimens if ceftriaxone is not available***

  Gentamycin..........................240 mg IM in a single dose PLUS

  Azithromycin........................2 g orally in a single dose PLUS

  Cefixime................................800 mg orally in a single dose

Management of Sex Partners: All sex partners of patients who have N. gonorrhea infection should be evaluated and presumptively treated if their last sexual contact with the patient was within 60 days before onset of symptoms or diagnosis. Most recent partner should be notified even if > 60 days prior. Partner therapy can be given with a single oral dose of 800 mg Cefixime (and 100 mg doxycycline PO BID for 7 days if chlamydia cannot be excluded).

Suspected treatment failures: In cases of suspected failure, obtain a specimen and submit for susceptibility testing. Report the case to the local health department <24 hours after diagnosis.

Disseminated Gonococcal Infection

Disseminated gonococcal infection (DGI) frequently results in petechial or pustular skin lesions, asymmetric polyarthralgia, tenosynovitis or oligoarticular septic arthritis, rarely perihepatitis, endocarditis or meningitis. Hospitalization and consultation with infectious disease specialist is recommended for initial therapy.

Treatment of Arthritis and Arthritis-Dermatitis Syndrome

- ***Recommended Regimens***

  Ceftriaxone............................1 g IM or IV every 24 hours, PLUS

  Doxycycline..........................100 mg orally 2 times per day for 7 days if chlamydia has not been excluded

- ***Alternative Regimens***

  Cefotaxime............................1 g IV every 8 hours OR

  Ceftizoxime...........................1 g every 8 hours PLUS

  Doxycycline..........................100 mg orally 2 times per day for 7 days if chlamydia has not been excluded

Treatment of Gonococcal Meningitis and Endocarditis

- ***Recommended Regimens***

  Ceftriaxone............................1-2 g IV every 24 hours PLUS

  Doxycycline..........................100 mg orally 2 times per day for 7 days if chlamydia has not been excluded

Recommended parenteral therapy for meningitis should be for 10-14 days and endocarditis for at least 4 weeks.

DISEASES CHARACTERIZED BY VAGINAL DISCHARGE

Management of Patients Who Have Vaginal Infections:

- Vaginitis is usually characterized by a vaginal discharge or vulvar itching and irritation; a vaginal odor may be present
- The three diseases most frequently associated with vaginal discharge are trichomoniasis (caused by T. vaginalis), bacterial vaginosis (BV) (caused by a replacement of a lactobacillus dominant flora by anaerobic microorganisms and Gardnerella vaginalis), and candidiasis (usually caused by Candida albicans)
- Mucopurulent cervicitis caused by C. trachomatis or N. gonorrhoeae can sometimes cause vaginal discharge
- Vaginitis is diagnosed by pH, KOH test, and microscopic examination of fresh samples of the discharge
- The pH of the vaginal secretions can be determined by narrow-range pH paper for the elevated pH typical of BV or trichomoniasis (i.e., pH of >4.5)
- One way to examine the discharge is to dilute a sample in one to two drops of 0.9% normal saline solution on one slide and 10% potassium hydroxide (KOH) solution on a second slide. Corner slips are placed on slides, then examined at low power and high power.
- An amine odor detected immediately after applying KOH suggests BV
- A cover slip is placed on each slide, which is then examined under a microscope at low and high-dry power. The motile T. vaginalis or the clue cells of BV usually are identified easily in the saline specimen. The absence of trichomonads or fungal elements should not rule out these infections.
- The yeast or pseudohyphae of Candida species are more easily identified on KOH specimen
- The presence of objective signs of vulvar inflammation in the absence of vaginal pathogens, suggests the possibility of mechanical, chemical, allergic or other noninfectious causes.

BACTERIAL VAGINOSIS (BV)

- BV is a clinical syndrome resulting from replacement of the normal H2O2 producing Lactobacillus sp. in the vagina with high concentrations of anaerobic bacteria (e.g., Prevotella sp., Mobiluncus sp., G. vaginalis)
- BV is the most prevalent cause of vaginal discharge or malodor
- Most women whose illnesses meet the clinical criteria for BV are asymptomatic
- Treatment of male sex partner has not been beneficial in preventing recurrence

Diagnostic Considerations: BV can be diagnosed by a Gram stain or the use of Amsels criteria meeting three of the following symptoms or signs:

a. A homogeneous, thin vaginal discharge that smoothly coats vagina
b. Clue cells on microscopic examination
c. A pH of vaginal fluid >4.5
d. A fishy odor of vaginal discharge before or after addition of 10% KOH (i.e., the whiff test)

Treatment: The principal goal of therapy in nonpregnant women is to relieve vaginal symptoms and signs of infection.

- ***BV, Recommended Regimens for Nonpregnant Women***
  Metronidazole .... 500 mg orally twice a day for 7 days, OR
  Clindamycin cream .... 2%, one full applicator (5 g) intravaginally at bedtime for 7 days OR
  Metronidazole gel.......... 0.75%, one full applicator (5 g) intravaginally, once daily for 5 days
- Clindamycin cream is oil-based and might weaken latex condoms and diaphragms for 5 days after use.
- Refraining from alcohol while on metronidazole is unnecessary
- ***BV, Alternative Regimens***
  Clindamycin..................... 300 mg orally bid x 7 days OR
  Clindamycin ovules....... 100 mg intravaginally once at bedtime x 3 days OR
  Tinidazole......................... 2 g orally once daily for 2 days OR
  Tinidazole......................... 1 g orally once daily for 5 days OR
  Secnidazole .... 2 g oral granules in a single dose

Follow-up: Follow-up visits are unnecessary if symptoms resolve. Persistence and recurrence are common, women should be advised to return is Sx recurs.

Management of Sex Partners: Routine treatment of sex partners is not recommended

Special Considerations:

- ***Allergy or Intolerance to the Recommended Therapy:***
  - Clindamycin cream is preferred in case of allergy or intolerance to metronidazole or tinidazole. Metronidazole gel can be considered for patients who do not tolerate systemic metronidazole, but patients allergic to oral metronidazole should not be administered metronidazole vaginally
- ***Pregnancy:***
  - BV has been associated with adverse pregnancy outcomes (i.e., premature rupture of the membranes, preterm labor, and intraamniotic infection)
  - Treat all symptomatic pregnant women when diagnosed

- Treatment of BV in high-risk pregnant women (i.e., those who have previously delivered a premature infant) who are asymptomatic has been evaluated but yielded mixed results
- Routine screening for BV in pregnant women at high or low risk for preterm delivery is not recommended
- The recommended regimen is metronidazole 250 mg orally three times a day for 7 days OR metronidazole 500 mg orally twice a day for 7 days OR clindamycin 300 mg orally twice daily for 7 days
- Tinidazole should be avoided during pregnancy

TRICHOMONIASIS

Diagnosis:

- Trichomoniasis is caused by the protozoan T. vaginalis, easily identified on a wet smear although sensitivity is low compared to culture. Most men who are infected do not have symptoms of infection, although a minority of men have nongonococcal urethritis
- Some women do have symptoms of infection, characteristically a diffuse, malodorous, yellow-green discharge with vulvar irritation; many women have fewer symptoms or appear asymptomatic
- NAAT are highly sensitive, and rapid poc tests are sensitive and efficient.

Treatment:

- ***Trichomoniasis, Recommended Regimen for women***
  Metronidazole...................... 500 mg 2 times per day for 7 days
- ***Trichomoniasis, Recommended Regimen for men***
  Metronidazole...................... 2 g orally in a single dose
- ***Trichomoniasis, Alternative Regimen for women and men***
  Tinidazole .... 2 g orally in a single dose
- In randomized clinical trials, the recommended metronidazole and tinidazole regimens have resulted in cure rates of approximately 84%-98% and 92% - 100% respectively
- Patients should abstain until they and their partners are treated. They should be tested for HIV, syphilis, gonorrhea and chlamydia.
- Metronidazole gel is not recommended due to its low efficacy

Follow-up:

- Retesting 3 months after treatment is recommended in sexually active women
- Infections with strains of T. vaginalis that have diminished susceptibility to metronidazole can occur; however, most of these organisms respond to higher doses of metronidazole or tinidazole
- If treatment failure occurs with metronidazole, the patient should be retreated with metronidazole (no reexposure has occurred) or tinidazole 2 g orally once daily for 7 days.

Management of Sex Partners: Sexual intercourse should be avoided until Rx is complete and both partners are asymptomatic. Partners should be referred for presumptive therapy

Special Considerations:

- ***Allergy, Intolerance, or Adverse Reactions:*** Effective alternatives to therapy with metronidazole or tinidazole are not available. Patients who are allergic to this class of drugs can be managed by desensitization

- ***Pregnancy:*** Symptomatic patients should be treated with metronidazole but not tinidazole
- Vaginal trichomoniasis is associated with adverse pregnancy outcomes, particularly premature rupture of the membranes and preterm delivery
- ***HIV Infection:*** Women with HIV should be treated with metronidazole 500 mg twice daily for 7 days

VULVOVAGINAL CANDIDIASIS (VVC)

- Vulvovaginal yeast infections (VVC) are caused by C. albicans or, occasionally, by other Candida sp. or other yeasts
- An estimated 75% of women will have at least one episode of VVC
- Typical symptoms of VVC include pruritus and vaginal discharge
- Other symptoms may include vaginal soreness, vulvar burning, dyspareunia, and external dysuria
- None of these symptoms is specific for VVC

Diagnostic Considerations:

- A diagnosis of Candida vaginitis is suggested clinically by pruritus and erythema in the vulvo-vaginal area; a white discharge may occur, as may vulvar edema
- The diagnosis can be made in a woman who has signs and symptoms of vaginitis, and when either a) a wet preparation or Gram stain of vaginal discharge demonstrates budding yeasts, hyphae or pseudohyphae or b) a culture or other test yields a positive result for a yeast species
- If culture cannot be done and KOH test is negative, empiric Rx can be considered for symptomatic women
- Candida vaginitis is associated with a normal vaginal pH (<4.5)
- Use of 10% KOH in wet preparations improves the visualization of yeast and mycelia by disrupting cellular material that might obscure the yeast or pseudohyphae
- Identifying Candida by culture in the absence of symptoms should not lead to treatment because 10%-20% of women usually harbor Candida sp. and other yeasts in the vagina. VVC can occur concomitantly with STIs

Treatment: Topical formulations effectively treat VVC. Treatment with azoles results in relief of symptoms and negative cultures in 80%-90% of patients.

- ***VVC, Recommended Regimens***
- ***Intravaginal agents:***

Butoconazole................2% cream 5 g (butoconazole 1-sustained release), single vaginal application
Clotrimazole*.................1% cream 5 g intravaginally for 7-14 days,OR
Clotrimazole*.................2% cream 5 g intravaginally for 3 days OR
Miconazole*...................2% cream 5 g intravaginally for 7 days, OR
Miconazole*...................4% cream 5 g intravaginally for 3 days, OR
Miconazole*...................200-mg vaginal suppository, one suppository for 3 days, OR
Miconazole*...................100-mg vaginal suppository, one suppository daily for 7 days, OR
Miconazole*...................1200-mg vaginal suppository, one time dose, OR
Tioconazole*..................6.5% ointment 5 g intravaginally in a single application, OR
Terconazole...................0.4% cream 5 g intravaginally for 7 days, OR

Terconazole .... 0.8% cream 5 g intravaginally for 3 days, OR
Terconazole .... 80-mg vaginal suppository, one suppository daily for 3 days, OR

- *Oral agent:*

Fluconazole..................... 150-mg oral tablet, one tablet in single dose.

* *Over-the-counter preparations*

These creams and suppositories are oil-based and may weaken latex condoms and diaphragms

Follow-up: Patients should be instructed to return for follow-up visits only if symptoms persist or recur

Management of Sex Partners: None; VVC usually is not acquired through sexual intercourse

Special Considerations:

- ***Pregnancy:*** VVC often occurs during pregnancy. Only topical azole therapies applied for 7 days should be used to treat pregnant women. Fluconazole should not be used.
- ***HIV Infection:*** Based on available evidence, therapy is same as seronegative women

PELVIC INFLAMMATORY DISEASE (PID)

- PID comprises a spectrum of inflammatory disorders of the upper female genital tract including any combination of endometritis, salpingitis, tubo-ovarian abscess, and pelvic peritonitis
- Sexually transmitted organisms, especially N. gonorrhoeae and C. trachomatis, are implicated in most cases; however, microorganisms that can be part of the vaginal flora (e.g., anaerobes, G. vaginalis, H. influenzae, enteric gram negative rods, and Streptococcus agalactiae) also can cause PID
- In addition, CMV, M. hominis, T. vaginalis and U. urealyticum may also be etiologic agents

Diagnostic Considerations: See complete CDC Guidelines (*www.cdc.gov*). Empiric treatment should be initiated in sexually active young women and others at risk for STIs if they are experiencing pelvic or lower abdominal pain, if no other cause can be identified and if ONE of the following minimum criteria are present on pelvic exam:

- Cervical motion tenderness OR
- Uterine tenderness OR
- Adnexal tenderness

Treatment: Must provide empiric, broad-spectrum coverage of likely pathogens including N. gonorrhea, C. trachomatis

- Suggested criteria for HOSPITALIZATION decision based on discretion of their provider and whether the woman meets any of the following criteria:
  - Surgical emergencies such as appendicitis cannot be excluded
  - Patient is pregnant
  - Patient does not respond clinically to oral antimicrobial therapy
  - Patient is unable to follow or tolerate an outpatient oral regimen
  - Patient has severe illness, nausea and vomiting, or high fever (>38.5° C or 101 ° F)
  - Patient has a tuboovarian abscess
- ***PID, Parenteral Regimen***

Ceftriaxone.................. 1 g IV every 24 hrs PLUS

Doxycycline................100 mg orally or IV every 12 hours PLUS
Metronidazole...........500 mg orally or IV every 12 hours OR
Cefotetan.....................2 g IV every 12 hours, PLUS
Doxycycline................100 mg IV or orally every 12 hours
OR
Cefoxitin........................2 g IV every 6 hours, PLUS
Doxycycline................100 mg IV or orally every 12 hours

- Because of pain associated with infusion, doxycycline should be administered orally when possible, even when the patient is hospitalized
- Both oral and IV administration of doxycycline provide similar bioavailability but oral treatment should continue through 14 days
- When tuboovarian abscess is present, many health-care providers use clindamycin (450 mg orally four times daily) or metronidazole (500 mg twice daily) with doxycycline for continued therapy (to 14 days) rather than doxycycline alone, because it provides more effective anaerobic coverage
- Parenteral therapy may be discontinued 24-48 hours after a patient improves clinically, and oral therapy should continue to complete a total of 14 days of therapy
- ***PID, Alternative Parenteral Regimens:***

Ampicillin / Sulbactam..... 3 g IV every 6 hours, PLUS
Doxycycline .... 100 mg IV or orally every 12 hours
OR
Clindamycin.......................... 900 mg IV every 8 hours, PLUS
Gentamicin............................ loading dose IV or IM (2 mg/kg of body weight) followed by a maintenance dose (1.5 mg/kg) every 8 hours. Single daily dosing (3-5 mg/kg) may be substituted.

IM or Oral Treatment: Can be considered for mild to moderate acute PID. Patients who do not respond to oral therapy within 72 hours should be reevaluated to confirm the diagnosis and be administered parenteral therapy on either an outpatient or inpatient basis.

- ***PID, Recommended Regimen***

Ceftriaxone....................500 mg IM once*, OR
Cefoxitin.........................2 g IM plus probenecid, 1 g orally in a single dose concurrently once, OR
Other parenteral third-generation cephalosporin (e.g.,ceftizoxime or cefotaxime), PLUS
Doxycycline ....100 mg orally twice a day for 14 days PLUS
Metronidazole.............500 mg orally twice a day for 14 days for anaerobic coverage

** For patients weighing >300 lbs with documented gonorrhea, 1 gm of ceftriaxone should be used.*

- ***PID, Alternative Oral Regimens:*** If parenteral cephalosporin therapy is not feasible (allergy), use of fluoroquinolones (levofloxacin 500 mg orally once daily or moxifloxacin 400 mg once daily for 14 days) with metronidazole (500 mg orally twice daily for 14 days) may be considered if the community prevalence and individual risk of gonorrhea is low. Tests for gonorrhea must be performed prior to instituting therapy and the patient managed as follows if the test is positive:

- If culture for gonorrhea is positive, treatment should be based on results of antimicrobial susceptibility. If strain is resistant or only NAAT available, consult and I.D. specialist.

Follow-up:

- Patients receiving oral or parenteral Rx should demonstrate substantial clinical improvement (i.e., defervescence; reduction in direct or rebound abdominal tenderness; and reduction in uterine, adnexal, and Cx motion tenderness) within 3 days after initiation of Rx
- Patients who do not improve within 3 days usually require additional diagnostic tests, hospitalization or surgical intervention
- Counsel to avoid sexual activity throughout the course of treatment
- If positive for GC or CT, retest in 3 months

Special Considerations:

- Pregnancy: Pregnant women who have suspected PID should be hospitalized and treated with parenteral antibiotics.
- Refer sexual partner for evaluation and presumptive treatment even if asymptomatic

HUMAN PAPILLOMAVIRUS INFECTION (HPV)

More than 40 types of HPV can infect the genital tract. Most HPV infections are asymptomatic, subclinical, or unrecognized. Visible genital warts usually are caused by HPV types 6 or 11. Oncogenic HPV types in the anogenital region (i.e., types 16 and 18) have been strongly associated with cervical and oropharyngeal cancers.

Prevention: HPV Immunization (preferable to vaccination)

HPV immunization may be recommended as early as age 9 in boy and girls through 26 years old. Gardasil-9 (the only form of HPV immunization currently) catch up vaccination may be used for ages up to 45 for men and women.

Cervical Dysplasia / HPV-Associated Cancers and Precancers

See chapter 5 for details on screening and treatment

Genital Warts:

Treatment:

- The primary goal is removal of genital warts and amelioration of symptoms
- Treatment can induce wart-free periods in most patients
- No evidence indicates that currently available treatments eradicate or affect the natural history of HPV infection. The removal of warts may decrease but not eradicate infectivity
- If left untreated, visible genital warts may resolve on their own, remain unchanged, or increase in size or number. No evidence indicates that presence of visible warts or their treatment is associated with the development of cervical cancer

Regimens:

- Treatment of genital warts should be guided by the patient's preference, the available resources, and the experience of the health-care provider.
- None of the available treatments is superior to other treatments, and no single treatment is ideal for all circumstances. The treatment modality should be changed if a patient has not improved substantially or has severe side effects. The majority respond within 3 months of therapy

- ***External Genital Warts, Recommended Treatments:***
- ***Patient-Applied***

  Podofilox........................0.5% solution or gel OR
  Sinecatechins* ....15% ointment OR
  Imiquimod*....................3.75% or 5% cream
  **Imiquimod and Sinecatechins may weaken condoms and diaphragms*
- Patients may apply podofilox solution with a cotton swab, or podofilox gel with a finger, to visible genital warts twice a day for 3 days, followed by 4 days of no therapy
- This cycle may be repeated as necessary for a total of four cycles
- The total wart area treated should not exceed 10 cm^2, and a total volume of podofilox should not exceed 0.5 mL per day
- If possible, the health-care provider should apply the initial treatment to demonstrate the proper application technique and identify which warts should be treated.
- Podofilox should not be used during pregnancy.
- Patients should apply imiquimod 5% cream with a finger at bedtime, three times a week for <16 weeks. If using imiquimod 3.75%, apply once at bedtime, but apply every night for <8 weeks.
- The treatment area should be washed with mild soap and water 6-10 hours after the application
- Data about the safety of imiquimod during pregnancy is limited
- Sinecatechin ointment should be applied three times daily using a finger to ensure covering with a thick layer of ointment until complete clearance of warts, but no longer than 16 weeks. Should not be washed off AND sex should be avoided while ointment on skin. Safety in pregnancy is unknown.
- ***Provider-Administered:***
- Cryotherapy with liquid nitrogen
- Trichloroacetic acid (TCA) or BCA 80%-90%. Apply a small amount only to warts and allow to dry, at which time a white "frosting" develops; powder with talc or NaHCO3 to remove acid if an excess amount is applied. Repeat weekly if necessary. OR
- Surgical removal by tangential scissor excision, tangential shave excision, curettage, or electrosurgery may be done
- ***External Genital Warts, Alternative Treatments (Provider administered)***

  Intra-lesional interferon OR photodynamic therapy OR topical cidofovir
- ***Cervical Warts***

Cryotherapy with liquid nitrogen. OR Surgical Removal OR TCA or BCA 80%-90%. For women who have exophytic cervical warts, biopsy to rule out high-grade squamous intraepithelial lesions should be performed before treatment.

Management of exophytic cervical warts should include consultation with an expert

- ***Vaginal Warts, Recommended Treatment***

Cryotherapy with liquid nitrogen. The use of a cryoprobe in the vagina is not recommended because of the risk for vaginal perforation and fistula formation. OR TCA or BCA 80%-90% applied only to warts. Repeat weekly if necessary OR Surgical Removal

- ***Urethral Meatus Warts, Recommended Treatment***

Cryotherapy with liquid nitrogen OR surgical removal

- ***Anal Warts, Recommended Treatment***

Cryotherapy with liquid nitrogen OR

TCA or BCA 80%-90% applied to warts OR surgical removal

- Management of warts on rectal mucosa should be referred to an expert

Management of Sex Partners: Persons should inform current partners since partners may have HPV despite no visible warts. No testing is recommended.

Special Considerations:

- ***Pregnancy:*** Sinecatechins, podophyllin, and podofilox should not be used during pregnancy. Imiquimod is low risk but should be avoided until more data available. Genital warts can proliferate and become friable during pregnancy, removal can be considered, but resolution may be incomplete. Rarely HPV types 6 and 11 can cause respiratory papillomatosis in infants and children. The route of transmission (i.e., transplacental, perinatal, or postnatal) is not completely understood. Vaginal delivery not contraindicated unless lesion size obstructive in labor (rare) or would result in excessive bleeding.

ECTOPARASITIC INFECTIONS

PEDICULOSIS PUBIS

Patients who have pediculosis pubis (i.e., pubic lice) usually seek medical attention because of pruritus or they notice lice or nits on their pubic hair. Usually sexually transmitted

Treatment:

- ***Pediculosis Pubis, Recommended Regimens***

  Permethrin.......................1% cream rinse applied to affected areas and washed off after 10 minutes OR

  Pyrethrins with piperonyl butoxide applied to the affected area and washed off after 10 minutes.

- ***Pediculosis Pubis, Alternate Regimens***

  Malathion.........................0.9% lotion applied to affected areas and washed off after 8-12 hours OR

  Ivermectin.......................250 mcg/kg body weight orally, repeated in 7-14 days

- Malathion can be used if treatment failure is believed to be due to resistance which is increasing and widespread

Other Management Considerations:

- The recommended regimens should not be applied to the eyes. Pediculosis of the eyelashes should be treated by applying occlusive ophthalmic ointment to the eyelid margins twice a day for 10 days
- Bedding and clothing should be decontaminated (either machine-washed and machine-dried using the heat cycle or dry-cleaned) or removed from body contact for at least 72 hrs
- Fumigation of living areas is not necessary

Follow-up: Patients should be evaluated after 1 week if symptoms persist. Retreatment may be necessary if lice are found or if eggs are observed at the hairskin junction. Patients who do not respond to one of the recommended regimens should be retreated with an alternative regimen

Management of Sex Partners: Sex partners within the last month should be treated
Special Considerations: Sexual contact should be avoided until patient and partners treated, bedding and clothing decontaminated, and re-evaluation performed.

- ***Pregnancy:*** Pregnant and lactating women should be treated with either permethrin or pyrethrins with piperonyl butoxide. Invermectin considered low risk and probably compatible with breastfeeding.

SCABIES

- Caused by a mite, the predominant symptom is pruritus; sensitization takes several weeks to develop; pruritus might occur within 24 hours after a subsequent reinfestation
- Scabies in adults is frequently sexually transmitted, although scabies in children usually is not
  - ***Scabies, Recommended Regimen***

    Permethrin cream........(5%) applied to all areas of the body from the neck down and washed off after 8-14 hours (safe in pregnancy) OR

    Ivermectin.......................200 mcg/kg orally, repeated in 2 weeks OR

    Invermectin ....1% lotion applied to all of body from neck down, washed off after 8-14 hours; repeat in 1 week if Sx persists
- ***Scabies, Alternative Regimens***

  Lindane....................................(1%) 1 oz. of lotion or 30 g of cream applied thinly to al areas of the body from the neck down and thoroughly washed off after 8 hours
- Lindane should not be used immediately after a bath, and it should not be used by a) persons who have extensive dermatitis, b) pregnant or lactating women, and c) children aged <10 years. Not first-line because of toxicity, d) as first-line therapy

Other Management Considerations: Bedding and clothing should be decontaminated (i.e., either machine-washed or machine-dried using the hot cycle or dry-cleaned) or removed from body contact for at least 72 hours. Fumigation of living areas is unnecessary
Follow-up: Pruritus may persist for several weeks. Retreatment after 2 weeks for patients who are still symptomatic; OR if live mites are observed. Patients who do not respond should be retreated with an alternative regimen
Management of Sex Partners and Household Contacts: Both sexual and close personal or household contacts within the preceding month should be examined and treated if infected

SEXUAL ASSAULT AND STIS: ADULTS AND ADOLESCENTS

Decisions to perform the following tests should be made on an individual basis. Initial examination after a sexual assault might include the following:

- NAATs for C. trachomatis and N. gonorrhoeae at the sites of penetration or attempted penetration should be performed
- Females should be offered NAAT testing for T. vaginalis from a urine or vaginal specimen. POC or wet mount with measurement of vaginal pH and KOH application for the whiff test from vaginal secretions should be performed for evidence of BV and candidiasis, especially if vaginal discharge, malodor, or itching is present.

- MSM should be offered screening for C. trachomatis and N. gonorrhoeae if they report receptive oral or anal sex during the preceding year, regardless of whether sexual contact occurred at these anatomic sites during the assault. Anoscopy should be considered in instances of reported anal penetration.
- A serum sample should be performed for HIV, HBV, and syphilis infection.
- ***Presumptive treatment:***
- An empiric antimicrobial regimen for chlamydia, gonorrhea, and trichomonas for women and chlamydia and gonorrhea for men.
  - Emergency contraception should be considered when the assault could result in pregnancy (see Emergency Contraception).
  - Postexposure hepatitis B vaccination (without HBIG) if the hepatitis status of the assailant is unknown and the survivor has not been previously vaccinated.
  - HPV vaccination for female and male survivors aged 9–26 years who have not been vaccinated or are incompletely vaccinated
  - Recommendations for HIV PEP are made on a case-by-case basis according to risk
- ***Recommended Regimen for Adolescents and Adult Female Sexual Assault Survivors***

  Ceftriaxone .... 500 mg IM in a single dose* PLUS
  Doxycycline .... 100 mg 2 times per day orally for 7 days PLUS
  Metronidazole .... 500 mg orally 2 times per day for 7 days
  **For persons weighing ≥150 kg, 1 g of ceftriaxone should be administered*
- ***Recommended Regimen for Adolescents and Adult Male Sexual Assault Survivors***

  Ceftriaxone .... 500 mg IM in a single dose* PLUS
  Doxycycline .... 100 mg 2 times per day orally for 7 days
  **For persons weighing ≥150 kg, 1 g of ceftriaxone should be administered*
- Clinicians should counsel persons regarding the possible benefits and toxicities associated with these treatment regimens; gastrointestinal side effects can occur with this combination.

Other Management Considerations:

At the initial examination and, if indicated, at follow-up, patients should be counseled about:

- Risk for pregnancy and possible use of emergency contraception
- Symptoms of STIs and the need for immediate examination if symptoms occur
- Abstinence from sexual intercourse until STI prophylactic treatment is completed

Risk for Acquiring HIV Infection:

- Although HIV antibody seroconversion has been reported among persons whose only known risk factor was sexual assault, the risk for acquiring HIV infection through sexual assault is low and depends on many factors
- These factors may include the type of sexual intercourse (i.e., oral, vaginal, or anal); presence of oral, vaginal or anal trauma; site of exposure to ejaculate; viral load in ejaculate; and presence of an STI
- The use of post-exposure prophylaxis (PEP) should be discussed and recommendations on initiation should consider (if considered, it is helpful to consult a specialist in HIV):
  - The likeliness of the assailant having HIV
  - Exposure characteristics that may increase risk

- Time elapsed after the event (should be initiated as soon after and up to 72 hours after the assault)
- The potential benefits and risks associated with nPEP

HIV INFECTION

Proper management of HIV infection involves a complex array of behavioral, psychosocial, and medical services. This information should not be a substitute for referral to a health-care provider or facility experienced in caring for HIV-infected patients.

Pregnancy: All pregnant women should be offered HIV testing at the first prenatal visit. Women at high risk of infection should be tested again in the third trimester. Women with no prenatal care should be tested at delivery. This recommendation is particularly important because of the available treatments for reducing the likelihood of perinatal transmission and maintaining the health of the woman. HIV-infected women should be informed specifically about the risk for perinatal infection. ART reduces the risk for HIV transmission to the infant from approximately 30% to <2% through use of antiretroviral regimens and obstetric intervention and by avoiding breastfeeding. ***ART TREATMENT SHOULD BE OFFERED TO ALL HIV-INFECTED PREGNANT WOMEN.***

STI screening for patients living with HIV:

- N. gonorrhea at genital sites at initial evaluation and annually
- C. trachomatis at genital sites at initial evaluation and annually
- Syphilis at initial evaluation and annually
- Trichomonas at initial evaluation and annually
- HAV (for MSM, HBV/HCV+, or IV drug users at initial evaluation
- HBV at initial evaluation (and consider vaccination)
- HCV at initial evaluation and annually

For MSM, more frequent testing can be considered, especially in the setting of rising rates of syphilis and antibiotic-resistant Gonorrhea.

EVALUATION & MANAGEMENT OF SEXUAL ASSAULT

Engage Rape Crisis Services. Have trained provider do the examination whenever possible. See SANE (Sexual Assault Nurse Evaluation) guidance

Legal: Report to authorities if required by your state. Contact child protective services if victim is a minor

Obtain informed consent before history, physical and treatment

History: circumstances of assault, whether victim had loss of consciousness (may want to test for rohypnol), date / time / location, use of weapons etc, specifics re: oral, vaginal or anal contact, penetration, ejaculation or condom use, areas of trauma, bleeding by victim or assailant, recent consensual sexual activity before or after assault including condom use, LMP, contraceptive use, use of drugs or alcohol, whether victim showered, changed clothing etc.

Physical exam: document any trauma with photographs (and patient's consent). Woods lamp (UV) may help identify semen or other debris. Colposcopy helps detect milder trauma.
Forensic exam done with a special "evidence collection kit" includes victim's clothing, swabs of buccal mucosa, vagina, rectum, combed (and pulled) specimens from scalp and pubic hair, fingernail scrapings and clippings, blood sample etc. Assure proper chain of evidence to legal authorities. PE may also include specimens for DNA, acid phosphatase, pregnancy, HIV, Hep B, syphilis, sperm, BV, Trich, GC/CT and Herpes.

Treatment: Offer emergency contraception. Empiric RX for STIs: ceftriaxone 500mg IM plus doxycycline 100mg PO BID x 7 days. Metronidazole 2g PO x 1 dose to treat trichomoniasis. HEP B vaccine and HPV vaccine if not immune and consider anti-retrovirals to decrease risk of HIV infection. Advise to abstain from intercourse until prophylaxis therapy completed and consider condom use until follow-up serologic testing complete (6 months)

Follow-up: Medical visit in 1-2 weeks. Ongoing psychosocial support and advocate services should be assessed. Do pregnancy test. Test for GC, CT, Trich and BV if woman declined prophylaxis or developed new symptoms or requests it. Follow-up tests for HIV and RPR at 6 weeks and 3 months. Follow up doses of Hep B vaccine.

COLOR PHOTOS

Combined and Progestin-Only Oral Contraceptives

POSTERS showing all pills can be ordered on form at end of book or at the website: www.managingcontraception.com

THE PILLS ARE ORGANIZED AS FOLLOWS:

Color photos of pills from lowest to highest estrogen dose

- Progestin-only pills with no estrogen
- ***NEWLY APPROVED Estrogen:*** Estetrol pill
- Lowest estrogen pills with 10-20 micrograms of the estrogen, ethinyl estradiol
- All of the 25-, 30- and 35-microgram pills (all ethinyl estradiol)
- All of the phasic pills
- Highest estrogen pills, with 50 micrograms of estrogen (ethinyl estradiol OR mestranol). Mestranol is converted in the body to ethinyl estradiol; 50 mcg of mestranol is equivalent to 35 mcg of ethinyl estradiol

Pills which are pharmacologically exactly the same are grouped within boxes. The color and packaging of pills dispensed in clinics may differ from pills in pharmacies.

PROGESTIN - ONLY PILLS

0.35 mg norethindrone

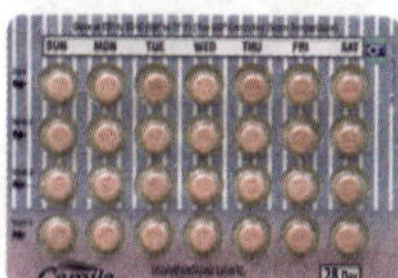

CAMILA®
Mayne Pharmaceuticals

JENCYCLA®
Lupin

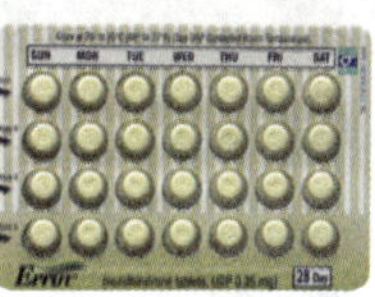

ERRIN®
Barr Laboratories

NORA-BE®
Actavis

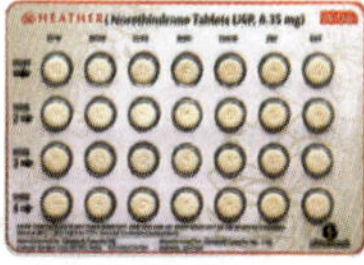

HEATHER®
Glenmark Pharmaceutical

JOLIVETTE®
Actavis

4 mg drospirenone

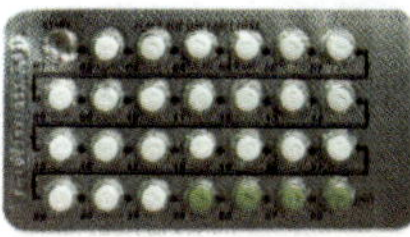

SLYND®
Exeltis USA, Inc.

The only estrogen-free oral contraceptive with a flexible 24-hour missed pill window and predictable bleeding profile.

COMBINED PILLS - ESTETROL PILLS

NEWLY APPROVED ESTROGEN - ESTETROL

3.0 mg drospirenone / 14.2 mg estetrol

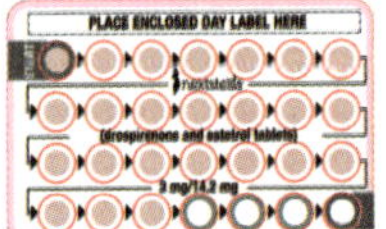

NEXTELLIS®
Mayne Pharma

COMBINED PILLS - 10 microgram EE PILLS

1 mg norethindrone acetate/10 mcg ethinyl estradiol/75 mg ferrous fumarate [7d]

MINASTRIN® FE 1/10 CHEWABLE
Actavis

(levonorgestrel/ethinyl estradiol/0.10mg/20 mcg and ethinyl estridol 0.01 mg

LoSEASONIQUE®
Duramed

CAMRESE®LO
Teva Women's Health

COMBINED PILLS - 20 microgram EE PILLS

NO SCHEDULED PERIODS - No inactive pills

90 mcg levonorgestrel/20 mcg ethinyl estradiol

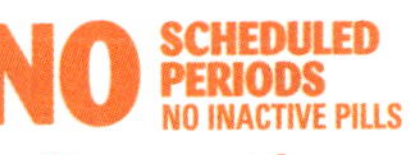

Hormones taken continously.

GENERICS AVAILABLE
(equivalent to the discontinued brand Lybrel®)
Various Manufacturers

3.0 mg drospirenone / 0.02 mg ethinyl estradiol

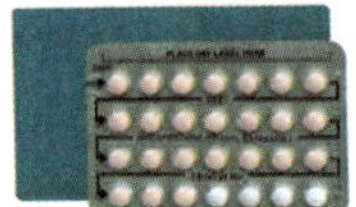

YAZ® 28 TABLETS → **BEYAZ® 28 TABLETS**
Bayer

Beyaz = Yaz + 451mcg folic acid
Bayer

GIANVI®
Teva Pharmaceuticals USA

YASMINELLE
BAYER

VESTURA® 3 X 28 TABLETS
(discontinued)
ACTAVIS

It is important for all reproductive age women to take folic acid daily

0.1 mg levonorgestrel / 20 mcg ethinyl estradiol

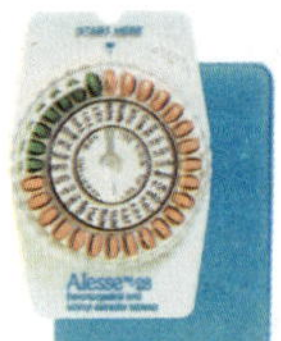

ALESSE® - 28 TABLETS
Wyeth

AMETHYST® - 28 TABLETS
ACTAVIS

SRONYX®
Mayne Pharmaceuticals

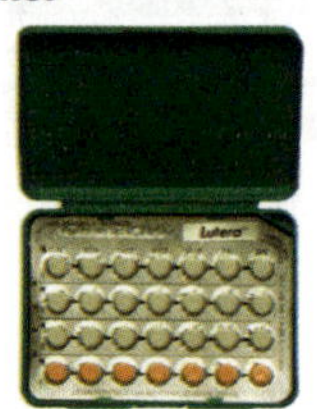

LUTERA™
Watson Pharmaceuticals

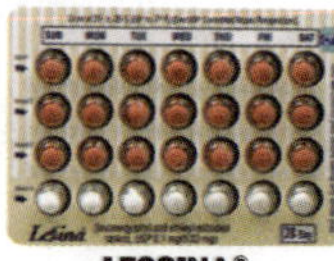

LESSINA®
Teva Pharmaceuticals USA

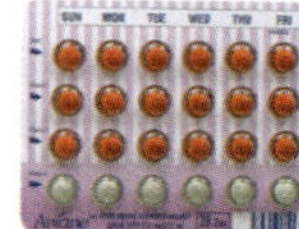

AVIANE®
Barr Laboratories

1 mg norethindrone acetate / 20 mcg ethinyl estradiol / 75 mg ferrous fumarate [7d]

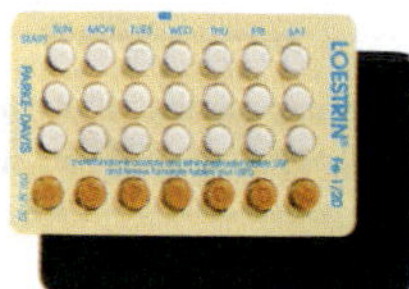

LOESTRIN® FE 1/20
DuraMed

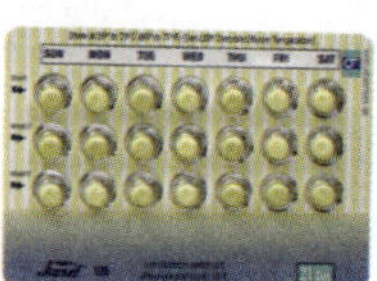

JUNEL ™
Barr Laboratories

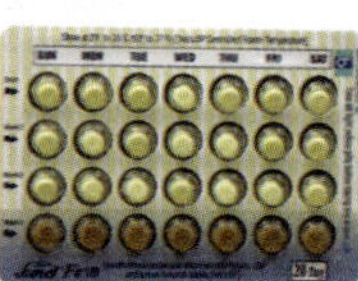

JUNEL ™ Fe
Teva Pharmaceuticals USA

MICROGESTIN® & MICROGESTIN FE®
Mayne Pharmaceuticals

TILIA FE® - 28 TABLETS
Mayne Pharmaceuticals

desogestrel / estradiol tablets 0.15 mg / 0.02 mg and ethinyl estradiol tablets 0.01 mg

AZURETTE® - 28 TABLETS
Mayne Pharmaceuticals

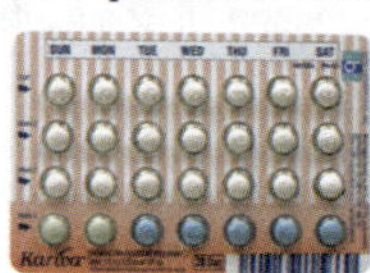

KARIVA®
Barr Laboratories

MERCILON®
Merck

COMBINED PILLS - ESTRODIOL VALERATE

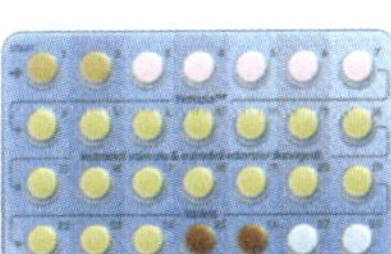

NATAZIA™

Natazia consists of 28 film-coated, unscored tablets in the following order:

- 2 dark yellow tablets each containing 3mg estradiol valerate
- 5 medium red tablets each containing 2mg estradiol valerate and 2mg dienogest
- 17 light yellow tablets each containing 2mg estradiol valerate and 3mg dienogest
- 2 dark red tablets each containing 1 mg estradiol valerate
- 2 white tablets (inert)

Bayer

COMBINED PILLS - NOMEGESTROL ACETATE

2.5 mg nomegestrol acetate / 1.5 mg estradiol

ZOELY

Theramex

COMBINED PILLS - 20 - 25 -30 microgram EE PILL

QUARTETTE

A 91 day ascending-dose, extended-regimen oral contraceptive for the prevention of pregnancy.

For each 91-day course, take in the following order:

1. Start the first light pink tablet (0.15 mg of levonorgestrel and 0.02 mg ethinyl estradiol) on the first Sunday after the onset of menstruation. take one light pink tablet once a day for a total of 42 consecutive days.
2. One pink tablet (0.15 mg of levonorgestrel and 0.025 mg ethinyl estradiol) once a day for 21 consecutive days.
3. One purple tablet (0.15 mg of levonorgestrel and 0.03 mg ethinyl estradiol) once a day for 21 days.
4. One yellow tablet (0.01 mg of ethinyl estradiol) once a day for 7 days. Bleeding should occur during yellow tablet use.

Teva Women's Health

COMBINED PILLS - 25 microgram PILL

CAZIANT™ 3X28 TABLETS

(0.1mg/0.025mg, 0.125mg/0.025mg, 0.15mg/0.025mg)

Each 28-day treatment cycle pack consists of three active dosing phases:

7 white tablets containing 0.100 mg desogestrel and 0.025 mg ethinyl estradiol;

7 light blue tablets containing 0.125 mg desogestrel and 0.025 mg ethinyl estradiol

7 blue tablets containing 0.150 mg desogestrel and 0.025 mg ethinyl estradiol.

Mayne Pharmaceuticals

COMBINED PILLS - 30 microgram EE PILLS

3.0 mg drospirenone / 30 mcg ethinyl estradiol

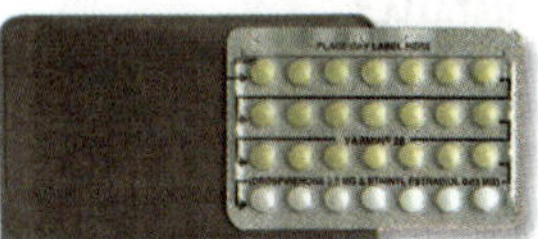

YASMIN® 28 TABLETS
BAYER

→ **SAFYRAL™**
Safyral = Yasmin + 451mcg Folic Acid
BAYER

ZARAH™
Mayne Pharmaceuticals

OCELLA™ 28 TABLETS
Teva Women's Health

It is important for all reproductive age women to take folic acid daily

0.15 mg levonorgestrel / 30 mcg ethinyl estradiol

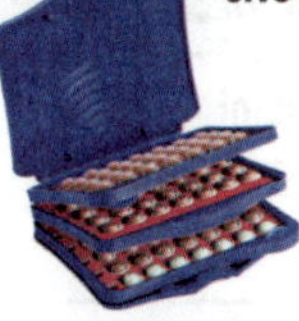

SEASONALE®
Barr Laboratories

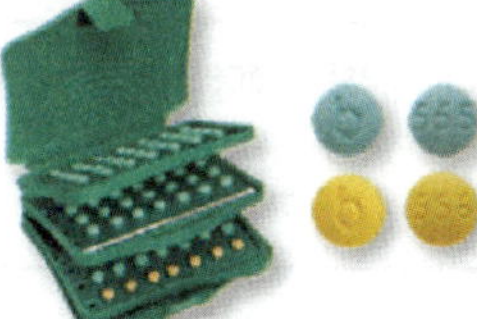

SEASONIQUE®
Barr Laboratories

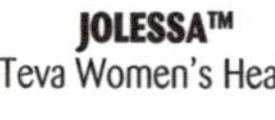

JOLESSA™
Teva Women's Health

CAMRESE™
Teva Women's Health

QUARTERLY PERIODS

0.15 mg levonorgestrel / 30 mcg ethinyl estradiol

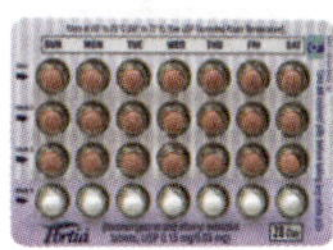

PORTIA®
Teva Pharmaceuticals USA

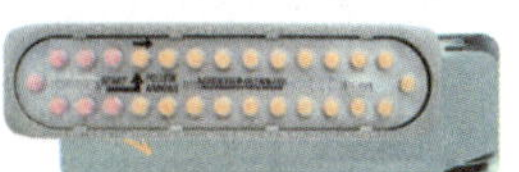

NORDETTE®-28 TABLETS
Teva Pharmaceuticals USA

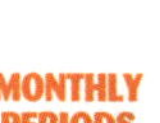

MONTHLY PERIODS

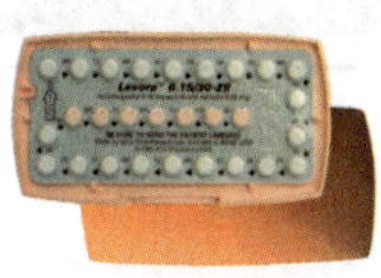

LEVORA TABLETS
Actavis

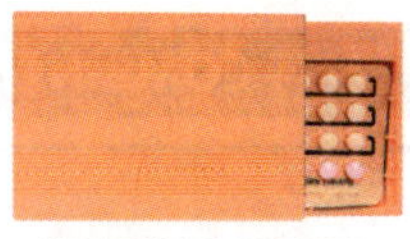

LEVLEN® 28 TABLETS
Berlex Laboratories

QUASENSE™
Actavis

COMBINED PILLS - 30 microgram EE PILLS cont.

0.3 mg norgestrel / 30 mcg ethinyl estradiol

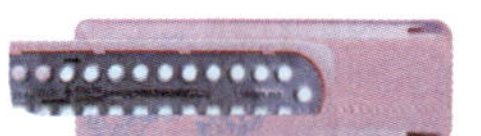

LO/OVRAL®-28 TABLETS
Wyeth

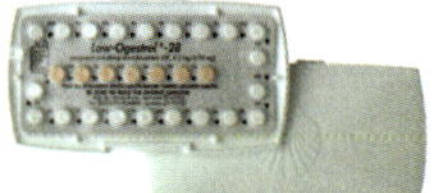

LOW-OGESTREL® - 28
Watson

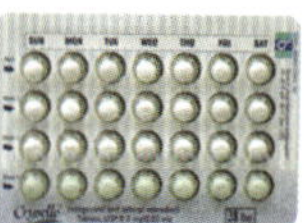

CRYSELLE®
Barr Laboratories

0.15 mg desogestrel/ 30 mcg ethinyl estradiol

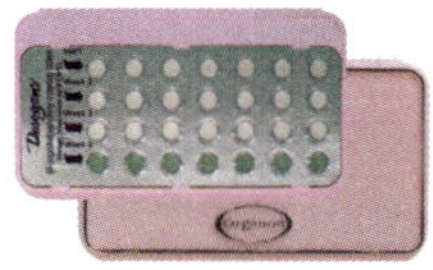

DESOGEN®
Merck

MONTHLY PERIODS

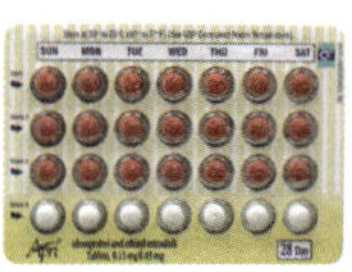

APRI®
Barr Laboratories

RECLIPSEN™
Teva Women's Health

SOLIA™
(discontinued)
Prasco

1.5 mg norethindrone acetate / 30 mcg ethinyl estradiol

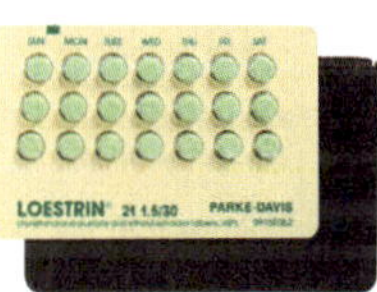

LOESTRIN® 21 1.5/30
DuraMed

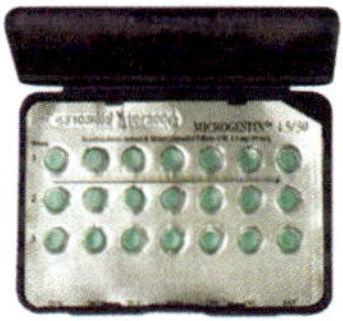

MICROGESTIN® 1.5/30 with or without Fe
Mayne Pharmaceuticals

MONTHLY PERIODS

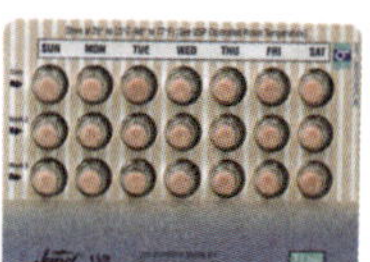

JUNEL ™
Barr Laboratories

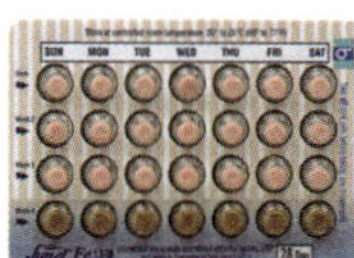

JUNEL ™ Fe
Barr Laboratories

COMBINED PILLS - 35 microgram EE PILLS

0.25 mg norgestimate / 35 mcg ethinyl estradiol

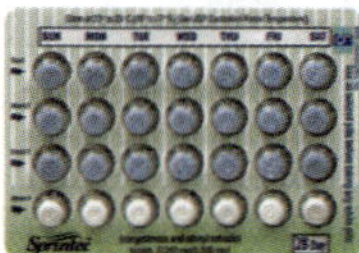

SPRINTEC®
Barr Laboratories

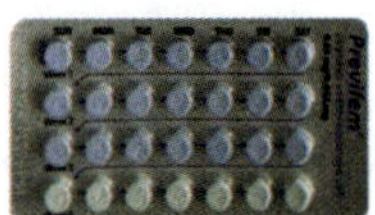

PREVIFEM™
Qualitest

Discount stores often carry generics for a few dollars per pack.

0.4 mg norethindrone / 35 mcg ethinyl estradiol

ZENCHENT®
(chewable)
Amneal Akyner

ZEOSA™
(chewable)
Teva Pharmaceuticals USA

FEMCON FE™
(chewable)
(discontinued)
Warner Chilcott

BALZIVA™ 1/35
Barr Laboratories

1 mg norethindrone / 35 mcg ethinyl estradiol

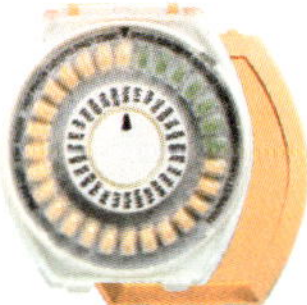

ORTHO-NOVUM® 1/35 28 TABLETS
Jannsen

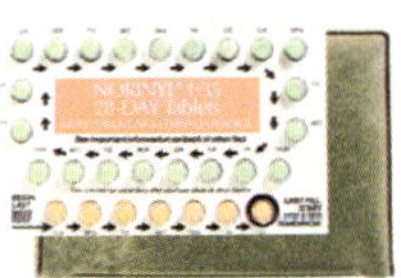

NORINYL® 1+35 28-DAY TABLETS
Allergan USA

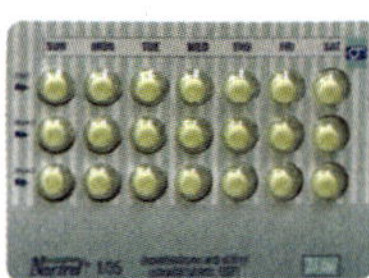

NORTREL®
Barr Laboratories

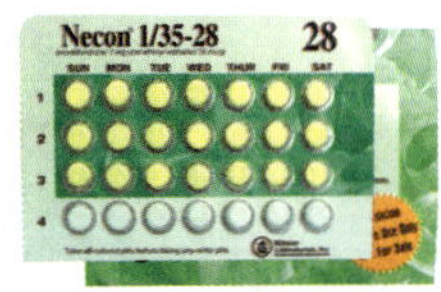

NECON® 1/35-28
Teva Pharmaceuticals USA

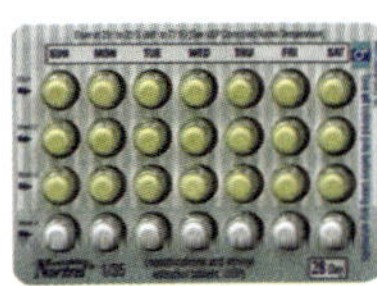

NORTREL®
Barr Laboratories

1 mg ethynodiol diacetate / 35 mcg ethinyl estradiol

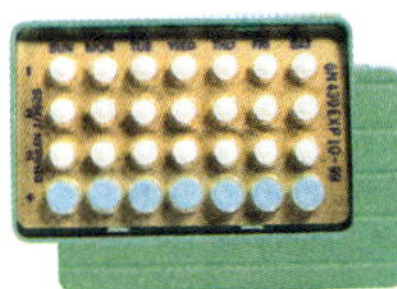

DEMULEN® 1/35-28
(discontinued in U.S.)
Pfizer

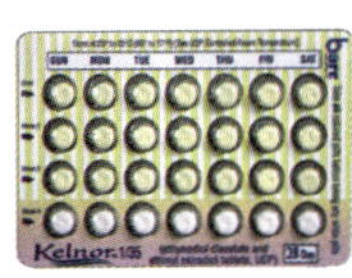

KELNOR ™
Teva Pharmaceuticals USA

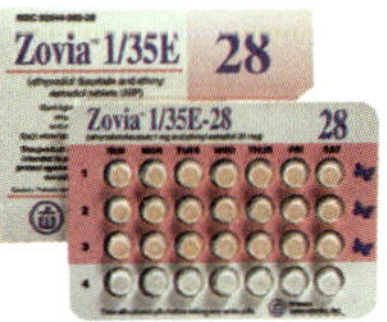

ZOVIA® 1/35E–28
Watson Pharmaceuticals

COMBINED PILLS - 35 microgram EE PILLS cont.

1 mg norethindrone / 35 mcg ethinyl estradiol

NECON 0.5/35®
Mayne Pharmaceuticals

COMBINED PILLS - PHASIC PILLS

desogestrel / ethinyl estradiol–triphasic regimen 0.1 mg/25 mcg (7d), 0.125 mg/25 mcg (7d), 0.150 mg/25 mcg (7d)

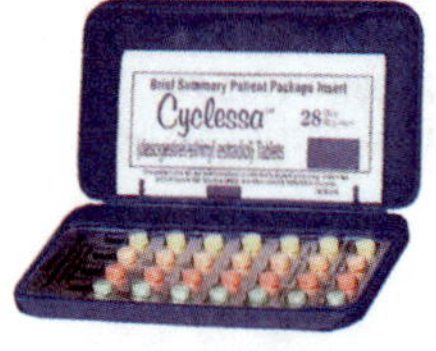

CYCLESSA®
Aspen Global Inc

CESIA™
Prasco

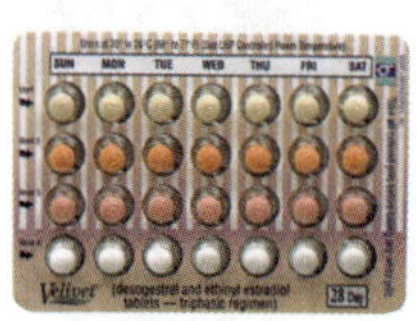

VELIVET™
Barr Laboratories

norethindrone / ethinyl estradiol 0.5 mg / 35 mcg (7d), 1 mg / 35 mcg (9d), 0.5 mg / 35 mcg (5d)

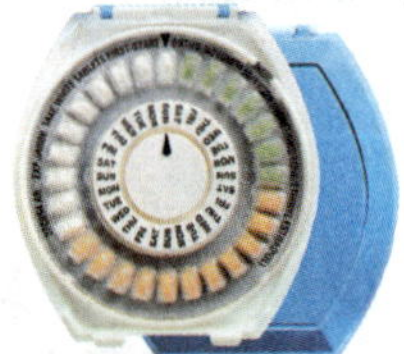

ORTHO-NOVUM® 10/11 - 28 TABLETS
(discontinued per FDA)
Jannsen

NECON® 10/11 - 28 TABLETS
(discontinued)
Actavis

ARANELLE™
Teva Pharmaceuticals USA

TRI-NORINYL®
Mayne Pharmaceuticals

LEENA®
Mayne Pharmaceuticals

COMBINED PILLS - PHASIC PILLS cont.

norethindrone acetate / ethinyl estradiol 1 mg / 20 mcg (5d), 1 mg/30 mcg (7d), 1 mg/35 mcg (9d), 75 mg ferrous fumarate (7d)

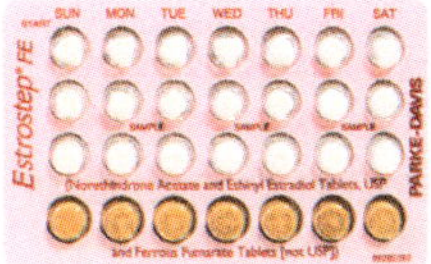

ESTROSTEP® FE - 28 TABLETS
Allergan

TRI-LEGEST® FE
Teva Pharmaceuticals USA

levonorgestrel / ethinyl estradiol–triphasic regimen 0.050 mg / 30 mcg (6d), 0.075 mg / 40 mcg (5d), 0.125 mg / 30 mcg (10d)

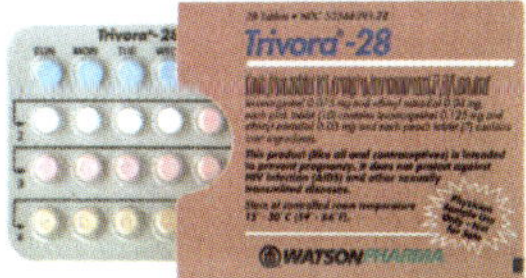

TRIVORA®
Watson Pharmaceuticals

TRI-LEVLEN® 28 TABLETS
MK Drughouse

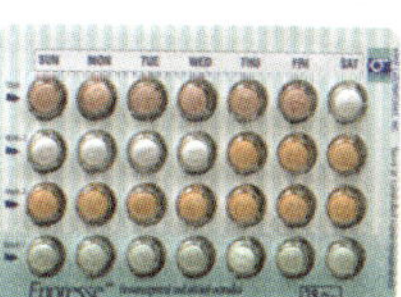

ENPRESSE®
Duramed

norgestimate / ethinyl estradiol
0.18 mg / 35 mcg (7d),
0.215 mg / 35 mcg (7d),
0.25 mg / 35 mcg (7d),
placebo (7d)

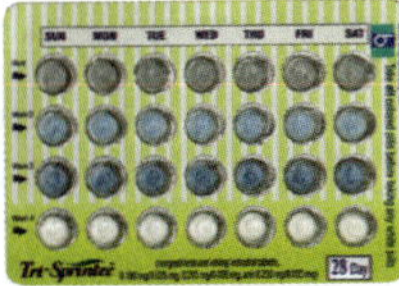

TRI-SPRINTEC®
Barr Laboratories

TRI-PREVIFEM™ - 28 TABLETS
Teva Pharmaceuticals USA

Discount stores often carry some generics for a few dollars per pack.

norethindrone / ethinyl estradiol
0.5 mg / 35 mcg (7d),
0.75 mg / 35 mcg (7d),
1 mg / 35 mcg (7d)

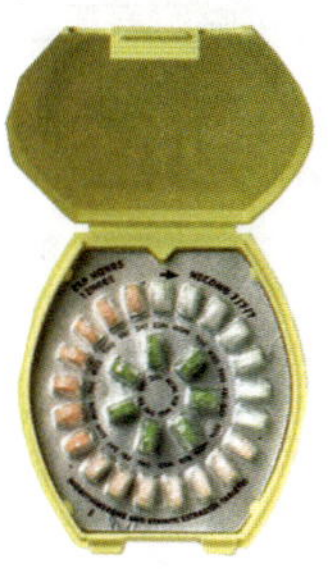

NECON® 7/7/7
Actavis

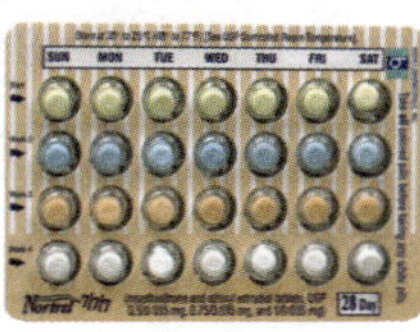

NORTREL® 7/7/7
Barr Laboratories

COMBINED PILLS - 50 microgram PILLS

Pills with 50 micrograms of mestranol are not as strong as pills with 50 micrograms of ethinyl estradiol

0.5 mg norgestrel / 50 mcg ethinyl estradiol

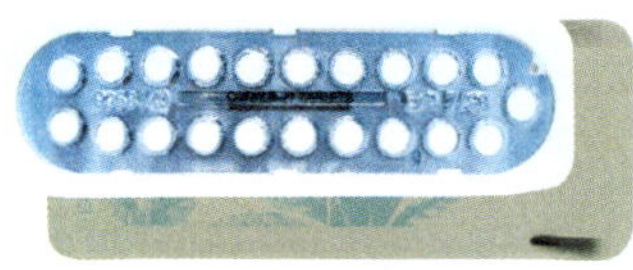

OVRAL® - 21 TABLETS
(discontinued per FDA)
Wyeth

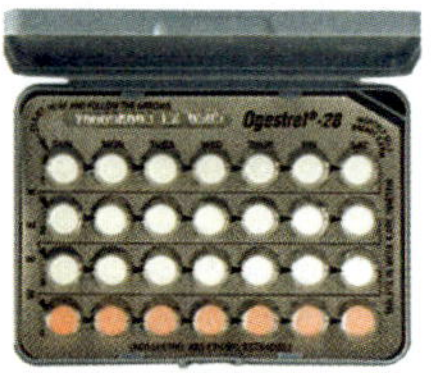

OGESTREL®
Mayne Pharmaceuticals

1 mg norethindrone / 50 mcg mestranol

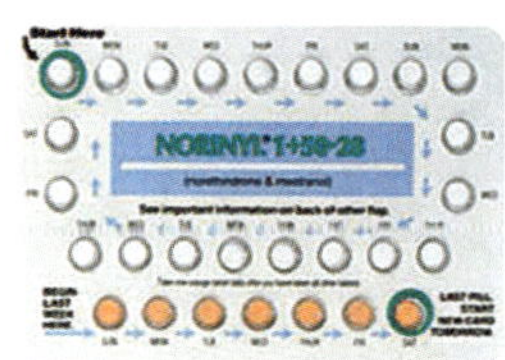

NORINYL® 1/50
(discontinued per FDA)
Actavis

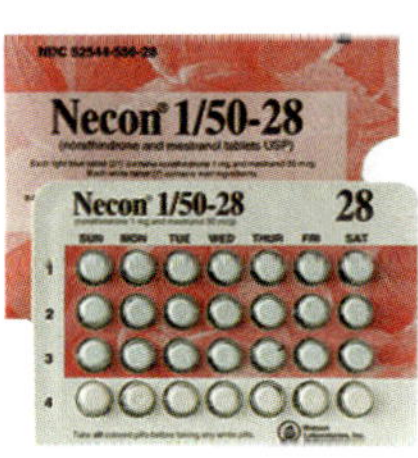

NECON® 1/50 - 28 TABLETS
Actavis

COMBINED PILLS - 50 microgram PILLS cont.

1 mg norethindrone / 50 mcg ethinyl estradiol

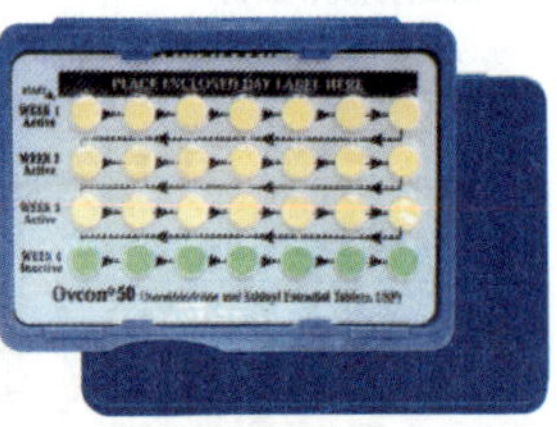

OVCON® 50 28-DAY
(discontinued per FDA)
Warner-Chilcott

1 mg ethynodiol diacetate / 50 mcg ethinyl estradiol

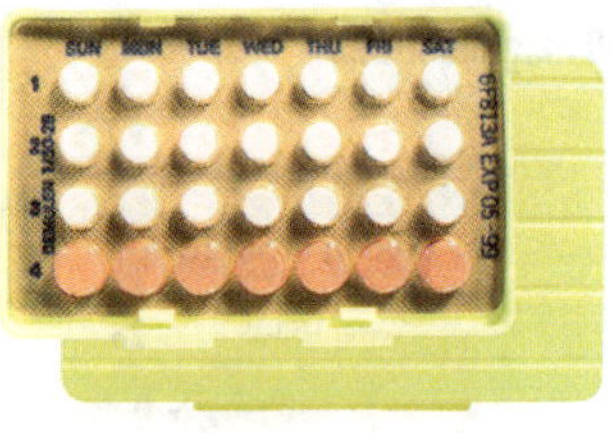

DEMULEN® 1/50-28
(discontinued per FDA)
Pfizer

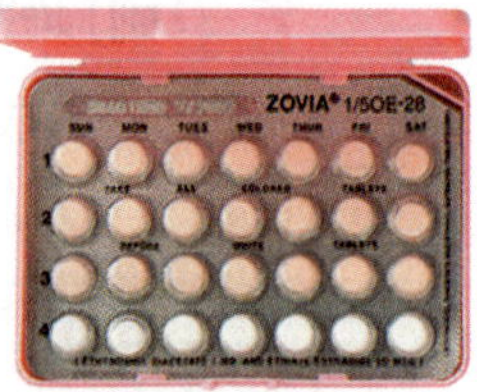

ZOVIA® 1/50
Actavis

REFERENCES

ACOG Committee Opinion 615, January 2015, Access to Contraception.

ACOG Committee Opinion 598. May 2014, The initial reproductive health visit.

ACOG CTE Opinion No. 518, Feb 2012

Alexander SC et. al., Jama Pediatrics, 2014 Feb: 168(2):163

Allmetal Hum Reprod. 2016; 31(11):2491

Amba J, Chandra A, Mosher V D et al. Fertility, family planning, and women's health: New data from 1995 NSFG. Vital Health Stat 1997; 23:62-63.

American College of Obstetrics and Gynecologists (ACOG). Emergency oral contraception. ACOG Practice Patterns 1996 (Dec. no. 3).

American College of Obstetrics and Gynecologists (ACOG). Committee Opnion No. 670: Immediate postpartum long-acting reversible contraception. Obstet Gynecol 2016; 128:e32-37

Anderson FD, Hait H, the Seasonale-301 Study Group. A multicenter, randomized study of an extended cycle oral contraceptive. Contraception 2003; 68; 89-96.

Anderson JE et al. Contraceptive Sterilization Among Married Adults: National Data on who Chooses Vasectomy and Tubal Sterilization. Contraception 85(2012):552-7

Anderson, et al, Contraception 49, 1994: 56.

Arevalo N, Jennings V, Nikula M. Efficacy of the new TwoDay method of family planning. Fertil Steril. 2004; 82:885-892.

Arevalo N, Jennings V, Sinai I. Efficacy of a new method of family planning: the Standard Days Method. Contraception. 2001; 65:333-338.

Artz, L, Demand M, Pulley LV, Posner SF, Macaluso M. Predictors of difficulty inserting the female condom. Contraception 65, 2002:151-157.

Association for Voluntary Surgical Contraception. Postpartum IUD insertion: Clinical and programatic guidelines (monograph) 1994 (AVSC has changed name to Engender Health).

Audet MC, Moreau M, Koltun WD, Waldbaum AS, Shangold G, Fisher AC, Creasy MD. Evaluation of contraceptive efficacy and cycle control of a transdermal contraceptive patch vs. an oral contraceptive: a randomized controlled trial. JAMA. 285; 2001:2347-2354.

A van Hylckamu Vlieg et al. The VTE risk of OCs, effects of oestrogendose and progestin type: results of the MEGA case-control study. BMJ 2009; 339: b2921.

Backman T, Huhtala S, Luoto R, Tuominen J, Rauramo I, Koskenvuo M. Advance Information Improves User Satisfaction with the Levonorgestrel Intrauterine System. Obstetrics and Gynecology 99, 2002: 608-13.

Ballagh SA. Sterilization in the office: the concept is now a reality. Contraceptive Technology Reports. February, 2003 supplement to the newsletter, Contraceptive Technology Update.

Bednarek PH, Creinin MD, Reeves MF et al. Immediate versus delayed IUD insertion after uterine aspiration N Engl J Med, 2011 Jun 9; 364(23): 2208-17.

Bonny AE, Ziegler J, Harvey R et al. Weight gain in obese and non-obese adolescent girls initiating depot medroxyprogesterone, OCPs and no hormonal method. Arch Pedi Adol Med. 160(1):40-5. 2006.

Barone MA, Nazerali H, Cortez M, et al. A prospective study of time and number of ejaculations to azoospermia after vasectomy by ligation and excision. J Urology 2003; 170:892-896.

Bartlett LA, et al. Risk factors for legal induced abortion related mortality risk by pregnancy outcome, U.S. 1991-1999. Obstet-Gynecol 2004; 103(4): 729-739.

Bearak et al. Contraception 2016

Beavis, Cancer 2017

Berel V, Hermon C, Kay C, Hannaford P, Darby S, Reeves G. Mortality associated with oral contraceptive use: 25 year follow-up of cohort of 46,000 women from Royal College of General Practitioners' oral contraceptive study; Br Med J 1999: 918:96-100.

Berga SL, Marcus MD, Loucks TL, Hlastala S, Ringham R, Krohn MA. Recovery of ovarian activity in women with functional hypothalamic amenorrhea who were treated with cognitive behavioral therapy. Fertil Steril 2003; 80:976-981.

Berlex Laboratories, Inc. YASMIN prescribing information: Physician Labeling and Patient Instructions; June, 2001.

Bjarnadottir R, Tuppurainen M, Killick S. Comparison of cycle control with a combined contraceptive vaginal ring and oral levonorgestrel/ethinyl estradiol. American Journal of Obstetrics and Gynecology. March 2002;186:389-95.

Brache V, Alvarez-Sanchez F, Faundes A, Tejada AS, Cochon L. Ovarian endocrine function through five years of continuous treatment with Norplant subdermal contraceptive implants. Contraception 1990;41:169.

Bradner, C.H., et al. Older, but Not Wiser: How Men Get Information About AIDS and Sexually Transmitted Diseases After High School. Family Planning Perspectives 2000; January/February.

Briggs GG, Freeman RK, Yaffe SJ. Drugs in Pregnancy and Lactation, Fifth edition. Lippincott Williams & Wilkins, Philadelphia. 1998.

BRITO Ferriani, et al. Contraception 2005

Burke HM, Chen M, Buluzi M et al. Effect of self-administration versus provider-administrated injection of subcutaneous depot medroxypregesterone acetate on contunuation rates in Malawi: A randomised controlled trial. Lancet Glob Health 2018; doi:10.1016/S2214-109X(18)30061-5

Canto-DeCetina TEC, Canto P, Luna MO. Effect of counseling to improve compliance in Mexican women receiving depot-medroxyprogesterone acetate. Contraception 63; 2001: 143-146. Cates W Jr., Steiner MJ. Dual protection against unintended pregnancy and sexually transmitted infections: What is the best contraceptive approach? Sex Transm Dis 2002;29:168-174.

CDC 2010. CDC US Medical Eligibility Criteria for Contraceptive Use, 2010

CDC 2013. Us Selected Practice Recommendations for Contraceptive Use 2013, CDC MMWR Recommendations and Reports/Vol. 62/No. 5, June 21, 2013

Cecil, Nelson, Trussell, Hatcher, Contraception 82. 2010; p489-490.

Centers for Disease Control and Prevention. 1998 Guidelines for treatment of sexually transmitted diseases. MMWR 1998:47(No. RR-1).

Centers for Disease Control Cancer and Steroid Hormone Study. Long-term oral contraceptive use and the risk of breast cancer. JAMA. 1983; 249:1591-1595.

Chi-Chem Contraception 1987;35:171-8

Cochrane Database of systemic reviews. Treatments for breast engorgement during lactation. 2008

Cochrane Database of Systematic Reviews. Vander Wijden et al. Lactational amenorrhea for family planning. 2008.

Colditz GA, Rosner BA, et al. Risk factors for breast cancer according to family history of breast cancer. J Natl Cancer Inst. 1996;88:365-371.

Cole JA et al. VTE, MI and stroke among transdermal contraceptive system users. Ob & Gyn 2007; 109(2) 339-346.

Collaborative Group; Lancet 1996

Collaborative Group on Hormonal Factors in Breast Cancer. Breast cancer and hormonal contraceptives: collaborative reanalysis of individual data on 53,297 women with breast cancer and 100,239 women without breast cancer from epidemiological studies. Lancet 1996; 347:1713-1727.

Connonlly, Thorpe, Pahel, Urogynecoly J. Pelvic Floor Disfunct 2005

Coutinho EM with Segal SJ. Is Menstruation Obsolete? Oxford University Press; Oxford; New York; 1999.

Cowman W.L. et al. Vaginal Misoprostol Aids in Difficult IUC Removal: a report of three cases. Contraception 2012;86:281-4.

Creinin MD, Burke AE. Methotrexate and misoprostol for early abortion: a multicenter trial. Acceptablity. Contraception 1996;54:19-22.

Creinin MD, Vittinghoff E, Schaff E, Klaisle C, Darney PD, Dean C. Medical abortion with oral methotrexate and vaginal misoprostol. Obstet Gynecol 1997;90:611-5.

Cromer BA, Lazebnik MD, Rome E et al. Double-blind controlled trial of estrogen supplementation in adolescent girls who receive depot medroxyprogesterone acetate for contraception. Am Jour Obstet Gynec 2005; 192:41-47.

Croxatto HB, Diaz S, Pavez M, et al. Plasma progesterone levels during long-term treatment with levonorgestrel silastic implants. Acta Endocrinol 1982;101:307-11.

Curtis et al. Contraception for Women in Selected Circumstances. Obstetrics and Gynecology, June 2002; 99 (6):1100-1112.

Curtis KM et. Al. Update to US SPR: Self-Administration of Subcutaneous Depo+Medroxyprogesterone Acetate. MMR May 21, 2021 / 70(20);739

Cundy T, Evans M, Roberts H, Wattie D, Ames R, Reid IR. Bone density in women receiving depot medroxyprogesterone acetate for contraception. BMJ 1991; 303: 13-16.

Daniels K, Mosher WD, Jones J. Contraceptive methods women have ever used: U.S. 1982-2020, National Health Statistics Report, 2013. No. 62

Davis KR, Weller SC. The effectiveness of condoms in reducing heterosexual transmission of HIV. Fam Plann Perspect 1999;31(6):272-279.

Davis TC et al. Patient Understanding and use of OCPs in a Southern Public Health Family Planning Clinic. Southern Medical Jnl 99(7) 713-8. 2006 Jul.de Abood M, de Castillo 2, Guerrero E, Espino M, Austin KL. Effect of Depo-Provera or Microgynon in the painful crises of sickle-cell anemia patients. Contraception 56; 1997:313.

Dermish et al. Contraception 2016

Diaz J, Bahamondes L, Monteiro I, Peta C, Hildalgo MM, Arce XE. Acceptability and performance of the levonorgestrel-releasing intrauterine system (Mirena) in Campinas, Brazil. Contraception 2000; 62: 59-61.

Dieben T, Roumen F, Apter D. Efficacy, cycle control, and user acceptability of a novel combined contraceptive vaginal ring. Obstetrics and Gynecology. Sept 2002; 100:585-93.

Dinger JC et al. The safety of DRSP-containing OC: final results from the EURAS on OCs based on 142, 475 women-years of observation. Contraception 2007; 75:344.

Dragoman et al. Contraceptive Vaginal Ring Effectiveness is Maintained during 6 Weeks of Use: a prospective study of BMI and obese women. Contraception 2013;87:432-436.

Duke JM et al. Contraception 75 (2007) 27-31.

Dunson D, Sinai I, Colombo B. The relationship between cervical secretions and the daily probabilities of pregnancy. Effectiveness of the TwoDay algorithm. Hum Repro 2001; 16: 2278-2282.

Edelman AB et al Contraception. 2016; 94(1):52

Edwards, S.R. The role of men in contraceptive decision-making: Current knowledge and future implications. Family Planning Perspectives 1994; March/April.

Farley TM, Rosenberg MS, Rowe PJ, Chen SH, Meirck O. Intrauterine devices and pelvic inflammatory disease: an international perspective. Lancet 1992; 339: 785-88.

Feldblum PJ, Morrison CS, Roddy RE, Cates W Jr. The effectiveness of barrier methods of contraception in preventing the spread of HIV. AIDS 1995;9 (suppl A):585-93.

Fehring et al., Randomized comparison of two Internet supplied fertility-awareness-based methods of family planning. Contraception 2013; 88:24-30.

Fine PM et al. Safety and acceptability with the use of a contraceptive vaginal ring after surgical and medical abortion. Contraception 75 (2007) 367.

Finer LB, Henshaw SK. Abortion incidence and service in the United States in 2000. Perspectives on Sexual and Reproductive Health 2003; 35(1): 6-15.

Fjerstad M, Trussell J, Lichtenberg ES. Severity of infection following the introduction of new infection control measures for medical abortion. Contraception 83 (2011), 330-335

Ford K, Labbok M. Contraceptive use during lactation in the United States: an update. American Institute of Public Health 1987; 77: 79-81.

Forrest JD. U.S. women's perceptions of and attitudes about the IUD. Obstet Gynecol Surv. 1996; 31:S30-34

Fox et al. 2013

Fox et al., Cervical preparation for surgical abortion prior to 20 weeks, Contraception 2014. Feb;89(2)75-84. Cervical Preparation for Surgical Abortion 20-24 weeks. SFP Guideline 20073, Contraception 2008. 308-314

Fraser SI, Affandi B, Croxatto HB, et al. Norplant consensus statement and background paper. Turku, Finland: Leiras Oy International, 1997.

Frezieres RG, Walsh TL, Nelson AL, Clark VA, Coulson AH: Breakage and acceptability of a polyurethane condom: A randomized controlled study. Fam Plann Perspect 1998;30;73-8.

Fu H Family Planning Perspectives 2009

Furlong LA. Ectopic Pregnancy risk when contraception fails. J Repro Med. 2002; Vol 47, No. 11.

Gallo I.D. et al. LNG-IUS Versus Oral Progestogen Treatment for Endometrial Hyperplasia: a long=term comperative cohort study. Hum Reprod 2013 Nov 28(11):2966-71.

Gallo MF, Grimes DA, Lopez LM et al. Non-latex versus latex male condoms for contraception. Cochrane Database Systematic reviews 2005.

Geere et al. Behind-the-counter status and availability of EC. AJOG 199(5): 478. 2008 Nov.

Glaser A. Can we identify women at risk of pregnancy despite using EC? Data from randomized trials of UPA and LNG. Contraception, 2011; 84(4):363

Glasier AF, Cameron ST, Fine PM, Logan SJ, Casale W, Van Horn J, Sogor L, Blithe DL, Scherrer B, Mathe H, Jaspart A, Ulmann A, Gainer Lancet. 2010; 375 (9714):

Glasier AF et al. Contraception 2003; 67:1-8.

Goldberg, Greenberg, and Darney-NEJM 2001

Goldstein M, Girardi S. Vasectomy and vasectomy reversal. Curr Thera Endocrinol Metab 1997;6:371-80.

Goodman S. et al. Increasing intrauterine contracption use by reducing barriers to post-abortal and interval insertion. Contraception 78 (2008) 136-142.

Grabrick DH, Hartmann LC, Cerhan FR, Vierkant RA, Therneau TM, et al. Risk of Breast Cancer with Oral Contraceptive Use in Women With a Family History of Breast Cancer. JAMA; 284:1791-1798.

Gray RH, Campbell OM, Zacur H, Labbok MH, MacRae SL. Postpartum return of ovarian activity in non-breastfeeding women monitored by urinary assays. J Clin Endocrinol Metab 1987;64:645-50.

Grimes DA. Health benefits of oral contraception: update on endometrial cancer prevention. The Contraception Report 2001;12(3):4-7.

Grimes DA. Modern IUDs: an update. The Contraception Report; November, 1998.

Grimes DA. Should first-time OC users be screened for genetic thrombophilia? The Contraception Report; 10:1, p.p. 9-11; March 1999.

Grimes DA. Transdermal contraceptive patch awaiting US approval. The Contraception Report; 12(4):12-14.

Grimes DA. IN Hatcher. Contraceptive Technology, 18th Ed. Intrauterine Devices (IUDS).

Grimes DA, Gallo MF, Halpein V. Fertility awareness-based methods for contraception. Cochrone Database of Systematic Reviews.

Grimes DA, Lopez L, Raymond EG et al. Spermicide used alone for contraception. Cochrane Database of Systematic Reviews 2005.

Guillebaud J. Contraception, your questions answered, 3rd edition. London, Churchill Livingstone, 1999.

Guillebaud J. Personal communication; October 14, 2001.

Gurtcheff SE, Turok DK, Stoddard G etal. Lactogenesis after early postpartum use of the contraceptive implant: A randomized controlled trial. Obstet Gynecol 2011;117:1114-1121

Guttmacher 2010 . US Pregnancies,Births, and Aboritons 2010: National and State Trends by Age, Race, and Ethnicity. 2014 https://www.guttmacher.org/pubs/USTPtrends10.pdf2]

Guttmacher 2014. Induced abortion in the United States. Guttmacher Institute, July 2014. http://www.guttmacher.org/pubs/fb_induced_abortion.html

Guttmacher Inst.- 2008

Hafner DW, Schwartz P. What I've Learned about Sex. A Perigee Book: New York: The Berkeley Publishing Group, 1998.

Hakim-Elahi E, Tovell HMM, Burnhill MS. Complications of first-trimester abortion: a report of 170,000 cases. Obstet Gynecol 1990;76:129.

Hall KS et al. Progestin-only contraceptive pill

Hall PE. New once-a-month injectable contraceptives, with particular reference to Cyclofem/Cyclo-Provera. Int. J Gynaecol Obstet 1998; 62: S43-S56.

Hausknecht R. Mifepristone and misoprostol for early medical abortion: 18 months experience in the United States. Contraception 2003; 67:463-465.

Haws, J.M., et al. Clinical Practice of vasectomies in the United States in 1995. Urology 1998; October.

Henshaw SK. Unintended pregnancy in the United States. Fam Plann Perspect 1998;30:24-9, 46.

Harris Interactive Inc. prepared for The National Women's Health Resource Center. Menstrual Management Survey Report. Aug. 29, 2008. Accessed at www.healthywomen.org/Documents/MenstrualManagementReport.pdf

Hartmann KE, Jerome RN, Lindegre ML et al. Primary Care Management of Abnormal Uterine Bleeding. ARHQ Comparative Effectiveness Reviews. Rockville, MD: Agency for Healthcare Research and Quality; March 2013

Hatcher RA, et al. Contraceptive Technology. 20th ed. New York: Irvington, 2011:37

Hatcher RA, Trussell J, Stewart F, Cates W Jr, Stewart GK, Guest F, Kowal D. Contraceptive Technology, 17th ed. New York NY, Ardent Media, 1998

Hayes J et al. A pilot clinical trial of ultrasound-guided postplacental insertion of a levonorgestrel intra-uterine device. Contraception 76(4): 292-6 2007 Oct.

Hynes J.S. et al. Interest in Multipurpose Prevention Technologies to Prevent HIV/STIs and Unintended Pregnancy Among Young Women in the United States; Contraception 97; 277-284 (2018)

Heinemann LA et al. Contraception 75 (2007) 328-336.

Heit et al. Ann Int Med 2005 143: 697-706.

Hennessy S., Berlin JA, Kinman JL et al. Risk of VTE from OCs containing desogestrel and gestodene versus levonorgestrel: a meta-analysis and formal sensitivity analysis. Contraception 64(2): 125-33, 2001 August.

Hilgers, T.W., Abraham, G.E., and Cavanagh, D. (1978), "Natural Family Planning. I. The Peak Symptom and Estimated Time of Ovulation", Obstetrics and Gynecology 52(5): 575-582.

Hofmeyer J. Sex Marital Therapy 2002

Hogue CJR, Cates W Jr, Tietze C. The effects of induced abortion on subsequent reproduction. The Johns Hopkins University School of Hygiene and Public Health. Epidemiol Rev 1982;4:66

Hubacher D., Grimes DA. 2002; Forest JD. 1996

Hynes J.S. et al., 2018

International Planned Parenthood Federation Handbook 1997.

Ito KE, Gizlice Z, Owen-O'Doud J. Parent opinion of sexuality education in a state mandated

abstinence education: does policy match parental preference? J Adol Health. 39(5): 634, 2006 Nov.

Jain J, Jakimiuk AJ, Bode FR, Ross D, Kaunitz AM. Contraceptive efficacy and safety of DMPA-SC. Contraception 2004; 70:269-275.

Jamieson DJ, Costello C, Trussell J, Hillis SP, Marchbanks PA, Peterson HB. The risk of pregnancy after vasectomy. Obstetrics and Gynecology 2004; 103:848-850.

Jatlaoui TC et al., Abortion surveillance—United States, 2013, Morbidity and Mortality Weekly Report,

2016, Vol. 65, No. SS-12.

Jerman J, Jones RK and Onda T, Characteristics of U.S. Abortion Patients in 2014 and Changes Since 2008, New York: Guttmacher Institute, 2016

Jick S, et al. Further results on the risks of nonfatal VTE in users of the contraceptive transdermal patch compared to users of OCs containing norgestimate and 35 mcg of EE. Contraception 2007; 76: 4-7

Johnson JV. et al Contraception 75 (2007) 23-26.

Jones RK, Coitus Interruptus IN Hatcher; RA Contraceptive Technology 21st edition. P 452

Jones RK, Dorroch JE, Henshaw SK. Patterns with socioeconomic charactericss of women obtaining abortions in 2000-2001. Perspectives in Sexual and Reproductive Health 2002,34:226-235.

Juliato CT et al. Usefulness of FSH measurements for determining menopause in long-term users of depot medroxyprogesterone acetate over 40 years of age. Contraception 76 (2007) 282-286.

Kapp N, Curtis K, Nanda K. Progestogen-only contraceptive use among breastfeeding women: Asystematic review. Contraception 2010:82;17-37

Kaunitz AM. personal communications; December 28, 1998 and February 24, 1999.

Kaunitz AM, Garceau RJ, Cromie MA. Comparative safety, efficacy, and cycle control of Lunelle monthly contraceptive injection (medroxyprogesterone acetate and estradiol cypionate injectable suspension) and Ortho-Novum 7/7/7 oral contraceptive (norethindrone/ethinyl estradiol triphasic). Contraception 1999; 60(4):179-187.

Kennedy KI, Trussell J. Postpartum contraception and lactation. IN Hatcher RA, Trussell J, Stewart F et al: Contraceptive Technology, 17th ed.; New York: Ardent Media Inc; 1998: 592-4. [The same data are presented in the Family Health International Module for the teaching of Lactational Amenorrhea]

Kirby D. (2001). Emerging Answers: Research Findings on Programs to Reduce Teen Pregnancy. Washington DC: The National Campaign to Prevent Teen Pregnancy

Kjos SL, Peters RK, Xiang A, Duncan T, Schaefer U, Buchanan TA. Contraception and the risk of type 2 diabetes mellitus in Latina women with prior gestational diabetes mellitus. JAMA 1998; 280: 533-38.

Klavon SL, Grubb G. Insertion site complications during the first year of Norplant use. Contraception 1990;41:27.

Kost K, Sigah, Contraception 2008

Krattenmacher R. Drospirenone: pharmacology and pharmacokinetics of a unique progestogen. Contraception 2000; 62:29-38.

Kuyoh MA, Toroitich-Ruto C, Grimes DA, et al. Sponge versus diaphragm for contraception: a Cochrane review. Contraception 2003; 67(1):15-18.

Kwiecien M et al. Contraception 2003; 67:9-13.

Lidegaard O et al. Hormonal contraception and risk of VTE: National follow-up study. BMJ 2009;339: b2890

Lipnick RJ, Buring JE, Hennekens CH, et al. Oral contraceptives and breast cancer: a prospective cohort study. JAMA. 1986; 255:58-61.

Lippes, J. Am J Obstet Gyn-1999; 180-265-9

Lippes J (Guest Editor). Quinacrine sterilization: reports on 40,252 cases. Intl J of Gynec & Obstet Volume 83, supl 2, October 2003.

R. Lyus, et. al. Outcomes with same-day cervical preparation with Dilapan-S osmotic dilators and vaginal misoprostol before dilatation and evacuation at 18 to 21+6 weeks' gestation. Contraception vol 87(1):71-75

R. Lyus, et. al. Same day cervical preparation with misoprostol second trimester D-E: a case series. Contraception vol 88 (2013):116-121

Marcell, A.V., et al. Where Does Reproductive Health Fit Into the Lives of Adolescent Males? Perspectives of Sexual and Reproductive Health 2003; 35(4):180-186.

Marguilies R, Miller L. Increased depot medroxyprogesterone acetate use increases family planning program pharmaceutical supply costs. Contraception 2001 (63):147-149.

Marrazzo JM and Cates W Jr. Reproductive tract infections. In: Hatcher RA, et al. Contraceptive Technology. 20th ed. New York: Ardent Media, 2011:573

Marrazzo JM and Park IU, Contraceptive Technology 21st edition, Ayer Company Publishing Inc. New York, p.58

Martin JA, Hamilton BE, Osterman MJ. Births in the United States, 2013. Hyattsville (MD): Centers for Disease Control and Prevention; 2014.United Nations. 2012 Demographic Yearbook. New York: UN; 2013.

McNicholas, 2017 IN PRESS

Medical Abortion Outcomes following quickstart of contraceptive implants and DMPA. ElizabethRaymond et al, Presented at the North American Forum on Family Planning, November 2015.

Michealsson-1998; Lancet, 353:1481-1484

Michaelson, M.D., Oh, W.K. Epidemiology of and risk factors for testicular cancer. Available from http://www.utdol.com [Accessed 10 October 2004]

Miller L, Verhoeven CH, Hout J. Extended regimens of the contraceptive vaginal ring: a randomized trial. ObGyn. 106(3): 473-82, 2005 Sep.

Miller L, Grice J. Intradermal proximal field block: an innovative anesthetic technique for levonorgestrel implant removal. Obstet Gynecol 1998;91:294-297.

Miller L, Hughes J. Continuous combination oral contraceptive pills to eliminate withdrawal bleeding: a randomized trial. Obstet Gynecol 2003;101:653-61.

MMWR, Vol 65, Number 4, July 29, 2016, U.S. Selected Practice Recommendations for Contraceptive Use, p19

Moreau C & Trussell J. Results from Pooled Phase III Studies of VPA for Emergency Contraception. Contraception 2012;88:673-80.

Monteiro I, Bahamondes L, Diaz J, Perotti M, Petta C. Therapeutic use of levonorgestrel-releasing intra-uterine systems in women with menorrhagia: a pilot study. Contraception 65; 2002; 325-328.

Morroni C et al. The Impact of Oral Contraceptive Initiation on Young Women's Condom Use in 3 American Cities: Missed Opportunities for Intervention. PloSOne 2014 July 8; 9(7):e101804. doi:10.1371/jpurnal

Mosher WD et al. Use of contraception and use of family planning services in the U.S.: 1982-2000. Advance data from vital and health statistics, No. 350. 2004.

Mulders TMT, Dieben TOM. Use of the novel combined contraceptive vaginal ring NuvaRing for ovulation inhibition. Fertility and Sterility 2001; 75:865-870

Mulders TMT, Dieben TOM, et al. Ovarian function with a novel combined contraceptive vaginal ring. Hum Reprod 2002;10:2594-2599.

Murray PP, Stadel BV, Schlesselman JJ. Oral contraceptive use in women with a family history of breast cancer. Obstet Gynecol. 1989; 73:977-983.

Narod-Lancet 357 (9267): 1467-70, 2001

Narod ST. The Hereditary Ovarian Cancer Clinical Study Group. Oral contraceptives and the risk of hereditary ovarian cancer. N Engl J Med 1998;339;424-8.

Narod ST. et al. Lancet 357 [9267]: 1467-70, 2001.

National FP and Repro Health Association April 2020

National Health Statistics Reports, No. 86, Nov. 2015

Nelson AL. Recent use of condoms and EC by women who selected condoms as their contraceptive method. AJOG 194(6): 1710-5, 2006 Jun.

Ness RB, Grisso JA, Klapper J, et al. Risk of ovarian cancer in relation to estrogen and progestin dose and use characteristics of oral contraceptives. Am J Epidemiol 2000;152:233-241.

Ness, R.B., et al. Do men become infertile after having sexually transmitted urethritis? An epidemiologic examination. Fertility and Sterility 1997; 68(2):205-213.

Nilsson CG, Haukkamaa M, Vierok H, et al. Tissue concentrations of levonorgestrel in women using lng-releasing IUD. Clinical Endocrinology 17(6):529-36, 1982.

O'Hanley K, Huber DH. Postpartum IUDs: keys for success. Contraception 1992; 45: 351-361.

Oddson et al. Efficacy & Safety of a Contraceptive Vaginal Ring (NuvaRing) Compared to a Combined Oral Contraceptive: a 1-year randomized trial. Contraception 2005; 70:176-182

Peipert JF, Gutman J. Oral contraceptive risk assessment: a survey of 247 educated women. Obstet Gynecol 1993;82:112-7.

Paulen ME, Curtis KM. Contraception 2009

Pazol K, et al., Trnds in use of medical abortion in the US: reanalysis of surveillance data from the CDC and Prevention, 2001-2008. Contraception 2012; 86:746-751.

Penfield JA, The Filshie clip for female sterilzation: A review of world experience. AJOG 2000; 182:485-489.

Peterson HB, Jeng G, Folger SG et al for the U.S. Collaborative Review of Sterilization Working Group. N Engl J Med 2000; 343:1681-7.

Peterson HB, Pollack AE, Warshaw JS. Tubal sterilization. In: Rock JA, Thompson JD, eds. TeLinde's Operative Gynecology. 8th ed. Philadelphia: Lippincott-Raven, 1997:541-5.

Petta LA, Ferriani RA, Abrao RA et al. Randomized clinical trial of a levonorgestrel-releasing IUS and a depot GnRH analogue for the treatment of chronic pelvic pain in women with endometriosis. Human Reprod 2005; 20(7):1993-8.

Pinkerton SD, Abramson PR. Effectiveness of condoms in preventing HIV transmission. Soc Sci Med 1997 May; 44(9):1303-1312.

Plichta, S.B., et al. Partner-specific condom use among adolescent women clients of a family planning clinic. Journal of Adolescent Health 1992; 13(6):506-511.

Polaneczky M, Guarnaccia, Alon J, Wiley J. Early experience with the contraceptive use of depot medroxyprogesterone acetate in an inner-city clinic population. Family Planning Perspectives 1996; 28: 174-178.

Porter, L.E., Ku, L. Use of reproductive health services among young men, 1995. Journal of Adolescent Health 2000; 27(3):186-194.

Postlethwaite D et al. IUC: evaluation of clinician practice patterns in Kaiser Permanente Northern California. Contraception 75 (2007) 177-184.

Preexposure Prophylaxis for the Prevention of HIV Infections in the United States - 2014; CDC Clinical Practice Guidline.

Raudaskoski TH, Lahti EI, Kauppila AJ, Apaja-Sarkkinen MA, Laatikainen TJ. Transdermal estrogen with a levonorgestrel-releasing intrauterine device for climacteric complaints: clinical and endometrial responses. Am J Obstet Gynecol 1995;172:114-9.

Raymond EG nad Grimes DA. The comparative Safety of Legal Induced Abortion and Childbirth in the US Obstet Gynecol 2012; 119:215-9

Raymond EG, Trussel J, Polis C. Population effect of increased access to ECP: A systematic review.ObGyn 109(1): 181-8. 2007.

Redmond G, Godwin AJ, Olson W, Lippman JS. Use of placebo controls in an oral contraceptive trial: methodological issues and adverse event incidence. Contraception 1999;60:81-5.

Reece et al., Sexually Transmitted Infections, 2009.

Reeves M et al., Prevention of infection after induced abortion. Contraception 83 (2011) 295-309

Rocca CH, Schwart EB, Stewart FH et al. Beyond access: acceptability, use and non-use of EC among young women. AJOG 196(1):29e 1-6, 2007.

Ropes ASW. Menstrual suppression survey, 2002.

Rosenbaum JE. Patient Teenagers? A comparison of the sexual behavior of virginity pledgers and matched non-pledgers. Pediatrics 2009; 123: 110-120.

Roumen FJ, Apter D, Mulders TM, et al. Efficacy, tolerability and acceptability of a novel contraceptive vaginal ring releasing etonogestrel and ethinyl estradiol. Hum Reprod 2001;16:469-475.

Santelli J et al. Abstinence-only education policies and programs: A position paper of the society for adolescent medicine. J Adol Health 38(2006) 83-87.

Santelli JS, Abma J, Ventura S, et al. Can changes in sexual behaviors among high school students explain the decline in teen pregancy rates in the 1990's? Journal of Adolescent Health, 2004, 35(2); 80-90.

Schafer JE, Osborne LM, Davis AR et al. Acceptability and satisfaction using Quick Start with the contraceptive vaginal ring vs. an OC. Contraception 73(5): 488. 2006.

Schwallie PC, Assenzo JR. Contraceptive use-efficacy study initializing medroxy-progesterone acetate administered as an intramuscular injection once every 90 days. Fertil Steril 1973; 24(5):331-339.

Secura G., Madden T. et al. Provision of no cost, long-acting contraception and teen pregnancy NEJM Oct. 2 2014

Seeger JD et al. Risk of thromboembolism in women taking EE/DRSP and other OCs. Obstet/Gynecol 2007; 110:587.

Segal SJ. Is menstration obsolete? Lecture in Atlanta, Georgia. November 1, 2001.

Sexual Activity and Contraceptive Use among teenagers in the U.S.., 2011-2015. NHS Report No.104

Shelton JD. Repeat emergency contraception: facing our fears. Contraception 66;2002:15-17.

Schmidt JE, Millis SD, Marchbanks PA, Jerg G, Peterson HB. Fertil Steril 2000; 74(5):892-8.

Sidney et al. Recent Combined Hormonal Contraceptives and the Risk of Thromboembolism and Other Cardiovascular Events in Users. Contraception 2013;87:93-100.

Silvestre L, Dubois C, Renault M, Rezvani Y, Baulieu E, Ulmann A. Voluntary interruption of pregnancy with mifepristone (RU-486) and a prostaglandin analogue. N Engl J Med 1990; 322:645-8.

Sivin I, Stern J et al. Prolonged intrauterine contraception: a seven-year randomized study of the levonorgestrel 20 mcg/day (LNG 20) and the Copper T 380Ag IUDs. Contraception 1991; 44:473-80

Shain IN Goldsmith 1986

Shulman LP, Oleen-Burkey M, Willke RJ. Patient acceptability and satisfaction with Lunelle monthly contraceptive injection (medroxyprogesterone acetate and estradiol cypionate injectable suspension). Contraception 1999;60(4):215-222.

Smith-McCune, Tvvesm JL, Rubin MM et al. Effect of Replens gel used with a diaphragm on tests for HPV and other lower genital tract infections. J of Lower Genital Tract Disease 10(4): 213-8, 2006 Oct.

Smith TW. Personal communication to James Trussell. December 13, 1993.

Sonalker S et al. OBSTET GYNECOL 2018; 132: 12-11-1211-21

Sonfield, A. Looking at Men's Sexual and Reproductive Health Needs. The Guttmacher Report on Public Policy 2002; November.

Sonfield, A. Meeting the Sexual and Reproductive Health Needs of Men Worldwide. The Guttmacher Report on Public Policy. 2004; March.

Speroff L, Darney PD. A Clinical Guide for Contraception. Third Edition. Lippincott Williams & Wilkins; Philadelphia; 2001.

Speroff L, Darney P. A Clinical Guide for Contraception. 6th ed. Baltimore: Lippincott, Williams & Wilkins, 2005:246

Speroff L, Glass RH, Kase NG. Clinical Gynecologic Endocrinology and Infertility. Sixth Edition. 1999; Lipincott Williams & Wilkins; Baltimore, Maryland.

Speroff L. The perimenospausal transition: maximizing preventive health care. In: Mooney B, Daughtery J, eds. Midlife Women's Health Sourcebook. Atlanta: American Health Consultants, 1995.

Steiner MJ. Cates W Jr, Warner L. The real problems with male condoms is nonuse. Sex Trans Dis 1999;26(8):459-61.

Steines M. et al. Decreased condom breakage and slippage rates after counseling men at a sexually transmitted infection clinic in Jamaica Contraception 75 (2007) 289-293

Stencheuer MA. Comprehensive Gynecology Fourth Edition. Mosby. 2001

Stewart FH, Harper CC, Ellertson CE, Grimes DA, Sawyer GF, Trussell J. Clinical breast and pelvic examination requirements for hormonal contraception: Current practice vs. evidence. JAMA 2001;285:2232-2239.

Strauss LT, Herndon J, Charg J et al. Abortion surveillance: U.S., 2002. In: CDC surveillance summaries, Nov 25, 2005 MMWR 2005; 54 no. 55-57.

Stuenkel CA, Davis SR, Gompel A, et al. Treatment of symptoms of the menopause: An Endocrine Society Clinical Practice Guideline. J Clin Endocrinol Metab 2015; 100:3975.

Sulak PJ et al. Am J Obstet Gynecol 2002; 186:1142-1149.

Sulak PJ et al. Obstet Gynecol 2000; 95:261-266.

Swica et al. Acceptability of Home Use of Mifepristone for medical abortion. Contraception 2013; 88:122-127.

Task Force on Postovulatory Methods of Fertility Regulation. Randomized controlled trial of levonorgestrel versus the Yuzpe regimen of combined oral contraceptives for emergency contraception. Lancet 1998; 352:420-33.

The Alan Guttmacher Institute. Sex and America's Teenagers. New York and Washington: 1994.

The Centers for Disease Control Cancer and Steroid Hormone Study- 1983

The Hereditary Ovarian Cancer Clinical Study Group. Oral contraceptives and the risk of hereditary ovarian cancer. N Engl J Med 1998;339;424-8.

Thomas MA et al. A novel vaginal pH regulator: results from the phase 3 AMPOWER Contraceptive clinical trial. Contraception 2020; 2:100031

Truitt ST, Fraser AB, Grimes DA, Gallo MF, Schulz KF. Hormonal contraception during lactation: a systematic reivew of randomized controlled trials. Contraception 2003; 68:233-8.

Trussell J. Contraceptive failure in the United States. Contraception 2018:83;397-404

Trussell J et al. Efficacy, Safety, and Pessimal Considerations. Contraceptive Technology 21st ed. P.118

Trussell J IN Contraceptive Technology 2018

Trussell J, Kowal D. The essentials of contraception. IN: Hatcher RA, et al. Contraceptive Technology. 20th ed. New York: Ardent Media, 2011:66.

Trussell J, Leveque JA, Koenig JD, London R, Borden S, Henneberry J, LaGuardia KD, Stewart F, Wilson TG, Wysocki S, Strauss M. The economic value of contraception: a comparison of 15 methods. Am J Public Health 1995;85:494-503.

Trussell J, Stewart F, Guest F, Hatcher RA. Emergency contraceptive pills: a simple proposal to reduce unintended pregnancies. Fam Plann Perspect 1992;24:269-73.

Tschugguel W, Berga SL. Treatment of functional hypothalamic amenorrhea with hypnotherapy. Fertil Steril. 2003; 80:982-985.

U.S. Collaborative Review of Sterilization. The risk of pregnancy after tubal sterilization. Am J Obstet Gynecol 1996; 174:1161-70.

U.S. Selective Practice Recommendations 2016, CDC MMWR, July 28, 2016

U.S. Selected Practice Recommendations for Contraceptive Use, 2016, MMWR July 29, 2016 p.35

Use of at-home semi-quantitztive pregnancy tests serve as a replacement for clinical follow-up of medical abortion? A US study. Contraception 2012; 86:757-762.

Valcencic M, Granitsiotis, Eur Urol 2003

Valle RF, Carignan CS, Wright TC, et al. Tissue response to STOP microcoil transcervical permanent contraceptive device: results from a prehysterectomy study. Fertil Steril 2001; 76:974.

Vander Wijden C, Kleijnen J, Vanden Berk T. Lactational amenorrhea for family planning. Cochrane Database Systematic Reviews 2005.

Vercellini P et al. Fertil Steril 2003; 80:560-63.

Vestergaard P, Rejnmark L., Mosekilde L. Oral contraceptive use and risk of fractures. Contraception 73; 2006: 571-576.

Von Hertzen H, Piaggio G, Ding J et al. Low dose Mifepristone and two regimens of levonorgestrel for emergency contraception: a WHO multicentre randomised trial. Lancet 2002; 360: 1803-10.

Youth Risk Behavior Survey-2003

Walsh T, Grimes D, Frezieres R, Nelson A, Bernstein L, Coulson A, Bernstein G. Randomized controlled trial of prophylactic antibiotics before insertion of intrauterine devices. Lancet 1998:351;1005-1008.

Warner DL, Hatcher RA, Boles J, Goldsmith J. Practices and patterns of condom usage for prevention of infection and pregnancy among male university students (Session PS-12). Proceeding of the Eleventh Annual National Preventive Medicine Meeting. March 1994.

Warner L, Hatcher RA, Steiner MJ. Male Condoms. IN Hatcher RA et al. Contraceptive Technology 18th Edition. 2004.

Warner L., Steiner M.J., 2017

Weidner, W., et al. Relevance of male accessory gland infection for subsequent fertility with special focus on prostatitis. Human Reproduction Update 1999; 5(5):421-432.

Weller S, Davis K, Condom effectiveness in reducing heterosexual HIV transmission. Cochrane Database System Rev. 2001

Westoff C, Kerns J, Morroni C, Cushman LF, Tiezzi L, Murphy PA. Quick Start: a novel contraceptive initiation method. Contraception 66; 2002:141-145.

Westhoff C et al. Changes in weight with depot medroxyprogesterone acetate subcutaneous injection 104 mg/0.65 ml Contraception 75 (2007) 261-267.

Whaley et al., Update on medical abortion: Simplifying the process for women. Current Opinions in Obstetrics and Gynecology Sept 2015

Whelton et al. 2017 ACC/AHA/AAPA/ABC/ACPM/AGS/APhA/ASH/ASPC/NMA/PCNA Guideline for the Prevention, Detection, Evaluation, and Management of High Blood Pressure in Adults: Executive Summary. Journal of the American College of Cardiology May 2018, 71 (19) 2199-2269; DOI: 10.1016/j.jacc.2017.11.005

White K, Teal SB, Potter JE. Contraception after delivery and short interpregnancy intervals among women in the United States. Obstet Gynecol 2015;125:1471-1477

White MK, Ory HW, Rooks JB, Rochat RW. Intrauterine device termination rates and menstrual cycle day of insertion. Obstet Gynecol 1980; 55:220-4.

White, Obstet Gynecol, 2015

WHO 2015 . Preventing Unsafe Abortion, World Health Organization, May 2015. http://www.who.int/reproductivehealth/topics/unsafe_abortion/magnitude/en/

WHO task force on Postovulatory Methods of Fertility Regulation. Lancet Aug 8, 1998

E. Wiebe, et. al., Can we safely avoid fasting before abortions with low dose procedural sedation? A retrospective cohort chart review of anesthesia-related complications in 47,748 abortions. Contraception 87(1) 2013:51-54.

Willett WC, Green A, Stampfer MJ, Speizer FE, Colditz GA, Rosner B, Monson RR, Stason W, Hennekens CH. Relative and absolute risks of coronary heart disease among women who smoke cigarettes. New Eng J Med 317:1303, 1987.

Winer RL, Hughes JP, Feng Q et al. Condom use and the risk of genital HPV infection in young women. NEJM 2006; 354:2645-54.

World Health Organization, Department of Reproductive Health and Research. Improving Access to Quality Care in Family Planning: Medical Eligibility Criteria for Contraceptive Use. Second Edition. Geneva. 2000.

World Health Organization. WHO Taskforce Postovulatory Methods of Fertility Regulation. Lancet Aug 8, 1998.

Writing Group for the Women's Health Initiative. Risks and benefits of estrogen plus progestin in healthy postmenopausal women. JAMA 2002; 288: 321-333.

Zhou et al. EC with Multiload Co-375 SL IUD: a multicenter clinical trial. Contraception 2001; 64:107-12.

Zieman M, Guillebaud J, Weisberg E, Shangold G, Fisher A, Creasy G. Integrated summary of contraceptive efficacy with the Ortho Evra transdermal system. Fertility and Sterility Supplement; Sept, 2001. S19

SPANISH/ENGLISH TRANSLATIONS

SPANISH / ESPAÑOL	ENGLISH / INGLES
• Abstinencia	• Abstinence
• Amamantar a Su Bebe	• Breast-feeding
• Tapa Cervical	• Cervical Cap
• Retraer el pene antes de ejecular	• Coitus Interruptus (Withdrawal)
• Injecciones Combinadas	• Combined Injectables
• La Pildora	• Combined Oral Contraceptives (COCs)
• Condones para hombres	• Condoms for Men
• Condones para Mujeres	• Condoms for Women
• La "T" o Dispositivo de Cobre	• Copper T 380-A
• Inyecciones de Depo-Provera	• Depo-Provera
• El Diafragma	• Diaphragm
• Contraceptivo de Emergencia	• Emergency Contraception
• Consciente Sobre Metodos de Fertilidad	• Fertility Awareness Methods
• Espuma Contraceptiva	• Foam
• Metodos para el Futuro	• Future Methods
• Dispositivos	• IUDs
• Gelatina Anticonceptiva	• Jellies
• El Dispositivo de "Levo Norgestrel"	• Levonorgestrel IUD
• Implantes de NORPLANT	• Norplant Implant
• El Dispositivo de "Progestasert"	• Progestasert IUD
• Contraceptives de Progesterona Solamente	• Progestin-Only Contraceptives
• Pildoras de Progesterona Solamente	• Progestin-Only Pills (POPs)
• Mifepristone	• Mifepristone
• Espermicidas	• Spermicides
• Ligadura o Estirilizacion de las Trompas	• Tubal Sterilization
• Tela Anticonceptiva	• Vaginal contraceptive film
• Vasectomia	• Vasectomy
• Todos los dispositivos	• All other IUDs at this time

INDEX

E

F

G

H

J

K

L

M

N

ManagingContraception.com

ADDITIONAL RESOURCES FROM MANAGING CONTRACEPTION INCLUDES:

- *Contraceptive Technology 21st edition*
- Contraceptive Options Wall Chart
- *Choices* in English and Spanish

VISIT

www.managingcontraception.com

Search Q&A archives for answers to your contraceptive questions.

VISIT

www.mimiziemanmd.com

to submit new questions.

16th Edition

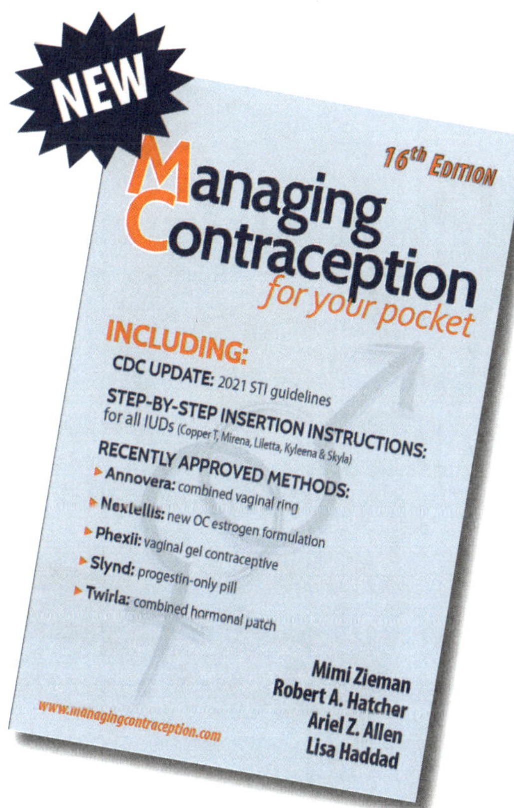

Completely Updated Edition

TO ORDER COPIES GO TO

managingcontraception.com

email info@managingcontraception.com or call 404-875-5001

NEW 21st Edition

Contraceptive Technology

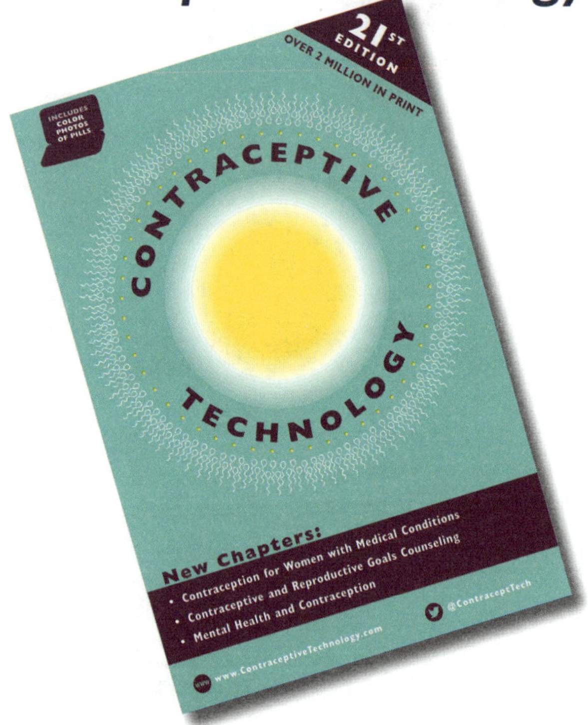

With over **2,000,000** copies distributed, this 1048 page book is a must in every office where family planning, contraception and women's health is dealt with! Also extensively used as a classroom text.

This is the 21st edition and started by Dr. Robert A. Hatcher MD, MPH over 30 years ago. Considered by many to be the bible on contraception.

TO ORDER COPIES GO TO

managingcontraception.com

email info@managingcontraception.com or call 404-875-5001

NEW 2021

Choices

Available in Spanish & English

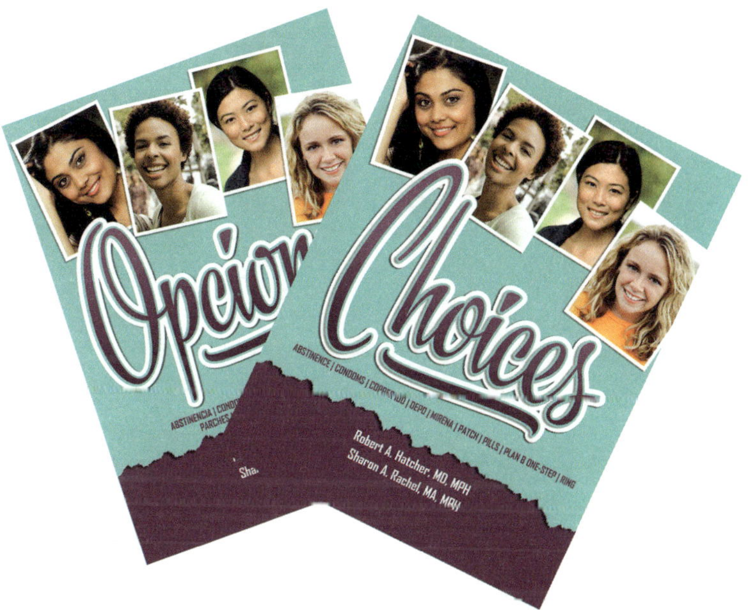

Written for teens and young adults!

CHOICES includes 21 updated descriptions of contraceptives (birth control methods). This completely updated book for 2021 gives a clear, concise overview of each method that is easily understandable by preteens to adults. It includes the most important information, including the advantages and disadvantages of each method, so the person reading can relate to their own situation. There is also a chapter on STI's.

It is our desire that young people have a choice, including abstinence, when it comes to their sexual health. Many **STATES** have ordered large quantities to give out to teens.

TO ORDER COPIES GO TO

managingcontraception.com

email info@managingcontraception.com or call 404-875-5001

Contraceptions Options

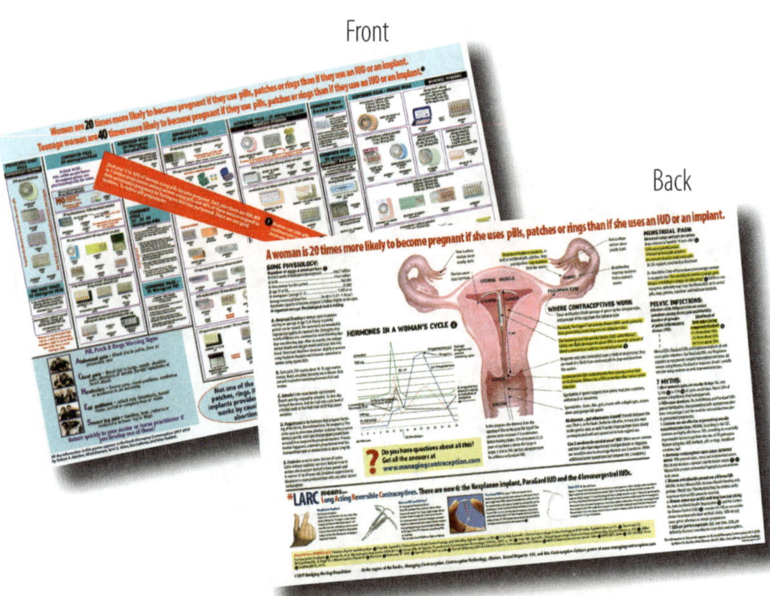

This large 24"x36" chart is printed and laminated both sides.Also available in smaller 11"x17" format for patient handout!

One side shows all the birth control pills from the lowest to the highest dosages. Great for the clinician determining which pill to prescribe and also very helpful for the patient that can't remember the name of the pill she is taking but can identify the package.

The other side chows **ALL** the contraceptive methods with emphasis on the LARC METHODS (Long Acting Reversible Contraceptives). It has an illustration of the uterus showing where and how contraceptives work. There is also an illustration of an IUD placement and MUCH MORE!!

GREAT TEACHING TOOL

TO ORDER COPIES GO TO

managingcontraception.com

email info@managingcontraception.com or call 404-875-5001

THE HISTORY OF CONTRACEPTION AND OF POPULATION GROWTH

2050: World population will reach 9.7 billion. By 2050, Africa's population is expected to be 2.4 billion, up from 1.1 billion in 2014. *[Population Reference Bureau, www.prb.org]*

2025: World population to reach 8 billion (this billion will take 14 years)

2017: World population at May 31: 12pm EST: 7,508,410,159 increasing at 3 new people per second
2016: FDA approves 19.5mg LNG IUD, Kyleena, for 5 years contraceptive use. Same size as Skyla but approved for more years
2016: 83% of people in the world are born in less developed countries [Population Reference Bureau, www.prb.org]
2015: **Liletta**, less expensive than Mirena
2013: **The mini-Mirena IUD called Skyla (13.5mg LNG) arrives** in the USA. Inserter barrel 15% smaller. Approved for 3 years of contraceptive use
2012: Brooke Winner, Peipert, Zhao, Buckel, Maddon, Allsworth, Secura published the classical paper on the effectiveness of long acting reversible contraceptive in the St. Louis Contraceptive CHOICE Project. *[NEJM May 24, 2012]*

2011: World population reaches 7 billion (this billion took 12 years)
2011: 20th Edition of *Contraceptive Technology*
2006: First HPV vaccine, Gardasil, released
2002 and 1996: Forest, Hubacher and Grimes point out A GLOBAL PARADOX. "Although the most common reversible contraceptive in the world, it (the IUD) has the worst reputation of all contraceptives... except among those using IUDs." *[Hubacher D., Grimes DA. 2002; Forest JD. 1996]*
2001: Ortho Evra Patch and NuvaRing approved
2000: Women can vote in all but 3 countries (see 1898)

1999: World population hits 6 billion (this billion took 12 years)
1997: FDA approves emergency contraception pills
1996: World Health Organization publishes evidence-based guidelines on the safety of contraceptives for women with over 150 characteristics and medical conditions
1992: FDA approve Depo Provera Injections
1992: First female condom, Femidom, marketed in Denmark (Reality in USA)
1991: Sivin describes 7 year cumulative failure rate of LNG IUD of 1.1%

1988: Five years after its approval marketing of Copper T-380A begins
1987: World population reaches 5 billion (this billion took 12 years)
1983: FDA approves Copper T-380A IUD in the United States
1983: **Implanon** implant developed by Population Council and first approved in Finland (leads to Nexplanon)
1983: **Jadelle** implant developed by Population Council and first approved in Finland
1982: Baulieu describes medical abortion using mifepristone followed by misoprospol
1981: First case of HIV/AIDS described in MMRW (CDC)
1981: Garret Hardin writes "nobody ever dies of overpopulation" after 500,000 die from flooding of an overcrowded East Bengal River delta
1980s: Per capita caloric consumption starts to fall (held off for decades by the green revolution)

1975: World population reaches 4 billion (this billion took 15 years)
1974: Al Yuzpe in Canada describes emergency contraception using Ovral pills
1973: FDA approves progestin-only pills (mini-pills)
1973: U.S. Supreme Court abortion decision: Roe v. Wade (TX) and Roe v. Bolton (GA)
1969: First edition of *Contraceptive Technology*
1969: Jaime Zipper in Chile describes suppression of fertility by intrauterine copper IUD
1968: Vatican pronouncement reaffirms opposition of Catholic Church to artificial contraception
1964: Dr. Alexander Langmuir makes family planning a public health priority at the Centers for Disease Control

1960: It took but 30 years to add the 3rd billionth person
1960: Combined birth control pills (Enovid) formally approved by FDA
1950s: Birth control pills taken continuously to treat endometriosis
1942: American Birth Control League renamed Planned Parenthood
1937: American Medical Association ends long standing oppistion to contraception
1936: German gynecologist Friedrich Wilde describes first cervical cap (fitted from a wax impression)
1936: John Rook opens rhythm birth control clinic in Boston

1930: World population now 2 billion (this billion took 100 years)
1930: Knaus (Austria) and Ogino (Japan) develop rhythm method
1930: Pope Pius XI in Of Chaste Marriage virulently attacks both contraception and abortion
1927: Novak (Hopkins) describes suction as means of performing an abortion
1920: Women can vote in the United States
1914: Margaret Sanger coins phrase "birth control" and fights for women's suffrage
1909: German surgeon Richard Richter reports success with silkworm-gut shaped into a ring
1898: **New Zealand** becomes the first country in the world where **women can vote**
1893: First vasectomy by Harrison in London
1882: First contraceptive clinic established in Amsterdam
1880: First tubal ligation and Dr. Wilhelm Mensinga invents a larger cervical cap eventually known as the diaphragm

1800: It took many thousands of years, perhaps 300 to 400 thousand years, for world population to reach 1 billion people
1798: Thomas Robert Malthus proposes dismal economic theory that population growth eventually will exceed the ability of the earth to provide food, resulting in starvation
Late 1770's: Casanova popularizes condoms for infection control and contraception. He recounts his attempts to use the shelled out rind of a lemon as a cervical cap. Lemon juice is a strong spermicide.

1 AD: 250 Million World population reaches 250 million, abstinence (particularly postpartum), withdrawal, lactation, intrauterine stones in camels, homosexuality and polygamy, lemons for their mechanical and spermicidal effect, unsafe abortion 5000 years ago using molokhia.

Nexplanon and Implanon Implants
The etonogestrel Implant
The most effective of all reversible methods. And for 4-5 years, more effective than most male or female sterilization procedures.

Jadelle Implant
The Levonorgestrel Implant
The least expensive of all implants.

The Copper T IUD

Harrison found that vasectomy made a vast difference in a man's vas deferens

2040: 9 Billion
2025: 8 Billion
2011: 7 Billion
1999: 6 Billion
1987: 5 Billion
1975: 4 Billion
1960: 3 Billion
1930: 2 Billion
1800: 1 Billion

Each 100 years in the millennia prior to Christ, the total population on our little spaceship Earth increased by one-half of 1%. Births virtually equaled deaths.

The Copper T IUD:

Paragard is the most effective emergency contraception. Less than 1 in 1,000 women receiving a Copper IUD as an emergency contraceptive becomes pregnant. The IUD may be left in place providing excellent contraception for 12 or more years.

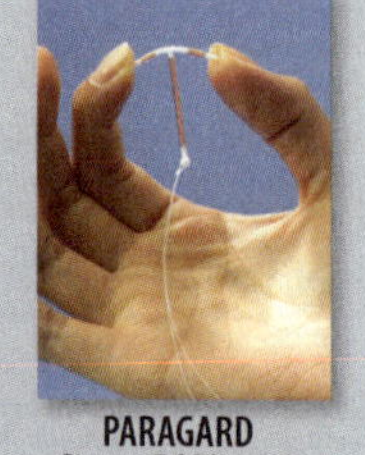

PARAGARD
Copper T 380-A IUD
The most commonly used reversible contraceptive in the world

One Plan B tablet:

contains 1.5 mg of levonorgestrel. It is available over-the-counter.

One Ella tablet:

contains 3.0 mg of ulipristal acetate. It is available by prescription only.

NOTE: Very over-weight women **should consider the** **Copper IUD rather than Plan B or Ella because of high failure rates in very over-weight women.**

This case may help you understand: Why 50% of all pregnancies in the U.S. are unplanned.

"I take a morning-after pill every month. When we have sex my boyfriend usually pulls out. We had unprotected sex twice one morning and each time he pulled out. My ovulation test became positive 3 days later (when sperm could still have been alive and well in me). I figure my risk of pregnancy is fairly low. Is it safe to use morning-after pills as often as I am using them?

I read on your site that I could get an IUD inserted for emergency contraception. I told an OB/GYN who said he had never heard of this."

OUR RESPONSE TO THIS WOMAN: If you were to receive an emergency Copper T IUD, it would be extremely effective both as an emergency contraceptive and as your ongoing contraceptive. Better yet, get that Paragard IUD placed when it is not an emergency.

Perhaps no single practice could more quickly lead to increased use of Long Acting Reversible Contraceptives as the use of IUDs for emergency contraception. This is underscored by the above person writing in to the www.managingcontraception.com website.

Who Can Use Which Contraceptive? The Question Clinicians Face Daily

2016 U.S. MEDICAL ELIGIBILITY CRITERIA FOR CONTRACEPTIVE USE

The table on the following pages summarizes the latest CDC medical eligibility criteria for starting contraceptives. These criteria are based on extensive reviews of available evidence. Please visit the CDC website to view the full document. There you will find more information on the evidence supporting MEC category assignment.

MEC categories for temporary methods:

1	**No restriction (*method can be used*)**
2	**Advantages generally outweigh theoretical or proven risks**
3	**Theoretical or proven risks usually outweigh the advantages**
4	**Unacceptable health risk (*method not to be used*)**

Simplified 2-category system for temporary methods

To make clinical judgment, the MEC 4-category classification system can be simplified into a 2-category system.

MEC Category	With Clinical Judgment	With Limited Clinical Judgment
1	Use the method in any circumstances	Use the method
2	Generally use the method	
3	Use of the method not usually recommended unless other, more appropriate methods are not available or acceptable	Do not use the method
4	Method not to be used	

To download most recent 2016 Medical Eligibility Criteria go to: www.cdc.gov

Summary Chart of U.S. Medical Eligibility

Condition	Sub-Condition	Cu-IUD I	Cu-IUD C	LNG-IUD I	LNG-IUD C	Implant I	Implant C	DMPA I	DMPA C	POP I	POP C	CHC I	CHC C
Age		Menarche to <20 yrs:**2**		Menarche to <20 yrs:**2**		Menarche to <18 yrs:**1**		Menarche to <18 yrs:**2**		Menarche to <18 yrs:**1**		Menarche to <40 yrs:**1**	
		≥20 yrs:**1**		≥20 yrs:**1**		18-45 yrs:**1**		18-45 yrs:**1**		18-45 yrs:**1**		≥40 yrs:**2**	
						>45 yrs:**1**		>45 yrs:**2**		>45 yrs:**1**			
Anatomical abnormalities	a) Distorted uterine cavity	4		4									
	b) Other abnormalities	2		2									
Anemias	a) Thalassemia	2		1		1		1		1		1	
	b) Sickle cell disease[‡]	2		1		1		1		1		2	
	c) Iron-deficiency anemia	2		1		1		1		1		1	
Benign ovarian tumors	*(including cysts)*	1		1		1		1		1		1	
Breast disease	a) Undiagnosed mass	1		2		2*		2*		2*		2*	
	b) Benign breast disease	1		1		1		1		1		1	
	c) Family history of cancer	1		1		1		1		1		1	
	d) Breast cancer[‡]												
	i) Current	1		4		4		4		4		4	
	ii) Past and no evidence of current disease for 5 years	1		3		3		3		3		3	
Breastfeeding	a) <21 days postpartum					2*		2*		2*		4*	
	b) 21 to <30 days postpartum												
	i) With other risk factors for VTE					2*		2*		2*		3*	
	ii) Without other risk factors for VTE					2*		2*		2*		3*	
	c) 30-42 days postpartum												
	i) With other risk factors for VTE					1*		1*		1*		3*	
	ii) Without other risk factors for VTE					1*		1*		1*		2*	
	d) >42 days postpartum					1*		1*		1*		2*	
Cervical cancer	Awaiting treatment	4	2	4	2	2		2		1		2	
Cervical ectropion		1		1		1		1		1		1	
Cervical intraepithelial neoplasia		1		2		2		2		1		2	
Cirrhosis	a) Mild *(compensated)*	1		1		1		1		1		1	
	b) Severe[‡] *(decompensated)*	1		3		3		3		3		4	
Cystic fibrosis[‡]		1*		1*		1*		2*		1*		1*	
Deep venous thrombosis (DVT)/Pulmonary embolism (PE)	a) History of DVT/PE, not receiving anticoagulant therapy												
	i) Higher risk for recurrent DVT/PE	1		2		2		2		2		4	
	ii) Lower risk for recurrent DVT/PE	1		2		2		2		2		3	
	b) Acute DVT/PE	2		2		2		2		2		4	
	c) DVT/PE and established anticoagulant therapy for at least 3 months												
	i) Higher risk for recurrent DVT/PE	2		2		2		2		2		4*	
	ii) Lower risk for recurrent DVT/PE	2		2		2		2		2		3*	
	d) Family history *(first-degree relatives)*	1		1		1		1		1		2	
	e) Major surgery												
	i) With prolonged immobilization	1		2		2		2		2		4	
	ii) Without prolonged immobilization	1		1		1		1		1		2	
	f) Minor surgery without immobilization	1		1		1		1		1		1	
Depressive disorders		1*		1*		1*		1*		1*		1*	

Key:	
1 No restriction (method can be used)	3 Theoretical or proven risks usually outweigh the advantages
2 Advantages generally outweigh theoretical or proven risks	4 Unacceptable health risk (method not to be used)

NOTES: (including cases you have seen)

Criteria for Contraceptive Use

Condition	Sub-Condition	Cu-IUD		LNG-IUD		Implant		DMPA		POP		CHC	
		I	C	I	C	I	C	I	C	I	C	I	C
Diabetes	a) History of gestational disease	1		1		1		1		1		1	
	b) Nonvascular disease												
	i) Non-insulin dependent	1		2		2		2		2		2	
	ii) Insulin dependent	1		2		2		2		2		2	
	c) Nephropathy/retinopathy/neuropathy‡	1		2		2		3		2		3/4*	
	d) Other vascular disease or diabetes of >20 years' duration‡	1		2		2		3		2		3/4*	
Dysmenorrhea	Severe	2		1		1		1		1		1	
Endometrial cancer‡		4	2	4	2	1		1		1		1	
Endometrial hyperplasia		1		1		1		1		1		1	
Endometriosis		2		1		1		1		1		1	
Epilepsy‡	(*see also Drug Interactions*)	1		1		1*		1*		1*		1*	
Gallbladder disease	a) Symptomatic												
	i) Treated by cholecystectomy	1		2		2		2		2		2	
	ii) Medically treated	1		2		2		2		2		3	
	iii) Current	1		2		2		2		2		3	
	b) Asymptomatic	1		2		2		2		2		2	
Gestational trophoblastic disease‡	a) Suspected GTD (immediate postevacuation)												
	i) Uterine size first trimester	1*		1*		1*		1*		1*		1*	
	ii) Uterine size second trimester	2*		2*		1*		1*		1*		1*	
	b) Confirmed GTD												
	i) Undetectable/non-pregnant ß-hCG levels	1*	1*	1*	1*	1*		1*		1*		1*	
	ii) Decreasing ß-hCG levels	2*	1*	2*	1*	1*		1*		1*		1*	
	iii) Persistently elevated ß-hCG levels or malignant disease, with no evidence or suspicion of intrauterine disease	2*	1*	2*	1*	1*		1*		1*		1*	
	iv) Persistently elevated ß-hCG levels or malignant disease, with evidence or suspicion of intrauterine disease	4*	2*	4*	2*	1*		1*		1*		1*	
Headaches	a) Nonmigraine (mild or severe)	1		1		1		1		1		1*	
	b) Migraine												
	i) Without aura (includes menstrual migraine)	1		1		1		1		1		2*	
	ii) With aura	1		1		1		1		1		4*	
History of bariatric surgery‡	a) Restrictive procedures	1		1		1		1		1		1	
	b) Malabsorptive procedures	1		1		1		1		3		COCs: 3 P/R: 1	
History of cholestasis	a) Pregnancy related	1		1		1		1		1		2	
	b) Past COC related	1		2		2		2		2		3	
History of high blood pressure during pregnancy		1		1		1		1		1		2	
History of Pelvic surgery		1		1		1		1		1		1	
HIV	a) High risk for HIV	1*	1*	1*	1*	1		1		1		1	
	b) HIV infection					1*		1*		1*		1*	
	i) Clinically well receiving ARV therapy	1	1	1	1	If on treatment, see Drug Interactions							
	ii) Not clinically well or not receiving ARV therapy‡	2	1	2	1	If on treatment, see Drug Interactions							

bbreviations: ARV = antiretroviral; C=continuation of contraceptive method; CHC=combined hormonal contraception (pill, patch, and, ring); COC=combined oral contraceptive; Cu-D=copper-containing intrauterine device; DMPA = depot medroxyprogesterone acetate; I=initiation of contraceptive method; LNG-IUD=levonorgestrel-releasing intrauterine device; NA=not pplicable; POP=progestin-only pill; P/R=patch/ring; SSRI=selective serotonin reuptake inhibitor; ‡ Condition that exposes a woman to increased risk as a result of pregnancy. *Please see the omplete guidance for a clarification to this classification: https://www.cdc.gov/reproductivehealth/contraception/contraception_guidance.htm.

NOTES:

Summary Chart of U.S. Medical Eligibility

Condition	Sub-Condition	Cu-IUD		LNG-IUD		Implant		DMPA		POP		CHC	
		I	C	I	C	I	C	I	C	I	C	I	C
Hypertension	a) Adequately controlled hypertension	1*		1*		1*		2*		1*		3*	
	b) Elevated blood pressure levels (*properly taken measurements*)												
	i) Systolic 140-159 or diastolic 90-99	1*		1*		1*		2*		1*		3*	
	ii) Systolic ≥160 or diastolic ≥100‡	1*		2*		2*		3*		2*		4*	
	c) Vascular disease	1*		2*		2*		3*		2*		4*	
Inflammatory bowel disease	(*Ulcerative colitis, Crohn's disease*)	1		1		1		2		2		2/3*	
Ischemic heart disease‡	Current and history of	1		2	3	2	3	3		2	3	4	
Known thrombogenic mutations‡		1*		2*		2*		2*		2*		4*	
Liver tumors	a) Benign												
	i) Focal nodular hyperplasia	1		2		2		2		2		2	
	ii) Hepatocellular adenoma‡	1		3		3		3		3		4	
	b) Malignant‡ (hepatoma)	1		3		3		3		3		4	
Malaria		1		1		1		1		1		1	
Multiple risk factors for atherosclerotic cardiovascular disease	(e.g., older age, smoking, diabetes, hypertension, low HDL, high LDL, or high triglyceride levels)	1		2		2*		3*		2*		3/4*	
Multiple sclerosis	a) With prolonged immobility	1		1		1		2		1		3	
	b) Without prolonged immobility	1		1		1		2		1		1	
Obesity	a) Body mass index (BMI) ≥30 kg/m^2	1		1		1		1		1		2	
	b) Menarche to <18 years and BMI ≥ 30 kg/m^2	1		1		1		2		1		2	
Ovarian cancer‡		1		1		1		1		1		1	
Parity	a) Nulliparous	2		2		1		1		1		1	
	b) Parous	1		1		1		1		1		1	
Past ectopic pregnancy		1		1		1		1		2		1	
Pelvic inflammatory disease	a) Past												
	i) With subsequent pregnancy	1	1	1	1	1		1		1		1	
	ii) Without subsequent pregnancy	2	2	2	2	1		1		1		1	
	b) Current	4	2*	4	2*	1		1		1		1	
Peripartum cardiomyopathy‡	a) Normal or mildly impaired cardiac function												
	i) <6 months	2		2		1		1		1		4	
	ii) ≥6 months	2		2		1		1		1		3	
	b) Moderately or severely impaired cardiac function	2		2		2		2		2		4	
Postabortion	a) First trimester	1*		1*		1*		1*		1*		1*	
	b) Second trimester	2*		2*		1*		1*		1*		1*	
	c) Immediate postseptic abortion	4		4		1*		1*		1*		1*	
Postpartum (*nonbreastfeeding women*)	a) <21 days					1		1		1		4	
	b) 21 days to 42 days												
	i) With other risk factors for VTE					1		1		1		3*	
	ii) Without other risk factors for VTE					1		1		1		2	
	c) >42 days					1		1		1		1	
Postpartum (*in breastfeeding or non-breastfeeding women, including cesarean delivery*)	a) <10 minutes after delivery of the placenta												
	i) Breastfeeding	1*		2*									
	ii) Nonbreastfeeding	1*		1*									
	b) 10 minutes after delivery of the placenta to <4 weeks	2*		2*									
	c) ≥4 weeks	1*		1*									
	d) Postpartum sepsis	4		4									

NOTES: (including cases you have seen)